Ghosts and The

MW01492785

Writing the Early Americas

Anna Brickhouse and Kirsten Silva Gruesz, Editors

Ghosts and Their Hosts

The Colonization of the Invisible World in Early America

SLADJA BLAŽAN

University of Virginia Press

Charlottesville and London

The University of Virginia Press is situated on the traditional lands of the Monacan Nation, and the Commonwealth of Virginia was and is home to many other Indigenous people. We pay our respect to all of them, past and present. We also honor the enslaved African and African American people who built the University of Virginia, and we recognize their descendants. We commit to fostering voices from these communities through our publications and to deepening our collective understanding of their histories and contributions.

University of Virginia Press
© 2024 by the Rector and Visitors of the University of Virginia
All rights reserved
Printed in the United States of America on acid-free paper

First published 2024

9 8 7 6 5 4 3 2 1

LIBRARY OF CONGRESS CATALOGING-IN-PUBLICATION DATA
Names: Blažan, Sladja, author.
Title: Ghosts and their hosts : the colonization of the invisible world / Sladja Blažan.
Description: Charlottesville : University of Virginia Press, 2024. | Series: Writing the early Americas | Includes bibliographical references and index.
Identifiers: LCCN 2024028946 (print) | LCCN 2024028947 (ebook) | ISBN 9780813952383 (hardback) | ISBN 9780813952390 (paperback) | ISBN 9780813952406 (ebook)
Subjects: BISAC: LITERARY CRITICISM / Subjects & Themes / Culture, Race & Ethnicity | LITERARY CRITICISM / Gothic & Romance
Classification: LCC RA544.C67 P854 2024 (print) | LCC RA544.C67 (ebook)
LC record available at https://lccn.loc.gov/2024028946
LC ebook record available at https://lccn.loc.gov/2024028947

Publication of this volume has been supported by *New Literary History*.

Cover art: Matthew McGinity
Cover design: Cecilia Sorochin

For Mila and Emíl, who remind me daily that life is full of magic

One need not be a Chamber—to be Haunted—
One need not be a House—
The Brain has Corridors—surpassing
Material Place—

Far safer, of a midnight meeting
External Ghost
Than its interior confronting—
That cooler Host—

Far safer, through an Abbey gallop,
The Stones a'chase—
Than unarmed, one's a'self encounter—
In lonesome Place—

Ourself behind ourself, concealed—
Should startle most—
Assassin hid in our Apartment
Be Horror's least—

The Body—borrows a Revolver—
He bolts the Door—
O'erlooking a superior spectre—
Or More—
        —Emily Dickinson

Contents

Acknowledgments

I am deeply indebted to everybody who was willing to chop off a chunk of their time and engage in a conversation with me. This book is a continuation of our discussions.

To begin, I'd like to thank my two anonymous reviewers for supporting this project and for their helpful suggestions. The first reviewer in particular gave me the necessary push to finish the book. Angie Hogan is the most wonderful editor and has accompanied and supported the publishing process from beginning to end. Thank you so much! The seeds for this topic were sown during the graduate classes I taught. I want to thank my students, whose curiosity and often surprising perspectives keep me exploring. I thank everybody at the English and American Studies department at the University of Würzburg, where I wrote a large part of the book: Catrin Gersdorf and MaryAnn Snyder-Körber for reading an early version of the manuscript and their valuable comments; Hannah Nelson-Teutsch, Rebecca Grözinger, and Nina Wintermeyer for agreeing to check my mistakes; for their support, willingness to discuss, and coffee breaks, I'd like to thank Heike Raphael-Hernandez, Molina Klingler, Sophie Renninger, Lena Pfeifer, Zeno Ackermann, Johannes Schlegel, Susanne Bayerlipp, Miriam Wallraven, and Jennifer Leetsch. I'd like to thank Roland Borgards and Andrew Gross for reading parts of the manuscript. Huge thanks to all my colleagues and participants at the faculty colloquium at Bard College Berlin, who made a space for me to present this (at the time unpresentable) book: Catherine Toal, Clio Nicastro, Kerry Bystrom, James Harker, Gale Raj-Reichert, Nina Tecklenburg, Ewa Atanassow, Nassim AbiGhanem, Matthias Hurst, and Boris Vormann.

I am deeply indebted to Becky Beetz for pushing me to go further, by reading the first draft and not giving up on me even at times when I wanted to do so myself. Thank you for making space for this book in the midst of your turbulent life. Endless thanks to all the numerous spiritual and intellectual advisors during the process of brooding, writing, thinking, debating, rejecting, and starting all over again. To name only a few: Sandy Alexandre, Kader Attia, Nicola Behrmann, Teri Boyd, Adam Butler, Eduardo Cadava, Bill Dixon, Simone Giostra, Aleksandar Hemon, Erica Kaufman, Christiane Kühl, Chris Kondek, Françoise Meltzer, Ana Teixeira Pinto,

Sean Patten, Berit Stumpf, Jörg Thomas Richter, Eleni Stecopoulos, Robin Trembley-McGaw, Jons Vukorep, Angi Vukorep, Lily Gurton-Wachter, Julia Weber, Brigitte Weingart, and so many more. Thank you for cooking, discussing, talking, walking, performing, and cocktail-mixing.

I want to thank the Alexander von Humboldt Foundation for supporting my interest in ghosts in its very early stages.

My dear parents, who never allowed themselves to dream and offered their lives so that I could live mine, I will never be able to thank them enough but will continue to do so for the rest of my life.

I want to thank Ocean Vuong for giving us all something to get back to when it looks like there is nothing else.

Most of all I thank Matthew McGinity for reminding me of the material power of the spirit every day. And for laughing with me.

Ghosts and Their Hosts

INTRODUCTION

Spectral Narratives

Ghosts are en vogue. From prize-winning novels like George Saunders' *Lincoln in the Bardo* (2017) to Hollywood blockbusters like David Lowery's *A Ghost Story* (2017), anthology television series like *American Horror Story* (Murphy 2011–21), Broadway musicals like *Ghost* (2012), and art exhibitions like *The Perfect Medium: Photography and the Occult* (2005) at the Met Museum, ghosts have infiltrated every cultural corner. *The Routledge Handbook to the Ghost Story,* published in 2018, only solidified their presence by changing the framework to scholarly discussions. What's more, a careful analysis of ghostly figurations throughout the history of US American literature and culture demonstrates that there has never been a time without ghosts. Most likely, there has never been a culture or a period without ghosts. And yet, despite this long genealogy, the contemporary abundance of ghosts confounds even the *New York Times,* which published a lengthy essay in October of 2018 with the title "The Ghost Story Persists in American Literature. Why?" (Sehgal). *Ghosts and Their Hosts* presents an answer to this pressing question.

   Ghosts are first and foremost figurations of power. With this statement, this book breaks with the established tradition of reading ghosts in the context of social critique. Giving form to intersubjective communication that disrupts the centrality of the (living) human, ghosts have the capacity to produce alternative histories. That quality can certainly be instrumentalized for recuperative purposes, but it can also be used as a narrative tool that aids the project of othering and exclusion and keeps unjust social structures in place. A ghost is a reminder that history is not the past, or as Faulkner famously put it: "The past is never dead. It's not even past." But who is reconfiguring the past in the present? This study is guided by the often-neglected question, who is hosting the ghost? While ghosts have the ability to expose the narrativity of history, they do not necessarily function as a corrective. Within the aforementioned *New York Times* article on the persistence of ghosts in US American literature and culture, the journalist Parul Sehgal repeats the much-promoted reading of ghosts as social critique: "ghosts protest norms—slavery, Jim Crow, mass incarceration—the norms that killed them" (2). Ghosts certainly have that power, yet they are not necessarily subversive concepts that are always summoned to present alternative histories. A ghost story can remedy injustice and present alternatives to the conventional linear representations of history; yet, it can also be instrumental in affirming existing power structures. Correcting historical memory might exhibit possibilities of restoration, but it can also contain a reconfiguration of social constellations necessary to validate existing hierarchies.

A ghost has no ontology—it is reasonable not to know what a ghost is. It is, therefore, only through the eye of the beholder that an understanding can be reached of the various reasons for the tireless engagement with spectral matters that has existed in US American literature and culture since its inception. Thus, rather than solely focusing on ghosts, this study also explores their hosts. This approach has exposed the inadequacy of the often-applied reduction of ghosts to Western gothic conceptualizations. It has been a humanities trope since the rise of postmodernism in the twentieth century to expose Western cultures' reliance on structures that suggest a progressive history from the past into the future. Accordingly, a ghost has been celebrated as an interruption, an abject appearance of the past in the present. This foremost European definition of a ghost, however, is far from universally valid, as it often appears in literary interpretations and critical theory alike. In most non-European cultures, a ghost bursts images of linearity and transforms them into an entangled, rhizomatic structure that points at numerous intersections and calls for reflection. Even in certain European conceptualizations—such as the one developed by the influential medieval scholar, physicist, and alchemist Paracelsus—ghosts are ever-present entities that share life with the living. As I demonstrate in this study, non-European cultures and European mysticism have been much more influential in establishing antebellum figurations of ghosts than has been acknowledged so far. In such nonlinear approaches, the ghost-seer is exposed as only one of many agents entwined within a larger web of relations. From the moment a ghost is perceptible, a network is exposed and an absolute autonomy of the ghost-seer is no longer possible. The sighting of a ghost is an interlocking, an inscription into deep history. The function of the ghost depends on the ghost-seer's entanglement within larger political, social, and psychological frameworks, all of which are exhibited in the sighting of a ghost and therefore examined here.

The invisibility of the ghost often marks the unacknowledged past, which now returns to haunt the present. Novels that seek to expose violently erased histories employ spectral characters for this reason. Kathleen Brogan even proposed a new subgenre, "cultural ghost stories" (3), which she subsumed under "ethnic literature" to demonstrate how ghosts could give a voice to those marginalized within mainstream cultures. In the context of US American literature, Toni Morrison provided a prime example with her novel *Beloved,* constructing one of the most intriguing figurations of ghosts to mark the circularity of the past in the present. In this novel, the ghost of a child who was killed by her enslaved mother to protect her from a fate similar to the one the mother had to suffer through, returns and initiates what was otherwise unimaginable. As Linda Krumholz and Blessing Diala-Ogamba have already observed: the ghost called Beloved "forces Sethe to confront her past in her incompatible roles as a slave and as a mother" (Krumholz 396). This "history-making is a healing process for the characters, the reader, and the author" (Krumholz 395). Their reading asserts the enormous capacity that a ghostly figuration can have. Ghosts have consequently been analyzed and employed as powerful rhetorical tools by scholars interested in questions of social justice such as Horkheimer and Adorno, Karl Marx, and more recently the sociologist Avery Gordon and the environmental studies scholars Elaine Gan, Anna Tsing, Heather Swanson, and Nils Bubandt, to name only a few.[1]

However, the movement in the other direction—the instrumentalization of ghosts and ghost stories to affirm power structures already in place—has not received much attention in current scholarship. Yet, reconfiguring the past as the present through figurations of ghosts can also serve the purpose of confirming the existing (unjust) order, as exemplified in interpretations offered here of spectral narratives in antebellum literature by Washington Irving and Nathaniel Hawthorne but also those by John Neal and Lydia Maria Child, authors who were invested in constructing emancipation narratives. I return to these early and markedly US American ghost stories because they have established a prototype for current narratives. What's more, they have inaugurated specific racialized images of spectral nature that continue to dominate contemporary screens and literature.

One of the most popular ghost stories written in the nineteenth century exemplifies this point. At the time, even Edgar Allan Poe considered the story first published in 1841 to be "the best ghost story we ever read" (275). William Gilmore Simms' "Grayling; or, 'Murder Will Out'"[2] opens with a typical statement intended to naturalize the presence of ghosts: "I very much doubt whether the poet, the painter, the sculptor, or the romancer, ever yet lived, who had not some strong biased leaning, at least, to a belief in the wonders of the invisible world. Certainly, the higher orders of poets and painters, those who create and invent, must have a strong taint of the superstitious in their composition" (1). Relegating spectral matters to the realm of the artistic, Simms proceeds with a traditional pattern. Here the ghost actually does materialize—it appears in the likeness of a former major who fought in the Revolutionary War and returned to seek revenge for his undignified murder. The tale offers a patriotic imaginary within which European settlers are marked as victims of English colonial power. The ghost, significantly, appears to one of the major's former subordinates in a South Carolina swamp. Through supernatural intuition, the ghost-seer eventually finds the murdered body in a bay "whose wall of thorns, vines, and close tenacious shrubs seemed to defy invasion" (29). The tightly entangled branches only seemingly resist incursion and are finally penetrated. Nature in this instance is, literally, torn apart, and order is reinstalled at the end of the narrative.

The story was published in a collection that Simms wrote with the attempt to establish US American themes as valid subjects for literary exploration, which, yet again, affirms the importance of reading ghost stories in the context of promoting specific US American literary topics. The story repeats a common pattern that had already been solidified by Washington Irving in what was to become the most famous US American ghost story, "The Legend of Sleepy Hollow" (1820). Whereas the land is said to be haunted by "native American" spirits, the ghost that appears is of European origin. In Simms' tale it is the ghost of a British-American general, in Irving's of a Hessian and therefore German soldier who fought on the side of the Americans. The role of nature in both tales is prototypical: when ghosts do materialize in early and antebellum American narratives, they are commonly those of male settlers of European descent who come to claim territory, history, and future. Nature is their antagonist.

I analyze this topos of antebellum literature as a signum of colonization, located at the intersection of racialization and environmental degradation. Simms' and Irving's ghost stories exemplify the settler colonial inscription into the remnants of what once was the Invisible World. Introduced in colonial North America by the European Puritan settler communities, this phrase referred to a hierarchical order that linked the natural world to the invisible realm of the spirits. Informed by this Puritan concept, the narrative structure of the ghost story is instrumentalized to shift the focus away from the colonial presence of European settlers, framing them as victims rather than as perpetrators. Nature is central to such exculpation narratives, as the material exhibition of the Invisible World. My close readings of depictions of haunted nature demonstrate that, particularly with respect to foundational periods marked by reconfigurations of the past, it is essential that scholars critically examine where the demarcation between life and death is erased and by whom. Taking a closer look into material aspects of spectral matters, I ask: How exactly has the past been reconfigured in the present and who is in control? What lasting effects are produced by this new constellation? What is marked as invisible and who could *see* it nevertheless? Why? Most importantly, what are the lasting effects of such agenda-setting?

Attempting to answer these and similar questions, I propose the following argument: struggling to extract the white, male subject while retaining a seemingly relational network, early American theories of subjectivity have often instrumentalized ghosts. In what follows, I trace the genealogy of this effort that in its erasure of non-European traditions faced significant challenges. Early American settler literature is structured around the public secret of slavery and the instrumentalization of the Indigenous population for purposes of establishing a national imaginary that could excuse genocide and dispossession. Yet, even in their erasure, North American Indigenous cultures and West African traditions have left significant marks on settler colonial storytelling. Ghosts appear rather often at the center of these exculpation narratives, as is demonstrated in the case of Washington Irving's tales. Charles Brockden Brown's and John Neal's texts express a sense of multivalent transcultural subjectivity and attempt to come closer to an inclusive view of the new republic, only to (re)produce racial subjugation. Lydia Maria Child instrumentalizes ghosts in the context of magic to create a feminist space of emancipation, but to the detriment of the Indigenous population. At the same time, all of these attempts at subjugation are opposed by powerful counternarratives, as is demonstrated in my reading of Hannah Crafts' *The Bondwoman's Narrative,* where ghosts initiate survival strategies for characters exposed to the atrocities of slavery.

It is therefore not a surprise that ghosts have played foundational roles in establishing the US cultural imaginary, with stories offering a medium for framing political ideologies, philosophical thought, racial anxieties, and social concerns.[3] *Ghosts and Their Hosts* is an inquiry into the effects of this powerful concept that collapses the past with the present and exposes the ghost-seer's entanglement with the human and nonhuman environment from the early Puritan era of colonial America to the beginnings of what came to be called the American Renaissance. The period covered by this inquiry begins in the late seventeenth century, because it is during this time that the modern understanding of ghosts developed its first contours. The influential if controversial English philosopher Thomas Hobbes shifted the discussion around ghosts from its religious context by exploring questions of imagination. By doing so, Hobbes put the ghost-seer on the philosophical map, initiating a discussion that produced a prominent opponent in Joseph Glanvill, one of the leading advocates of natural philosophy in the late seventeenth century. With two such influential public intellectuals engaging in a heated debate, the transatlantic community was sure to respond. Their philosophical approach to spectral matters managed to transfigure even Puritan ways of ghost-seeing, as is demonstrated in the first chapter by a reading of the ways in which the prominent ministers Increase and Cotton Mather redefined apparitional tales as natural phenomena and in doing so racialized the ghost story genre. The opening chapter demonstrates ways in which the Puritan concept of the Invisible World intersects with questions of race, adding to the larger Enlightenment project of manufacturing Man in the face of the Other. Ghost stories in US American literary history have been complicit in the construction of this huMan, which Denise Ferreira da Silva calls "the transparent I" and explains as a construct that came to symbolize whiteness. This conjecture has left lasting marks on the literary output not only of all of the writers of the early US American period analyzed in this study but far beyond.

The late seventeenth century marks the beginning of a transatlantic secularization of spectrality in literature and philosophy that continued throughout the eighteenth century. This is demonstrated in the second chapter of this study, which analyzes treatises on ghosts written by philosophers and writers such as Immanuel Kant, Christoph Martin Wieland, and Comte de Volney. Above all, the latter two have received much attention in the United States. Analyzing this transatlantic discourse on spectrality demonstrates its elemental function in the formation of a modern subjectivity via morality, which, while posing as universal, established racialized exclusionary premises. From this outset, *Ghosts and Their Hosts* offers a revised reading of texts by what are today considered representative US American writers from the early period, namely Charles Brockden Brown, Washington Irving, Lydia Maria Child, Nathaniel Hawthorne, and Harriet Beecher Stowe, combined with interpretations of nearly forgotten texts such as the anonymously published *St. Herbert—A Tale* (1796, considered by some scholars to be the first US American gothic novel), seldom-interpreted texts such as John Neal's epic novel *Logan* (1822) and Child's "She Waits in the Spirit Land" (1846), as well as recently discovered texts such as Hannah Crafts' *The Bondwoman's Narrative* (ca. 1852). Moreover, numerous stories, pamphlets, newspaper articles, and philosophical treatments relating to the concept of ghosts serve as a source to analyze how modern subjectivity emerged in relation to spectrality and, more to the point, to the racialization of the same. This work is important because it demonstrates how ghosts and ghost stories simultaneously aided the colonial project of dehumanization and land appropriation in the United States and provided stories of recuperation, carving out an established and permanent place for ghosts in US American literature and culture.

In particular, the often-employed images of sentient forests carry the mark of the Puritan supernatural into modern representations of spectral power. Therefore, this study gives due attention to an exploration of nature possessed by the spirits of the dead. Within this discourse, ghost stories slowly developed into racialized, gendered, and sexualized narratives, giving ghosts a material presence and aiding the project of naturalizing and fixing these categories. The study ends in the 1840s with the emergence of the so-called American Renaissance—a US American historical literary phenomenon commonly understood to be part of transatlantic Romanticism. Ghosts are established as cultural and narrative figurations on both sides of the Atlantic by the 1840s, as is expressed most succinctly in the writings of Edgar Allan Poe.[4] Concurrently, American spiritualism—a popular religious and cultural practice conducted through communication with the spirits of the dead—took the country by storm.[5] These two important developments in the cultural makeup of the United States—the American Renaissance, commonly understood to begin with Poe's writing around 1840, and American spiritualism, initiated with the experience of spirit-rapping by the Fox sisters in 1848—changed the perception and presentation of ghosts in literature and culture and thus provide a logical endpoint to this study.

Spanning a period roughly between the mid-seventeenth and the mid-nineteenth centuries, the present study demonstrates how hostility toward ghosts collapses in the maxim of the Enlightenment: "know thyself." What Andrew Spira called the "invention of the self" in the eighteenth century increasingly included rather than shunned the many ghosts that populated the transatlantic world. As a marker of the mysterious, including ghosts in the makeup of the Self exposed the unknown as an integral part of the psyche. Literary figurations of the spectral Self served the narrative function of integrating the irrational. The spectral in fictional texts repeatedly provides the form that enables a negotiation of what is present but not understood. This use of the irrational as a present absence opens a space for speculation over the organization of reality. Caroline Levine most convincingly explained the importance of forms for the perception of reality. In *Forms: Whole, Rhythm, Hierarchy, Network,* she writes: "it is the work of form to make order. And this means that forms are the work of politics" (3). Levine's conclusion, that any arrangement or form of reality has political and philosophical relevance in that it inherently gives a certain shape to human experience, is crucial to understanding the complex ways in which power works through spectral narratives.

Ghosts have proven resilient to the Age of Reason, and the institutionalization of knowledge based on the dialectics between the rational and the irrational particularly, because of their missing ontology, which positions them between the two. If there are no ghosts, why do people see them? The attempt to answer this question has led various scholars to consider the effects a human life might have on posterity after death, which immediately situates ghosts at the center of ethics. The corresponding theories, in turn, have been central to defining an atemporal sense of the Self in relation to the Other. The sighting of a ghost initiates a conversation with an externalized sense of the Self that in this moment joins a community of disembodied souls. To sight a ghost is a direct inscription into a larger community of thinking beings. Immanuel Kant therefore develops a theory of personhood that relies on the will not only of the living but also of those who are dead. As I demonstrate in the second chapter, Kant's community of "all thinking beings," however, does not include *all* human beings but only those with the capacity for reason. Death in life, therefore, became an important topic particularly within eighteenth-century moral theory, for reasons that have nothing to do with the philosophers' interests in the occult. Rather, moral theory at the time is driven by an interest in how death shapes life, an ethical discourse that only grew over the centuries. Even when posing as universal, these philosophical discussions on morality and ethics are exclusive. The elusive quality of the ghost makes this possible. Addressing science in the twenty-first century, Donna V. Jones writes in *The Racial Discourses of Life Philosophy:* "Even if not mysterious, life remains what is both most intimate and opaque to us. [...] Just as we have no word that expresses the unity of day and night, the unity of life and death is not easily expressible" (3). Classifying this lasting oscillation between life and death under the concept of vitalism, Jones continues by asserting a constitutive relation between vitalism and racialism. Ghostly figurations that are analyzed in this study are an expression of this racialized death-in-life sentiment that took hold with the Enlightenment. Affirming Jones' theory, this study demonstrates that ghosts in a settler colonial North American context cannot be understood separately from racial and colonial discourses.

Apart from feminist, postcolonial, and critical race studies, this book is indebted to more recent developments within New Materialism. Recalling sources that influential scholars in this field reference illustrates that redefining life through death is entangled with the study of ghosts. The central claim of material studies is that objects possess agency and are thus, in certain ways, alive. Redefining life through what was perceived to be dead is thus a central tenant of New Materialism. Looking at the research published in this field by one of its originators, Jane Bennett, reveals a long list of cited scholars who embrace the idea of ghosts to promote their theories of life. Bennett acknowledges that the history of vitalism is central to current ideas in new materialist thinking. In an interview, they explain that philosophers such as Henri Bergson and Hans Driesch gave "philosophical voice to the vitality of things" and "came close to a vital materialism" (J. Bennett, "Agency" 95). Henri Bergson not only developed an interest in ghosts but also served as the president of the Society for Psychical Research in 1913. The German biologist and philosopher Hans Driesch proposed life as an organizing power and published a methodology of parapsychological research focused on ghosts as intrapsychic subjectivity. Agency certainly does not equal life in New Materialist theories, nor can ghosts be described in terms of vital materialism, yet the history of parapsychological research promotes various attempts at defining life through death, thus effectively paving the way for innovative materialist theories to emerge. My study demonstrates ways in which the spectral came to constitute subjectivity that in its modern outing is racialized even before vitalism. These congruencies between racialized colonial spectral theory and new vitalist attempts to explain the world in terms of nonhuman agency demonstrate the potential that ghosts hold for future scholarship. Rather than simply a trace of the past that happens to appear in the present, ghosts are an elemental part of any "now" and therefore determine the future. As Molly McGarry asserts in her book on spiritualism, the dead are not only a means of connecting with the past but also a road into "worldly and otherworldly futures" (2).

Influenced by current developments in New Materialism, the phrase *spectral narratives* is adopted here to address the material aspects of perceiving a ghost. The ghost-seer *sees* something. "The specter is first and foremost something visible. It is of the visible, but of the invisible visible, it is the visibility of a body which is not present in flesh and blood," explains Jacques Derrida in an interview with Bernard Stiegler (Derrida and Stiegler 115). This is a much-quoted but contextless definition of the ghost. As I demonstrate in this study, the visibility of bodies not present in the United States is a space where colonialism intersects with nature. I use *spectrality* to encompass the multifunctionality and variety of stories featuring ghosts in their diverse manifestations. To some, they are not even recognizable as ghosts, appearing in natural forms and behaviors. In fact, in its early stages, the history of US American literature records surprisingly few supernatural sightings of the dead returning to haunt the living as visions of a deceased person. Instead, early cultural figurations of ghosts established a strong genealogy of spectral intrapsychic connections, not only between the living and the dead but also between humans and a type of nonhuman agency that is often represented as perceptible in forests. As common in numerous non-European traditions, ghosts need not come in human forms. Trees and stones repeatedly feature in antebellum narratives that indicate their sentient forces. Analyzing ghosts in now often-taught and -adapted texts by Irving, Neal, Child, and Hawthorne, reveals how nature turns into an agent that interferes, even communicates, with human protagonists. What does it say? To answer this question, it was necessary to expand the definition of *ghost* to spectrality—therefore, materiality.

The complexity of the question—who and what will survive as a trace, reminder, or influence even after death—is therefore reflected in this study in a careful analysis of presences. Shifting to materialist methodologies exposed that the non-Christian genealogy of ghosts and spirits—representing a sense of the biological and nonbiological world as vital and alive through the concept of death—is elemental not only for an understanding of modern representations of ghosts but also for the advent of modern subjectivity that in its transatlantic rendition establishes itself in close affiliation to racialization. So far, US American ghost stories in the context of literature have been studied mainly in relation to their European counterparts within gothic and psychological frameworks, often stripped of ethnic or racial insights. This study argues that the high number of enslaved people in the United States at the turn of the nineteenth century and the ubiquitous tradition of animism among them left a strong mark on the literary and cultural makeup of the early republic. Animism is a philosophy that subjectivizes rather than objectivizes nature and objects and by doing so blurs the line of demarcation between life and death. Moreover, the writings of missionaries and travelers to the North American continent attest to a strong interest in Indigenous cosmologies, which rely on the coexistence of ancestral spirits. These two traditional channels of communication with the dead were more influential in establishing the centrality of spectrality in US American literature than has been acknowledged by literary scholarship so far. The reason for this omission can be found in the ghost stories themselves. Antebellum writers demonstrate a pronounced effort to conceptualize an alternative form of death-in-life, often reverting back to pagan traditions or medieval mystics rather than spelling out their indebtedness to West African and Indigenous North American cultures. All of these traditions clash with Puritan visions and Protestant revisions of ghost-seeing and fuse into a modern version of US American spectral narratives. Retracing this complex genealogy in *Ghosts and Their Hosts* amounts to a transcultural definition of the US American spectral narrative beyond the human.

A well-researched and important, if mostly overlooked, contribution to the field of spectrality is Christopher Peterson's *Death, Mourning and American Affinity*. Peterson proposes the qualification of spectrality as implicated in but not reducible to "the social effects of racism, sexism and homophobia that engender a field of unlivable, abject beings" (10). Taking this proposition as a starting point, it is argued here that spectrality—even in cases where people are consigned to an existence described by Orlando Patterson as social death—does not allow for erasure. Spectrality can mark a perceptible absence or an imperceptible presence not bound to spatial and temporal restrictions. A ghost is never a metaphor for social death. The appearance of a ghost demonstrates that even enslaved people could never be erased from social life. The ontological insecurity inscribed in the appearance of a ghost functions as a trace. It is therefore significant to note that Indigenous spirits did not materialize in the form of ghosts in early American narratives written by European settler writers.

The focus on the materiality of spectrality and the inclusion of non-European perspectives in this study also led to a reconsideration of the US American gothic. The analyzed period overlaps with the emergence of the gothic novel in England of the 1760s, its peak in the transatlantic context in the 1790s, and its waning in the 1830s. Ghosts have always been central to gothic concerns, yet they have served purposes that have not been acknowledged so far. Suppressed trauma, ancestral guilt, and hidden depravities are identified as central to the US American gothic by influential scholars such as Leslie Fiedler, Charles L. Crow, Teresa Goddu, Agnieszka Soltysik Monnet, Carroll Smith-Rosenberg, or Jason Haslam. One of the most quoted scholars in this field, Teresa Goddu, writes in *Gothic America* that slavery is America's unique "historical haunting" (10). The gothic in Goddu's study is a way of coping with this haunting, and a critique of the national myth of New World innocence: "Significantly, when race is restored to the *darkness* of American literature, the gothic reappears as a viable category" (7–8). Yet, as I demonstrate, it is public and conscious secrets that structure the ghost story in the colonies and early republic alike, rather than the subconscious dominated by questions of guilt as has been suggested before. Following Toni Morrison, Maisha L. Wester rightly puts race at the center of the American gothic. In her reading, the genre is "loaded with ghostly 'monsterizings' or racial otherness" ("Gothic" 10). In fact, ghost stories have provided the form to occlude the presence of slavery and the genocide of the Indigenous population. This also explains why early American literature has produced surprisingly few ghosts proper, in the meaning of the vision of a dead human body and its reappearance among the living. At the same time, the trope of the US American forest haunted by spirits of Indigenous provenance is established. Extending the concept of ghosts to material manifestations in the forest more broadly exposes the long history of instrumentalizing literary narratives to produce a national imaginary of purification. As a meticulous practice that in Bruno Latour's theory serves the purpose of separating nature from culture, nonhumans from humans, and the objective from the subjective, purification narratives have structured some of the most important US American ghost stories. Rather than gothic, early American literature is ecogothic. The missing ecogothic perspective has occluded what has been at the heart of early American literature, the racialized forest.

The argument put forward in this study is that ghosts are not symptoms of the return of the repressed as has often been suggested in previous scholarship. Rather, ghosts expose that history is not the past and thus create a space in settler colonial narratives for unwanted and unaccounted-for yesterdays. In place of an eruptive imposition on the present, ghosts are often summoned or conjured. Sometimes their appearance is even prevented. The oft-repeated argument that slavery and genocide structure early American literature and provide its gothic contours led to the assumption that ghosts must be the harbingers of justice. Seeing ghosts would thus equal a repentance for the sins of slavery and of the genocide of the Indigenous population. Rather than the suppressed or repressed, ghosts in literature often occupy the domain of the sanctioned, the excluded from perception, and the rejected from public domain—the occluded, not necessarily the occult. A careful reading of ghost stories exposes what was left unsaid and what type of communities have been constructed around those secrets. Locating ghosts within the aesthetics of secrets is what makes them so appealing to both those who veil and those who want to unveil certain social structures. For a secret to exist, it needs to be known by someone. For a ghost to exist, it needs to be *seen* by someone. It was not the psychological suppression of slavery that made the early US susceptible to spectral matters but the public secret of slavery, a conscious—even legal—decision, rather than a subconscious inaccessible truth looming to materialize and wreak havoc.

What is more, even if understood as a symptom of the return of the repressed, ghosts would imply a progressive working-through of a traumatic experience. The interpretation of early US American spectral narratives presented in this study demonstrates that ghosts in literature have been deployed in the service of exculpation and justification as much as they have been helpful for processes of healing or collective therapy. Psychological readings of ghosts have obscured the precariousness of lives affected by colonial structures of the early republic. Still dominant today, the tendency to psychologize anything ghostly obscures the necropolitics of ghosts, a concept that allows us to formulate how the meaning of death emerges through interpretations of embodiment and the ways in which lives of some parts of the population are justified by the deaths of others (Mbembe, *Necropolitics;* Holland). Subjectivity as a function of reciprocity is highly questionable, particularly in colonial circumstances. Acknowledging the diasporic and multicultural quality of life in the postrevolutionary United States, *Ghosts and Their Hosts* proposes that rather than unity, multivalence is central to subjectivity in the early republic. And this multiplicity of voices includes those that are erased.

To conclude, the antebellum ghost story is a colonial tool for justifying land appropriation and the exploitation of human labor. As scholars such as the philosopher Judith Butler have convincingly argued: "The public sphere is constituted in part by what cannot be said and what cannot be shown. The limits of the sayable, the limits of what can appear, circumscribe the domain in which political speech operates and certain kinds of subjects appear as viable actors" (*Precarious Life* xvii). Settler colonial writers of the early republic found themselves in an awkward situation in which they needed to address the injustice happening at their doorsteps without writing about it. Spectral narratives are often configurations of this secret but public sphere. In fact, structuring the new republic around the public secret of slavery was even made official with the passage of the so-called gag rules in 1836, which banned the US House of Representatives from considering antislavery petitions. Passing those rules paradoxically exposed the necessity to forcefully keep slavery a community-structuring secret. It is therefore not a surprise that most canonical early American writers knew not to mention slavery, while encoding the secret in their writings. Ghosts and particularly haunted forests became a welcome instrument that could express and promote this topical veiling.

The focus on spectrality in early American narratives demonstrates the entanglement of North American Indigenous epistemologies, European literature, and West African knowledge, and in so doing transforms European traditions rather than merely replicating them. This multivalence makes interpreting literary figurations of ghosts as a symptom for a collective mourning over the sins of slavery untenable, as it takes into consideration only one strand of influence. Instead, this study of ghosts registers an epistemology of relationality. Encompassing non-European knowledge systems into the makeup of US American early literature in this study led to a new theory of ghosts within and outside of the scope of the gothic novel around 1800. The present study is therefore a renegotiation of the relation between cosmology and aesthetics. Spectral voices are elemental to relationality, as they create room for alterity and entanglement by either including or announcing a necessary elimination of certain subjectivities for the purposes of promoting others. Most importantly, this ontological mandate was produced not apart from but within European moral theory. As Denise Ferreira da Silva explains in *Toward a Global Idea of Race:* "historical and scientific symbolic tools both produce the national subject as a self-determined being and circumscribe the subaltern (outer-determined) moral region inhabited by the non-European members of the national polity" (xiv). In what follows, I read moral philosophy formed by spectrality, tracking actual practices through which linkages with the past are established in what is marked as absent. This spectral realism brings to the fore what history has systematically obliterated, and hopefully can repurpose these gaps for future ghosts to find a home.

1

Instrumentalizing Ghosts
"Free Philosophy" in the Seventeenth Century

Spectrality concerns the rendering visible of what would otherwise be invisible; it demands an act of perception, the seen and the seer, accompanied most often by the transmission of a sign that demands interpretation. *Spectrality* is thus helpful as an operative term when attempting to interpret ghosts in view of their materializations. The Puritan period in what is today the United States has left a particularly deep and long-lasting mark when it comes to spectral matters. The Salem witchcraft crisis—a series of witchcraft accusations, hearings, and legal persecutions that took place in colonial Massachusetts from 1691 to 1693—continues to attract scholarly and popular attention even into the twenty-first century.[1] This chapter highlights the importance of an often-neglected albeit elemental aspect of the supernatural in the Puritan context in the North American colonies—the manifestation of ghosts. For ghosts to be recognized as such, they need to materialize, either by borrowing the body of another human or object or by making themselves perceptible to someone by appealing to their senses. Whereas witches are imagined as embodied, ghosts rely on a borrowed physicality. This chapter takes a close look at whose bodies (do not) materialize within the Puritan spectral narrative.

Gillian Bennett has pointed out that ghosts and witches were not only regularly treated together in the literature of the supernatural throughout the seventeenth century, they "were so closely allied" as to "constitute virtual synonymity" (3). It is perhaps for this reason that the scholarship on the supernatural in Puritan America tends to treat ghosts and witches as interchangeable entities that lead to joint conclusions.[2] Yet, while witches have received lots of attention in current scholarship, ghosts are seldom mentioned in the context of the Puritan supernatural. Disentangling ghosts from this close embrace in analyzing specifically scenes of ghost-sightings reveals that influential Puritan scholars actively suppressed the idea of ancestral spirits in favor of stories of satanic possession. Paradoxically, materialist teachings such as the analysis of spectral sightings in Thomas Hobbes'

Leviathan (1651) only fueled the Puritan attempt to cleanse the country of "heathen believes" in the earthly presence of the spirits of the dead, with stories of "more sensible Demonstrations of an *Enchantment* growing very far towards a POSSESSION by Evil Spirits" (C. Mather, *Memorable* 12). The chapter demonstrates how Enlightenment attempts at elucidating the population feed right into white supremacist fantasies. Bodies marked as inhabited by a foreign spirit are presented as demonic and corrupted. But who are they corrupted by? In tracing the transatlantic travel of one of the first and most retold poltergeist narratives in Anglo-American culture, "The Daemon of Tedworth," this chapter demonstrates how particular performative steps involved in the process of spectral embodiment created a cultural blueprint for marking racialized bodies as satanic.

The chapter begins with an analysis of the connection between ghosts and imagination in Hobbes' *Leviathan* and Joseph Glanvill's response. In his famous collection of supernatural phenomena, *Saducismus Triumphatus* (1681), Glanvill functionalized ghost stories in order to fight the atheistic materialism of Hobbes. The transatlantic scope of this debate is exemplified in the collection published by the Puritan minister Increase Mather, published in 1684 under the title *An Essay for the Recording of Illustrious Providences*. Mather partially rewrote stories published in Glanvill's compendium, adjusting them to specifically North American colonial purposes. Tracing this history of functionalizing ghost stories from Hobbes to Glanvill to Mather exposes specific racialized and gendered materializations of one of the most important concepts that helped structure life in Puritan colonial America, the Invisible World. The construction of the Invisible World that materializes mainly in the forest owes much more to the presence of Indigenous cultures and their philosophies than has been acknowledged so far. Given that this Puritan spectral landscape set the ground for the first generation of professional writers in the United States, it will be necessary to analyze it first.

The seventeenth century marks not only the establishing and institutionalization of Enlightenment ideals, it is also a period that introduced what in retrospect can be termed ghost studies. Historian Keith Thomas extensively describes the importance and influence of divine providence in Puritan circles, the belief that an ultimate being determines the course of events. Every layperson was expected to keep track of providences, "any fortunate coincidence could be recognized as 'providence' and any lucky escape might be seen as a 'deliverance'" (Thomas 108). Tracing ghosts in late seventeenth-century New England, particularly within the genre of the so-called apparitional tale, demonstrates that this also meant that every layperson was continually on the lookout for "the Black man" (*Wonders* 37). Spectrality during this initial period of transatlantic exchange in US American cultural history is increasingly secularized, establishing nontheological moral imperatives instead. Observing these processes demonstrates the construction of race and gender within imagined materializations of spirits in seventeenth-century North America as well as ways in which narratives that focus on satanic spirits could be instrumentalized for justification of land appropriation.

From Ghosts to Imagination with Thomas Hobbes

Brian Easlea argued that the separation of the magical world from the scientific or mechanical world advanced only at a very slow pace and persisted from 1450 until at least 1750. The numerous publications with the aim of either confirming or discrediting the concept of ghosts that can be found throughout the long seventeenth century prove his point. From Reginald Scot's attack on magical beliefs as deception and fraud in *Discoverie of Witchcraft* (1584) to Cotton Mather's defense in *The Wonders of the Invisible World* (1692),[3] the scholarly debate around ghosts tightened the Enlightenment tension between reason and superstition as the once disqualified opponents became increasingly able to confront each other on equal grounds. Publications on the supernatural turned away from questions of affirmation or debunking efforts toward more scientific inquiries of the applied vocabulary or structural questions. Numerous post-Reformation publications such as most notably John Wagstaffe's *The Question of Witchcraft Debated* (1669) turned their attention to the language of the supernatural in order to disprove its applicability in the context of reason. Wagstaffe's instrumentalization of wit and ridicule was particularly successful and came to be a common style for writers who sought to expose what in their opinion was a false belief. In a countermove, publications in support of the supernatural turned to the vocabulary of reason. Paradoxically, it was the late seventeenth-century focus on Enlightenment methods such as logic, criticism, and freedom of thought that shifted the supernatural into the realm of morality. Shifting the focus from questions of existence to questions of perception acknowledged the status of the supernatural as an appropriate rival for the Enlightenment. In what follows, I examine examples of this tension in the writing by two prominent philosophers with opposing views, Thomas Hobbes and Joseph Glanvill.

Supporters of the belief in ghosts and witches in the seventeenth century had a serious opponent in the English philosopher Thomas Hobbes (1588–1679), who dedicated considerable passages to the debate in the last section of *Leviathan*. In his seminal publication, Hobbes openly attacked clerics who taught in schools for using apparitional tales for their own self-serving purposes in order to keep "common people" under their control (397).[4] While close bonds with the dead in the form of ghosts walking the earth were effectively cut with the spread of the Reformation and the theological elimination of purgatory in England, apparitional sightings during the seventeenth century were often converted into narratives that center on the devil. In Hobbes' opinion, clerics who used scripture to interpret Satan as the cause of "phantasms that appear in the air," built by nothing but "a confederacy of deceivers, that to obtain dominion over men in this present world, endeavor by dark, and erroneous doctrines to extinguish in them the Light both of Nature and of the Gospel" (393). To prove his assertion, Hobbes analyzes a number of passages from the Bible where the language of magic is, in his opinion, misused and abused. Consecration was mistaken for "*conjuration* or *incantation*" (398), whereby ghosts were needed to keep man in "Spiritual Darkness" (393).

Leviathan was written under the influence of a growing concern with the "corruption" of people, which was propelled by the events of the Civil War that raged from 1642 to 1651. Particularly language and its abuses were at the center of Hobbes' attention. In his attempt to expose rhetorical techniques of humanism, Hobbes delivers a careful examination of narrative elements, such as for example metaphors and similes, as tools that help create political disorder.[5] His treatment of ghosts is also a study of the language of spectrality and its functionalization. The fact that Hobbes dedicated a whole chapter in a text firmly grounded in political philosophy to demonology demonstrates the effect spectral matters could have in politics and culture in general at the time. Often referred to as the Age of the Enlightenment, the 1660s mark the highest presence of trials concerning witchcraft along with the inauguration of the Royal Society of London, an institution that dedicatedly promoted reason and acquiring knowledge through experimentation.[6] The period in which Hobbes wrote and distributed his manuscript was marked by a tension between religious supernaturalism and scientific realism. It is within this divide that Hobbes presents one of the first materialist critiques of ghosts and demons, shifting the discussion away from theology towards philosophical and political considerations.

Hobbes' investigations of the nature of ghost-seeing are spread throughout the pages of his most famous work, but they culminate in chapter 45, titled "Of DEMONOLOGY, and Other Relics of the Religion of the Gentiles." This chapter is particularly important for an understanding of literature, as there, thinking about the abuses of the human tendency to believe in magic and ghosts, Hobbes was led to an analysis of the nature of "imagination." If those who see ghosts imagine them, they can do so only in relation to "sight," a certain form of visualization (Hobbes 414). A ghost is what "living creatures" believe they have seen, as in a dream (Hobbes 414). This is the first modern definition of ghosts, as it does not concern the ghost as much as it focuses on the ghost-seer. Interchangeably using demons and ghosts, in chapter 45, Hobbes explains that they have been perceived as "things really without us: Which some (because they vanish away, they know not whither, nor how) will have to be absolutely incorporeal, that is to say immaterial, or forms without matter; color and figure, without any colored or figured body; and that they can put on airy bodies (as a garment) to make them visible when they will to our bodily eyes" (Hobbes 415). A ghost is therefore a presence that can make itself visible if it wants to. Making a distinction between what can be seen with "our bodily eyes" and something "seen as in memory or a dream," Hobbes traces the sources of such "erroneous" thinking in the demonology of the Greeks, the philosophy of Aristotle, and the theories of possession found among the Jewish population, therefore naturalizing the presence of imagined ghosts throughout history. He, furthermore, describes the reliance on spirits in everyday life as a form of gentilism—a heathen or pagan activity, which spread not by belief but contagion.[7] Thinking about what this might imply, he continues about the pagans' supposed ghost-seeing:

> As if the dead of whom they dreamed were not inhabitants of their own brain, but of the air, or of heaven, or hell; not phantasms, but ghosts; with just as much reason as if one should say, he saw his own ghost in a looking-glass, or the ghosts of the stars in a river; or call the ordinary apparition of the sun, of the quantity of about a foot, the *demon* or ghost of that great sun that enlightens the whole visible world: And by that means have feared them, as things of an unknown, that is, of an unlimited power to do them good or harm. (Hobbes 415)

Interpreting ghosts as something unreal but really *seen* as if in memory or a dream, Hobbes acknowledges the power of imagination as a means of exercising control; and men of letters—be they poets or priests—he identifies as the main executors. This passage, central for any study of ghosts, lays out the relation between ghosts and imagination, and their potential not only in a religious but also in a secular context. For Hobbes, a ghost implied materiality, even if the human faculties were not sufficient to feel its presence. Human imagination that relies on replicas and deformations of what is visible can conceive of a ghost as a possibility. This possibility of ghostly existence can be threatening, and this threat can be felt as real. As such, the imagined figuration can be abused for manipulation. Shifting the agency away from divinity to "the governors of the heathen commonwealths," who now have an "occasion" to install laws with the help of demons or ghosts, Hobbes exposes the necessity of understanding ghosts and the power of those who have control over this knowledge (Hobbes 415). From here, he concludes that fiction is a powerful tool for the governing classes. This line of thinking cemented the promise of studying the apparitional tale as a form of expression for human imagination, and its place at the origin of what is today understood as literature.[8]

The publication of Hobbes' *Leviathan* introduced a shift in the scholarly study of ghosts in the middle of the seventeenth century, as it ventured away from questions of belief towards the world of imagination. Hobbes' organizing device in the understanding of ghosts became vision: "And these are the images which are originally and most properly called *ideas*, and IDOLS, and derived from the language of the Grecians, with whom the word εἰδω signifies *to see*. They also are called PHANTASMS, which is in the same language, *apparitions*. And from these images it is that one of the faculties of man's nature is called the *imagination*. And from hence it is manifest that there neither is, nor can be, any image made of a thing invisible" (Hobbes 422). To do justice to the hundreds of reported cases of ghost-seeing, Hobbes introduced a discussion about the reactivation of once-"seen" images within the mind's eye. As his theory of seeing what is not there was prompted by the study of ghosts, Hobbes' text also exposed the significance of ghosts for the study of imagination.

Aware of the necessity to express a position for or against the existence of spirits, Hobbes remained the materialist who opted for the existence of spirits that are not sensible to human faculties: "To conclude, I find in Scripture that there be angels and spirits, good and evil; but not that they are incorporeal, as are the apparitions men see in the dark, or in a dream or vision; which the Latins call *spectra*, and took for *demons*. And I find that there are spirits corporeal (though subtle and invisible) but not that any man's body was possessed or inhabited by them; and that the bodies of saints shall be such, namely, spiritual bodies, as St. Paul calls them" (Hobbes 418). Hobbes found an effective way to avoid questions of ghostly existence and the danger of being marked as an atheist in acknowledging the existence of incorporeal angels and spirits and corporeal saints. And even if "spectra" did exist, humans did not have the faculties to perceive them. But they did have the faculties to imagine them.

Hobbes called for awareness of the existence of these faculties because of the power relations implied. As I will demonstrate in the subsequent chapter, this assertion was affirmed by Puritan ministers in colonial North America and repeated throughout the next centuries, most notably by Immanuel Kant in *Dreams of a Spirit-Seer* (1766) and by Charles Brockden Brown in *Wieland; or, The Transformation* (1798). In the sections dealing with ghosts, Hobbes introduced the idea that imagination is a powerful, potentially political tool and certainly a functional asset. Ghost-seeing from this moment on was increasingly discussed as a cultural phenomenon, a part of being human, and, thus, in need of analysis.

From Imagination to Ghosts with Joseph Glanvill

Those who argued in support of ghosts in the seventeenth century found a worthy advocate in the writer and cleric Joseph Glanvill (1636–1680).[9] As a member of the Royal Society, an intellectual association that promoted scientific views and claimed to reject superstition, Glanvill surprisingly broke with convention and militantly defended the study of witches and ghosts against his contemporaries. The mission statement of the Royal Society at its inauguration in 1660 was to promote and advance experimental knowledge (Skouen 23).[10] Glanvill explained his move toward the supernatural by redefining the aim of the Royal Society in an address drafted specifically for this purpose. In *Scepsis Scientifica* (1665), he explained that the aim of science was "*the searching out the true* laws *of* Matter *and* Motion, *in order to the securing of the* Foundations *of* Religion *against all attempts of* Mechanical Atheism" (53).[11] Writing about ghosts was therefore a scientific task. Not concerned with the actual existence of spirits, Glanvill nonetheless proposed that the denial of their existence was the first step towards atheism. In *Saducismus Triumphatus; or, Full and Plain Evidence Concerning Witches and Apparitions*—which he wrote until his death in 1680 and was published the following year by his mentor, Cambridge Platonist Henry More—Glanvill explains his reasons for shifting toward the supernatural more clearly. Building tension in the form of thesis and antithesis, as was typical for his period, he writes in his most famous publication:

> The NOTION of a Spirit is impossible and contradictious, and consequently, so is that of Witches; the Belief of which is founded on that Doctrine.

To which OBJECTION I answer,
(1) If the *Notion* of a *Spirit* be *absurd*, as is pretended, that of a GOD and a SOUL *distinct* from *matter*, and *immortal*, are likewise *absurdities*. (Glanvill, *Saducismus* 6–7)

In the preface, More pronouncedly names Hobbes and Spinoza as the opponents and spells out his reasons for publishing the book in a letter to Glanvill that addressed their adversaries, referred to as "Hobbians [*sic*] and Spinozians":

> I look upon it as a special piece of Providence, that there are ever and anon such fresh examples of Apparitions and Witchcrafts as may rub up and awaken their benummed and lethargick Mindes into a suspicion at least, if not assurance that there are other intelligent Beings, besides those that are clad in heavy Earth or Clay. In this, I say, methinks the Divine Providence does plainly outwit the Powers of the dark Kingdom, in permitting wicked men and women, and vagrant spirits of that Kingdom, to make Leagues or Covenants one with another; the Confession of Witches against their own Lives being so palpable an Evidence, (besides the miraculous Feats they play) that there are bad Spirits, which will necessarily open a Door to the Belief that there are good ones, and lastly that there is a God. (16)

In his letter, More marks a transition, from bad spirits that lead to good spirits, which in turn lead to God. This simple proposal met with a large number of followers on both sides of the Atlantic, who quickly helped establish *Saducismus Triumphatus* as an influential study of ghosts and witchcraft that became equally important in Puritan circles in the American colonies.

Both Glanvill and More followed a rather explicit intention. In the course of the abolishment of purgatory by the Reformation, ghosts were banned. Marking death as the hour of entrance to Heaven or Hell left no space for the undead or the in-between. Yet, as a wave of atheism and religious skepticism began spreading in the wake of the Reformation, Protestant and non-Protestant clergy rediscovered the use of spectral matters. The denial of the existence of spirits was seen as a direct way into atheism. As a consequence, the late seventeenth century witnessed a renaissance of stories that promote supernatural power, many of which revert back to apparitional entities. In 1697, a vicar of Walberton in Sussex, England, expressed the sentiment most succinctly. He was recorded as having proclaimed the collecting of providences that feature ghosts as "one of the best methods that can be pursued against the abounding atheism of this age" (quoted in Thomas 112). Glanvill in *Saducismus Triumphatus,* thus, instrumentalized the spread of apparitional narratives for exactly the opposite purpose than Hobbes did a few years before. While Hobbes claimed ghosts were used to misinterpret the Bible, Glanvill used stories of ghosts to fight the spread of atheism and, thus, confirm teachings of the Bible.[12] The success of both demonstrates the enormous potential of ghosts.

In need of a concise publication that would stop the rapid spread of rationalism and recollect the remains of supernatural belief still in existence, *Saducismus Triumphatus* marks a peculiar period of skepticism in the history of Anglo-American thought, and a shift in the discussion on ghosts. The aggressive title that was to demonstrate the "triumph" of superstition over rational thought, or so-called Sadducees—a name used for materialists, after a Jewish sect that rejected the idea of the afterlife during the time of Jesus—already suggests a struggle.[13] Arguing that, in fact, any kind of science would be impossible if firsthand observation and the occasional imposture were dismissed, Glanvill countered Hobbes' accusations of the clergy by proposing a tentative suspension of disbelief. Promoted by Glanvill and More, printing ghost stories in the seventeenth century acquired significance within the realm of reason.

In *Hamlet in Purgatory,* Stephen Greenblatt writes about the afterlife of ghosts even upon the abolishment of purgatory. He interprets the English Protestant attack on the purgatory as an attack "on the imagination," which, in turn, facilitated "Shakespeare's crucial appropriation" of the very purgatory in *Hamlet* (3). Shakespeare was certainly not alone in instrumentalizing ghosts to defend imagination. One of the widely circulated and representative ghost stories at the time was printed in *Saducismus Triumphatus* with the title "The Demon of Tedworth." The site of Tedworth's house was first featured in Glanvill's *A Blow at Modern Sadducism, in Some Philosophical Considerations about Witchcraft,* published in 1668. It remained equally prominent in *Saducismus Triumphatus,* in which Glanvill claims to have been encouraged by More to investigate this case.[14] The publication was soon to become one of the most famous studies of ghosts and witchcraft, and the Tedworth occurrence detailed there remains an often-repeated ghost story all the way into our own times.[15] In his cultural study of ghosts, Colin Wilson even suggests that "The Demon of Tedworth" is "perhaps the best-known of all poltergeist hauntings" (120). The widespread dissemination of the text established a structure that became prototypical. I will use this popular tale to exemplify the centrality of materialization for the formation (in Caroline Levine's sense) of spectral narratives.

In 1661, the English "gentleman" John Mompesson of Tedworth and an "idle Drummer" became engaged in a serious dispute (Glanvill, *Saducismus* 89). Irritated by the sound of drumming, and looking for any means to stop it, Mompesson discovers that the energetic musician was busking on a counterfeit permit. He confiscates the drum kit and stores it securely in a dark corner in the back of his house. The drummer is arrested and sent to prison; the story is laid to rest. Months later, Mompesson heard a "great knocking at his doors," and a "Thumping and Drumming on the top of his house, which continued a good space, and then by degrees went off into the Air" (91). The sound of drumming becomes a constant nocturnal companion for months, but this time there was neither a permit to disclaim nor a drummer to be imprisoned. The inexplicable sound eventually spreads throughout the house until other mysterious occurrences join the already established disorder: "Another Night, Strangers being present, it purr'd in the Childrens Bed like a Cat, at which time also, the Cloaths and children were lift up from the Bed, and six Men could not keep them down. Hereupon they removed the Children, intending to have ript up the Bed. But they were no sooner laid in another, but the second Bed was more troubled than the first" (106–7). "It" proves to be persistent, and further "disturbances" worried the Mompesson family: a "hurling in the Air over the House," "scratching under the Childrens Bed," levitating of furniture, offensive sulphurous smells, frequent "silly tricks," unaccounted lights, doors opening and shutting without an apparent agent, sounds of steps but no visible presence of a body, a rustling sound that recalls silk garments, "panting like a Dog out of Breath," and the rattling of chains (102). "This was in the day time, and seen by a whole Room full of People," as "strangers" were continually invited to witness and report on the mysterious occurrences (104).

The scene described above already contains significant modern elements of a ghost story that are still common; the unaccounted swishing and whispering, the sound of rattling chains, the possessed body of a child, levitation, and even "the motion of Boards and Chairs of themselves" (Glanvill *Saducismus* 114) and the astonished observers will remain popular throughout the centuries to follow. Most important in this narrative structure is the gradual materialization, which remains the source of narrative tension and the audience's fascination alike. The first step involves a narrator who is forced to reasonably conclude that the unseen occupant was a "Spirit" (96), an immaterial presence of undefined character affecting the body of others without having one of its own. The spirit in this text appears to be an invisible entity that can see and influence living beings and objects. Being invisible and perhaps immaterial itself, it is difficult to battle. Gradually, the angry presence begins taking hold of Mompesson's body: "And now and then he [Mompesson] should find himself forcibly held, as it were bound Hand and Foot, but he found that whenever he could make use of his Sword, and struck with it, the Spirit quitted its hold" (100). While the spirit remains invisible, the narrator gradually adds characteristics that account for an entity, even if without a shape. "It" now is named a "spectre," as its presence was felt by the way it affected the inhabitants (97): "The Man presently reached after his Sword, which he found held from him, and 'twas with difficulty and much tugging that he got it into his power, which as soon as he had done, the Spectre left him, and it was always observed that it still avoided a Sword" (97). Unlike the earlier spirit, the "spectre" appears to have a body of its own, even if it is conceivable solely in the way it affected another. Marking the unknown with a name and a borrowed physicality allows the narrator to literally fight it. The materiality of the "spectre" is inscribed in its fear of the sword, as this fear is associated with a body that could be hurt.[16] This prompts a "Gentleman of the Company" to logically conclude that if a presence is felt, one should talk to "it" (98). Entering into a conversation with the mysterious visitor might lead to an agreement, possibly a positive outcome for both sides. Eventually, the "Gentleman," who is introduced as yet another "stranger," performs a public address of the Unknown, during which the specter becomes the devil himself: "*Satan,* if thee Drummer set thee to work, give three knocks and no more" (98). The drummer—which before becoming Satan or at least his vassal, was first termed "it," then a spirit that turned into a specter—finally responds. Three knocks are heard and a Bible is discovered in the ashes, lying open at the third chapter of Saint Mark, which contains the passage where Jesus transfers power to his disciples to cast out unclean spirits. Having created a body step-by-step, Mompesson and his numerous visitors discovered how to dispose of it. This process of embodying and addressing a problem now can safely be folded into a dénouement: the real drummer was consulted and freed from prison, and the evil disturbance was put to rest.

It is during the late seventeenth century in tales like "The Daemon of Tedworth" that ghost stories in Western cultures receive their recognizable narrative form. At the same time, ghosts are increasingly acknowledged as powerful ideological entities. The unwillingness of a growing number of natural philosophers to condemn the supernatural, and their inclusion

of ghosts within intellectual discussion, shifted the debate beyond questions of belief. The poltergeist event in Tedworth was published within
a philosophical treatise that set itself the task of scientifically proving
the authenticity of supernatural occurrences without verifying the *true* character of the event. Fluctuating between a scientific inquiry and a fictional
story, "The Daemon of Tedworth," with its central placement in *Saducismus
Triumphatus,* was never proved or disavowed. It did not take an enlightened scholar to unveil the mysteries of deception: in the very introduction,
the reader is informed by More that both Glanvill and Mompesson "had
confess'd the whole Matter to be a Cheat and Imposture" (More quoted in
Glanvill *Saducismus* "To the Reader," n.p.).[17] Glanvill followed his interest
in ghosts, not to enter a conversation with adversaries of the occult but
to advance his understanding of metaphysical questions and the ideas of
the new sciences. Only seemingly opposing materialists like Hobbes, he allowed himself to dwell on the possibilities of the immaterial and the power
of imagination. As we will see in what follows, his search for divinity is
paved with very real bodies incorporating what was presented as evil spirits. The late seventeenth century, thus, temporally marks the beginning of
performative ghost-seeing in a European Anglo-American cultural context.

Embracing the idea of an ongoing scientific experiment on ghosts that
is prone to failure as much as it is to success arguably marked the birth of
the modern ghost story.[18] Glanvill and More's text succinctly expressed the
ideology that drove the discussion around ghosts toward a scholarly
analysis of spectrality as a cultural occurrence. Instead of the prevailing
dogmatism of disbelief, both proposed an open-minded investigation, or,
as Glanvill would later call it, "Free Philosophy" (Glanvill, *Essays* 63). In his
collection *Essays on Several Important Subjects in Philosophy and Religion,*
Glanvill titled essay 7 "Anti-Fanatical Religion, AND Free Philosophy." Free
philosophy is also mentioned in essay 4 as a cure against "a defect in clearness of Thoughts" (2) as well as against "Notional Knowledge" (4). Glanvill's mentor More himself had already published a defense of witchcraft
before promoting Glanvill's writing, in which he forwards his theories as a
"mere Naturalist" who follows his goal to "vanquish *Atheisme*" (More B4).
Both of these scholars claimed that their idea of free philosophy implies
free thinking, skepticism, and criticism and, therefore, is an enlightened
effort put in the service of promoting Christian religion. In this way, when
ghosts seemed to have reached the end of their earthly reign in England,
they returned more fervently than ever, supported and functionalized by
prominent voices of scientists and rationalists.

The Puritan Apparitional Tale as Democratic Natural History

Hobbes' warning about the power of the ghost story and Glanvill's application of the same did not go unacknowledged on the other side of the
Atlantic. In the manuscript that preceded *Saducismus Triumphatus,* published under the title *A Blow at Modern Sadducism, in Some Philosophical
Considerations about Witchcraft* (1668), Glanvill had already proposed the
study of spirits and ghosts to the Royal Society by comparing the land of
spirits to "America": "Indeed, as things are present, the LAND of SPIR-
ITS is a kind of AMERICA, a not well discover'd *Region;* yea, it stands
in the *Map* of *humane Science* like *unknown Tracts,* fill'd with *Mountains,
Seas,* and *Monsters.* For we meet with little in the *Immaterial Hemisphere,*
but *Doubts, Uncertainties,* and *Fables;* and whether we owe our ignorance
in these matters, to the *nature* of the *things* themselves, or to the *mistakes*
and *sloth* of those that have enquired about them I leave to your Lordship's
happy sagacity to determine" (preface, n.p.). Exploring ghosts is presented
as uncharted territory that calls for more inspection. Yet, unexplored
"America" was a rich and uncharted land of spirits itself. The missionary
work of the Irish natural scientist Robert Boyle—one of the principle
founders of the British Royal Society and one of the most important figures
in the history of modern science—helped establish the North American
colonies as a haven for ghost stories. Boyle shared with Glanvill the conviction that promoting stories related to ghosts and witchcraft would secure the dominance of Christianity. From 1661 to 1689, he took over the
governorship of the newly inaugurated "Company for the Propagation of
the Gospel in New England." According to Michael Hunter, throughout
his life Boyle retained an at times covert interest in ghosts and witchcraft,
which was expressed in his effort to collect and commission others to collect what he himself called "supernatural phenomena" (*Robert Boyle* 224).
Although Boyle had never set foot in the New World, Hunter provides
ample evidence of Boyle actively commissioning missionaries to collect
"supernatural phenomena" among the Indigenous population in New
England (*Decline of Magic* 12, 14). Sarah Rivett's research also affirms that
missionaries at the time were collecting stories about ghosts. For example,
Rivett quotes a letter that a Puritan missionary has sent to Boyle in 1670
asking for money to compensate a group of "Indians" who use "a particular
'root' that allows them to 'read' spiritual phenomena" ("Empirical Desire"
16). Boyle's documents relating to the supernatural were collected in a
manuscript entitled *Strange Reports,* and stories concerning ghosts, spirits,

and witches were to comprise the second part of this text. Only the first part, with a focus on natural occurrences, was published; the second part is lost. Yet, in spite of this missing record, Rivett and Hunter documented that Boyle was actively promoting collecting ghost stories and related phenomena on both sides of the Atlantic and that he commissioned assistants to collect supernatural phenomena among the Indigenous population in the colonies.

It is, therefore, not a surprise that by the end of the seventeenth century, the so-called New World was directing its own "wary, and luciferous enquiries towards the World of Spirits" (Glanvill, *Blow*, Preface, n.p.). Boyle's and Glanvill's hopes of enlarging the philosophical horizon through the study of ghosts and witchcraft were shared by many of their American contemporaries, most prominently by the Puritan clergyman Increase Mather. Mather was yet another member of the Royal Society, and the founder of its American counterpart, the now almost forgotten American Scientific Society.[19] He followed the already beaten path of spectral experimentation, although he adjusted the rules to the needs of his own country.

The narrative form that most prominently expresses this sentiment is the providence tale of the seventeenth century, which was, next to the sermon, the most common literary genre in New England. Narratives with what was interpreted as providential plots came to represent a medium that God uses to speak to his subjects in Puritan America. There, God's language became a collection of natural acts that were interpreted as paranormal, such as floods and lightning. Within this genre, natural disasters were conjoined with scenes of possession, haunting, and witchcraft, creating a powerful tool against atheistic tendencies. A combination of the supernatural, the sublime, and the transcendent was accordingly tightened within a scientific framework that was perfectly suited to the idea of a promised land offering freedom of religious expression. James Hartman demonstrated in his key study *Providence Tales and the Birth of American Literature* how the New England providence tale went through a dramatic change at the end of the seventeenth century, becoming a tool to persuade atheists, skeptics, and materialists of the power and compassion of God. The apparitional tale, which Hartman convincingly considers to be a subgenre of the providence tale in Puritan America, had a significant role in facilitating this connection.

The story of the Daemon of Tedworth's journey across the ocean demonstrates how aspects of vague or erroneous knowledge can be instrumentalized and turned into a productive source of national importance. Following Glanvill's example, and unfazed by his knowledge of the story's fictitious nature, Mather wrote in his *An Essay for the Recording of Illustrious Providences* (1684) about "the disturbance" in the house in Tedworth, "which was by wise men judged to proceed from conjuration" (I. Mather, *Essay* 156).[20] Keeping his sources secret and the "wise men" anonymous, Mather collected similar stories in New England, however, he significantly chose to exclude narratives collected among the Indigenous population. And even the ghost stories imported from England serve only as a reference: "A parallel Story of a House at Tedworth in England. Concerning another in Hartford. And of one in Portsmouth in New-England lately disquieted by Evil Spirits. The Relation of a woman at Barwick in New-England molested with Apparitions, and sometimes tormented by invisible Agents" (135). The "invisible Agents" in most of the examples collected by Mather demonstrate a preference for molesting settler colonial women and children. Mather suggests that divine providence is at work, while assuring the reader that "as yet no place, nor any person in *New-England* (excepting the instances before mentioned) have been troubled with *Apparitions*" (202). Drawing a fine line between believing and doubting, Mather confirms: "Nevertheless, that spirits have sometimes really (as well as imaginarily) appeared to Mortals in the World, is amongst sober men beyond controversie" (203). Thus, while the possibility of ghosts was approved, the American readership was assured that none were walking the earth of New England, even if sometimes it seemed like they were. Aware of the accessibility of spiritual matters beyond questions of proof or belief, Mather meandered together with his readers through "providential" scenes gathered from "wise men" without developing a theory or discussing questions of authenticity.

In contrast to Hobbes, whose analysis of ghost stories led to an attempt at a theory of imagination, Mather focused on the value of ghost stories as proof of the providential nature of the (new) world. The one problem he faced was how to acknowledge the existence of ghosts without affirming their presence. Apart from paraphrasing the occurrence in Tedworth, Mather offered numerous similar stories that were gathered by anonymous Puritan ministers from England and Ireland, but avoided acknowledging the local presence of similar stories. In the preface, he explained that the collected material was the result of a meeting of Massachusetts ministers in 1681 who decided to compile a register of providences influenced by the English Presbyterian minister Matthew Poole. He, in turn, was to collect providential accounts throughout the country and analyze them in a concise publication. Part of Poole's script made it into Mather's text rewritten and polished; the rest consists of stories borrowed from Glanvill, providential episodes related by New England ministers, and Mather's own observations, comments, and speculations. Prior to publishing the collection, a call for submissions was sent out to ministers in all North American colonies to collect their own regional tales. Those were subsequently approved "at some meeting of the elders" and integrated in the final version of Mather's publication (I. Mather, *Essay,* Preface, n.p.). Ceremonial approval by figures of authority vouched for authenticity, while the result resembles a catechism of American wonders presented as natural history. Yet, the collection pronouncedly excludes materializations of ghosts and stories collected among the Indigenous population.

Oscillating between fact and fiction, incredible stories are established as credible possibilities. Mather even promotes the obscure origin of his book: "the composer whereof is to me unknown" (I. Mather *An Essay* Preface). This element in no small degree adds to the interpolation of known and unknown, rational and irrational, realism and magic, rumor and fact. In classic ghost-story manner, Mather took care to accumulate sources that could be tracked only with great difficulty. Shifting the responsibility away from the author to "notable" references, he explained the provenance of one of the stories: "The relator had this from the mouth of Mr. Beaumond, a minister of note at Caen in Normandy, who assured him that he had it from one of the ministers that did assist in carrying on the day of prayer when this memorable providence hapned. Nor is the relation impossible to be true; for Luther speaks of providence, not unlike this, which hapned in his congregation" (I. Mather, *Essay,* Preface, n.p.). The individual tales are bracketed by narrative frames within which the reader is informed that the unknown is mediated through rumors, the origin of which drowns in a sea of voices. The multiplication of references reduces or eradicates the need for a traceable source. Instead, the act of witnessing dominates the narrative within a generic publication, which is presented as a collection resembling an anthropological field study. Excusing himself on account of his ill health and age, Mather expresses the hope that another person, preferably "born in this land," would "do such a service to his country" and continue where he left off. In the preface, he added that while his collection remained a transatlantic conglomeration of similar occurrences on both sides of the ocean, his publication would hopefully serve as a first step in writing "the Natural History of New-England" (I. Mather, *Essay,* Preface, n.p.).

Collecting stories about "divine judgements, tempests, floods, earthquakes, thunders as are unusual, strange apparitions, or whatever else shall happen that is prodigious, witchcrafts, diabolical possessions" was offered as natural history and a matter of national importance and scientific inquiry (I. Mather, *Essay*, Preface, n.p.).[21] Mather hoped that this work would develop into a relevant body of science based on guidelines proposed by the already famous scientist Boyle. Choosing Boyle was not a coincidence, for the famous chemist and preeminent member of the Royal Society was a resolute spokesperson for the spread of the gospel among the world's heathen. Yet, rather than simply collecting ghost stories, Mather went to great lengths to divorce ghosts from the belief in a return of the dead. Like the clerics accused by Hobbes, he shifted the focus to the devil's business instead. Thus, the idea of a revenant is completely banned. Mather repeatedly urges his readers to comprehend that magicians and necromancers were said to cause dead persons to appear, but "those apparitions were caco-daemons, which feigned themselves to be the spirits of men departed" (*Essay* 211). The rich tradition of Indigenous spirits is carefully avoided during this project. Chapter after chapter, Mather vehemently rejects the idea of the return of the dead and the presence of ancestral spirits, insisting rather that while God sent his angels, the devil assumes the shape of deceased people. In doing so, he confirms what was already proposed by Hobbes, namely that imagination simply plays tricks on the ghost-seer's mind. Mather concludes that it was "a cursed and lying art" to propose that it is possible for men to cause "the souls of dead persons to be brought back again" (*Essay* 212). Or again: "That the ghosts of dead persons have sometimes appeared, that so the sin of murder (as well as that of theft) might be discovered, is a thing notoriously unknown" (*Essay* 220). In this way, one of the most common assumptions about ghosts is discarded: the reanimation of the dead for purposes of reinstalling justice. Instead, justice was regulated by the voice of God alone, who communicated with Puritan America through providential sign language. In one of his later publications, *Cases of Conscience concerning Evil Spirits Personating Men, Witchcrafts, Infallible Proofs of Guilt in Such as Are Accused with That Crime* (1693), Mather for the purposes of replacing ghosts with the devil even reinterpreted the much-discussed and only story of necromancy in the Bible: the conjuring of the prophet Samuel. In Mather's interpretation, "the Devil by the Instigation of the Witch of Endor appeared in the likeness of the prophet Samuel" (*Cases of Conscience,* n.p.); a very peculiar interpretation indeed, as the devil's motivation remains occluded. This rewriting of ghost stories all the way back to the Bible proved programmatic in Mather's oeuvre. His insistence on providing a semiscientific framework without leaving the confines of religion turned ghosts into a powerful rhetorical figure in North America. Puritan settlers were now free to interpret the providential signs they collected in whichever way they pleased.

Thus, during the seventeenth century, the methodology of the new sciences promulgated by the Royal Society of London is not only appropriated for the study of ghosts but also for the conversion of the pagan belief in ancestral spirits into a Christian ghost story genre based on providence. The "land of spirits" did, indeed, become "a kind of America" as anything spectral became recodified as providence. This colonial measure framed by science, more than anything else, explains the sudden animation and interest in anything ghostly in the colonies. Following the lead of Glanvill and More and adopting ideas developed by Hobbes and Boyle, Mather suggests that some of the episodes presented in his compendium might be true while others might not and marks the realm of rumors or what Shibutani in his now classic definition described as "improvised information that emerges out of a collective process of discussion" as a significant scientific source of information.[22] The preface calls for experimentation and openness— the general method of Aristotelian scholasticism. In this way, the very nature of the publication, placed somewhere in between the triangle of natural science, public history, and sensational fiction before it was established, allowed for a cogent policing of spirits in colonial America. Opening a semisecular space populated by spirits, ghosts, and witches, Mather claimed to provide a neutral forum where the voice of the people could be heard. Everybody was invited to practice free philosophy in the colonies, as long as they were of European descent and willing to convert their stories into providential tales.

The transformation of ghosts into the devil that represents the shift of individual responsibility to divine providence received full acknowledgment in one of the most curious episodes of Puritan history in New England: the introduction of so-called spectral evidence. The phrase refers to a legal claim that was invented in Salem during the notorious witchcraft trials of 1692 and used in the Court of Oyer and Terminer.[23] In court, spectral evidence referred to the assumption that if a devil made a contract with a person, the devil received permission to assume the person's shape to either recruit further vassals or simply to carry out his satanic deeds. In this way, a person could appear in one place even if evidence proved that the actual body had been seen in another. The many stories of satanic contracts could be used in court as evidence. In spite of Increase Mather's later rejection of this concept, his writings were corroborated in supporting this type of testimony, as he repeatedly insisted that North American colonies had never been sites for apparitions. Paradoxically, the concept of spectral evidence grew out of his previous promotion of satanic possession in place of ghostly sightings. According to the logic in his writing, so-called ghost sightings could only be explained as incidents in which the devil takes the shape of human bodies or remotely controls their actions. The devil could possess anybody—or any body. This idea was to replace the "heathen" belief in spirits of the dead returning to the realms of the living. In Puritan America, thanks to, among others, Increase Mather's tireless promotion, the devil was to replace ghosts in the form of material bodies.

Just as ghosts entered scientific discourse without their existence having to be proved, the devil infiltrated the courtroom without needing to be verified.[24] The fiction behind witnessing a case of possession opened the doors to sensation-thirsty storytellers in the seventeenth and eighteenth centuries, while the possibility of punishment was extended to anyone who opposed the teachings of influential Puritan ministers. Indeed, the devil was now to be expected on each and every street corner. People seen in places where they should not have been became suspects. In this way, the devil's radius extended limitlessly. In Puritan American courts, the English colonists adopted the rhetoric of spectrality that they had previously rehearsed in the omnipresent providential narratives. Using simple sentences and a reporting style concerned with verification and authentication, most of the narratives circled around serious atrocities that remained unchallenged. Visible violence on the bodies of women or children or less dramatic stories of adultery could now be explained as the result of possession. When "a noble person" was frequently seen going out of an empress' chamber, it "appeared that the suspected noble person had not been there, only a daemon in his shape" (I. Mather, *Essay* 214). Puritan America found a new way to close its eyes by looking carefully; and spectral evidence spread like a wave throughout the Boston area, quickly becoming the most common means of accusation in court.[25] The extent to which ghosts that are devils had taken over New England is recognizable in the decision of the Governor of Salem at that time, William Phips, to create a special court in October 1692, specifically charged with dismantling or rather ignoring spectral evidence. Increase Mather followed his lead and used his authority to end the abuse of this type of witnessing by making spectral evidence unusable as legal testimony. However, the concept was already so widely spread that no judicial proposal could stop it.

The Spectral Settler Colonial Palimpsest

Ghosts that turned out to be the devil went through another significant transformation in Puritan North America of the late seventeenth century. To enforce a claim to authenticity, which was formed from rumors nestled within a scientific discourse, Increase Mather repeatedly insisted on his use of "found" material. His findings proved that ghosts, or the devil, related to matters concerning the Indigenous population. Consequently, new versions of the story of the Daemon of Tedworth emerged with significant changes; in the most prominent one, the disturbance of the inhabitants was explained by "cobs of Indian corn" that fell on the haunted house in New England (*Essay* 159). The Christianization of the ghost story remained the same and strengthened the chain of divine power wrapped around colonial America. John Mompesson of Tedworth, just like in the European version, was rescued from the supernatural disturbance with the help of the Bible. In fact, the story was already so established in the North American colonies that the narrator in Mather's providence tales simply reduced the story to an outline of the Tedworth story, which served to establish a precedent and move on to "similar occurrences" in New England; one of which concerned a certain Nicholas Desborough from Hartford, who experienced commotion comparable to that seen in the Mompesson household. However, in this case, the inhabitant was molested by "stones, pieces of earth, *cobs of Indian corn,* & c., falling about him, which sometimes came in through the door, sometimes through the window, sometimes down the chimney; at other times they seemed to fall from the floor of the chamber, which yet was very close, sometimes he met with them in his shop, the yard, the barn, and *in the field at work*" (*Essay* 159; emphasis added). This seemingly minute element proved important, as it placed the occurrence within a North American context. Indeed, Indian corn cannot be found in any of the European versions of poltergeist stories. Drawing from mostly European tales, Mather needed an exclusively North American element. Given the heavy symbolic weight that corn carried at that time, this narrative addition begs interpretation. Native to Mexico and later the Americas, corn was cultivated as the most important food crop by hundreds of different Indigenous cultures. As such, the presence of "Indian corn" would inevitably have been understood as an Indigenous element by readers on both sides of the Atlantic. In this way, borrowed stories from "the Old World" transformed the unknown sources of "evil" within passages from colonial America into a quite specific source of distress. Yet, corn is only one element in this influential compendium that marks the presence of the Native population as the source of evil.

As Mather explains: "It would fill a volume to give an account of all the memorable preservations in the time of the late war with the Indians" (*Essay* 39). The longest episode in the American version of the Glanvillian wonder compendium is the narrative of one Quintin Stockwell, who claimed he was captured by "the Indians" and then set free. With this narrative, a sudden move to personal storytelling creates a sense of urgency. An almost adventurous character is introduced, and a tale more of captivity than providence was recounted by a survivor of the incident: "The enemy espying us so near them, ran after us and shot many guns at us; three guns were discharged upon me, the enemy being within three rods of me, besides many other, before that" (*Essay* 40). The use of asyndeton in this tale marks the desperation of the narrator. Whereas the agent of evil was unknown before, now there was suddenly an enemy "within three rods" confronting "me," while the providential tale takes on the narrative structure of an adventure. For the first time, a first-person narrator joins the providential assortment, as a face-to-face encounter is recounted: "and whilst I was going, I fell right down lame of my old wounds that I had in the war, and whilst I was thinking I should therefore be killed by the Indians, and what death I should die, my pain was suddenly gone, and I was much encouraged again" (42). The tales involving unspecified characters that are referred to only as "Indians" in this collection are without exception testimonials of European Puritan settlers who had seen evil and can now report on it to future generations. Next to mainly female bodies which suffered from levitation and pinches from "invisible hands," Mather's publication collects domestic stories of settlers who lived in fear of "the Indians." The providential accounts could easily morph into captivity narratives and similar frontier tales. Every time Stockwell escaped a seemingly life-threatening situation, the author suggested a divine providence as his source of strength and rescue from "the devil" or "the Indian" or both. Even when Stockwell was but recapitulating the emotional and physical support that came from that very same "Indian," the author manufactured evil. Stockwell reports: "This Indian now was kind, and told me that if he did not carry me I would die, and so I should have done sure enough; and he said I must tell the English how he helped me" (56). Unaffected by the display of camaraderie, the omniscient narrator of the report concludes: "No doubt but others are capable of declaring many passages of Divine Providence no less worthy to be recorded than these last recited" (58). This convincing mixture of providence tale, captivity narrative, and apparitional tale, in turn, allowed the author, Increase Mather, to propose that with divinity's help, benevolence could be exchanged for evil. Placed as yet another example of remarkable providence, Mather's local additions replaced unknown immaterial disturbance in the European precedent cases with the short-lived physicality of the North American Indigenous population. "It," which became a spirit, which became a specter, which turned into a devil, now had a visible presence—a specific racial identity. The stones falling on haunted houses were now Indian corn; "It" was an "Indian"; "It" could be battled with a sword and exterminated or exorcized once and for all. Before race was invented, the Puritans had ghosts. Wonders take inexplicable turns, indeed, and Mather concluded that European settlers must be the chosen nation, since God decided to save them from the hands of "the Indian." In this way, a sense for victimization, destiny and retribution was created within the settler colonial North American imaginary with the help of a European ghost story template. In a second step, this newly established forum was marked with racial identity insignia. With the "Indian," the evil in Puritan America finally received a body that could be exorcized. And the pattern was so effective that it could be applied to other narrative frameworks.

Increase Mather's *An Essay for the Recording of Illustrious Providences* opened the door to numerous epigones. Stories of evil as "Indians" embedded within providential tales mushroomed even before the typical captivity narratives were established as a genre.[26] Soon they were to support the idea that the war against "Native Americans" was just and that the army existed purely "to execute the vengeance of the Lord upon the perfidious and bloody Heathen."[27] Cotton Mather, Increase Mather's son, emerged as one of his father's most fervent proponents, continuing and refining the narrative tradition his father had domesticated. By the time the second Mather published *The Wonders of the Invisible World* (1693), the connection between the Indigenous people of North America and the devil was not a question of subtle tales anymore. In one of the most famous passages of his infamous collection, Mather explains that colonial settlers had a religious responsibility to cleanse the newly acquired territory, since it had been in the hands of the devil: "The New-Englanders are a people of God settled in those, which were once the Devil's territories; and it may easily be supposed that the Devil was exceedingly disturbed, when he perceived such a People here accomplishing the Promise of old made unto our Blessed Jesus, that he should have the Utmost parts of the Earth for his Possession" (C. Mather, *Wonders* 20). With passages such as this one, Mather marked the Puritan providential project in North America as land appropriation.

Later, Mather explicitly spelled out how this project was to be carried out most pronouncedly in the collection of essays *Good Fetch'd Out of Evil* (1706), in which he replaced with divine intervention any positive interpretation of cultures native to the territories that became the colonies: "Tis a wonderful Restraint from God upon the Brutish Salvages, that no *English Woman* was ever known to have any Violence offered unto her *Chastity*, by any of them. [. . .] Tis wonderful, that when many of the *Captives* have been just going to be Sacrificed, Some strange Interposition of the Divine Providence has put a Stopp to the Execution, and prevented their being made a Sacrifice. The Stories are Numberless. Take a few of them" (*Good Fetch'd Out of Evil* 26). In what follows, Cotton Mather offers a long list of captivity narratives in which nameless Indigenous characters decide to spare the lives of European settlers. These stories were then used to propose that divine providence rescued the captives from the "Hands of the Barbarous Indians, a Subject of wondrous Afflictions, of wondrous Deliverances" (C. Mather, *Wonders* 35), thus actively suppressing even the possibility of benevolence. In a prototypical story, a man who "valiantly kill'd an Indian or two" is captured by an undefined group of "Indians" (*Wonders* 35), who propose that the widow of one of the killed men should decide upon the future of the captive. The woman orders him to be released, since no revenge can bring back her husband. Of this, Mather concluded: "One cannot well imagine any other than *Supernatural* and *Angelical* Assistances" (*Wonders* 37). Conjuring ghosts in North America would never again be far removed from drawing magic circles around Indigenous protagonists.

The main agent within this narrative construction was and remains the devil, who now regularly oscillates between depictions of "an Indian" or "a black man." In fact, already in *An Essay for the Recording of Illustrious Providences* the narrator reports "disturbances" in the Morse house in New England and relates them to a "*Blackmore* Child" (I. Mather, *Essay* 154). The incident is first compared to the story from Tedworth. While most "disturbances" were presented as "undoubtedly preternatural and not without diabolical operation," the narrator assured his readers that their earthly presence was commonly not identifiable (*Essay* 113). However, an alteration can be found in the following version, which depicts the sight of the devil:

All this while the Devil did not use to appear in any visible shape, only they would think they had hold of the Hand that sometimes scratched them; but it would give them the slip. And once the Man was discernably beaten by a Fist, and an Hand got hold of his Wrist which he saw, but could not catch; and the likeness of a Blackmore Child did appear from under the Rugg and

Blanket, where the Man lay, and it would rise up, fall down, nod and slip under the clothes when they endeavored to clasp it, never speaking any thing.
(I. Mather, *Essay* 154)

In later reprints, a "Blackmore Child" is closer identified with a footnote
that reads "Blackamoor, negro" (I. Mather, *Essay* 1914, 30). Thus, while the
devil "did not used to appear in any visible shape," it now showed itself
to the Euro-American settler family pronouncedly, in the shape of a racialized child.

While the anthropomorphized vision of the devil as a "Blackmore
Child" in providential tales might have been a single occurrence, the figure
appears repeatedly as an adult. In *The Wonders of the Invisible World* (1693),
in a curious passage that is part of the "report" about the first Salem witchcraft trial,[28] Cotton Mather reports on the "Black man" who walked the
earth asking "Sufferers" to sign his "Book" (*Wonders* 37). Later, the same figure was identified as "a little Black hair'd man," who was "bragging that he
was a Conjurer" (*Wonders* 71). Furthermore, in his sketch of the first trial,
Mather concluded that the "*Black man* (as the Witches call the Devil; and
they generally say he resembles an Indian)" is in possession of preternatural
strength (*Wonders* 75). The "Black man," who generally resembled an "Indian," and implicitly was the devil, not only kept returning throughout the
younger Mather's account of the Salem witch trials, but also became one of
the most frequent characters in his oeuvre. As Norton explains in her study
In the Devil's Snare: "the frequent references to the 'black man' by confes-
sors and the afflicted establish a crucial connection between the witchcraft
crisis and the Indian wars" (59).

Just as in his father's writing, the "Black man" in the younger Mather's
work surrounded himself with specters (C. Mather, *Wonders* 75). He also
preferred the company of young women still in their bodies. Mather introduced his record "Account of the Sufferings of Margaret Rule" as "a
very entertaining story" and continued with a letter in which he agreed
to write "some things which [he] would have omitted in a farther publication" (*Wonders* 18). While the story of Margaret Rule has been interpreted
by various feminist scholars, the opening incident has been widely omitted
from analysis.[29] Yet, it is in the introductory section that an emphasis on ra-
cializing apparitional tales comes to the fore. There, the reader is introduced
to a "converted Indian" who is a zealous preacher of the gospel in his neighborhood and "to whose conduct was owing very much of what good order
was maintained among these proselyted savages" (19). The "Indian" buried

his son and then died. Setting a stereotype, the Indigenous character only receives a voice through the settler narrator and posthumously—a narrative structure that later turned canonical in the literature of the early republic. It is at this connecting point between life and death, between speech and silence, that Mather introduces his reader to "the black man": shortly before the Indian died, "the black man" appeared to him while he was working in the forest. He urged the Indian to stop preaching, yet the latter refused. The "black man" vanished, and shortly after "the Indian" died, a certain woman named Margaret Rule fell sick to bed. Cotton Mather's narrative immediately moves on to the "black man," who was now assumed to be controlling Rule's body. In this narrative, the devil moves from trying to corrupt the converted Indigenous man to possessing the body of the woman, while Mather remains close to both in order to control his itinerary and report about it to posterity. The fact that the markedly Indigenous character was not saved, in spite of his dedication to Christianity, proves that the role of this character differs from already established providential paths.

It is often in front of the possessed body of young women that Mather claimed to encounter this invisible character repeatedly referred to as "the black man." In the account of supposed possession, Mather explains:

> Sometimes, but not always, together with the Spectres there look't in upon the Young Woman (according to her account) a short and a Black Man, whom they call'd their Master, exactly of the same Dimensions and Complexion and Voice, with the Divel that has exhibited himself unto other infested People, not only in other parts of this Country but also in other Countrys, even of the European World, as the relation of the Enchantments there inform us, they all profest themselves Vassals of this Devil, and in obedience unto him they address themselves unto various ways of Torturing her; accordingly she was cruelly pinch't with Invisible hands very often in a Day, and the black and blew marks of the pinches became immediately visible unto the standers by. (C. Mather, *Wonders* 25)

Specters that serve the black man and appear to be controlling the body of a woman proved to be a frequent constellation in Mather's writing. The bruised body described in the scene above belonged to Margaret Rule. Increase and Cotton Mather often visited Margaret Rule and regularly reported that "the black man" and his helpers were the perpetrators who injured and marked her body, insisting that the wounds on her body proved the existence of the devil and his specters. In spite of the many witnesses,

the torture of Margaret Rule and the obvious physical abuse were never resolved. The incident, however, did lead to a controversy even while it was
happening, during which not only the integrity of both Mathers was questioned but also their insistence on "the black man" and his specters.

In a controversial publication that first appeared in England under the
telling title *More Wonders of the Invisible World* (1700), the Boston mer-
chant Robert Calef introduced himself as a witness and confronted Cotton Mather directly, indicating that "the black man" was an invention by
Mathers rather than an apparition seen by Puritan Americans. In a scene
that was to cause quite a disturbance in the Mathers' household, Calef depicted father and son leaning over the body of the supposedly possessed
Margaret Rule and pushing her to *see* the "black man." Encircled by some
thirty or forty people, Calef, who called himself the witness, describes
"Mr. M (father and son)" asking questions:

> Do you know that there is a hard master? Then she was in a fit. He laid his
> hand upon her face and nose, but as he said without perceiving breath; then
> he brushed her on the face with his glove, and rubbed her stomach (her breast
> not being covered with the bed-clothes) and bid others to do so too, and said it
> eased her—then she revived. *Q.* Don't you know there is a hard master? *A.* Yes.
>
> Then he asks about the black man. *Q.* You have seen the black man,
> have you not? *A.* No. *Reply;* I hope you never shall. *Q.* You have had a Book
> offered you, hant you? *A.* No. *Q.* The brushing of you gives you ease, don't it?
> *A.* Yes. She turn'd her self and a little Groan'd. (44)

Calef's chronicle entry from September 19, 1693, a short time after the first
encounter, reads as follows: "This Night I renew'd my Visit, and found her
rather of a fresher Countenance than before, about eight Persons present
with her, she was in a Fit Screaming and making a Noise: Three or four
Persons rub'd and brush'd her with their hands, they said that the brushing
did put them away, if they brush'd or rub'd in the right place; therefore they
brush'd and rub'd in several places, and said that when they did it in the
right place she could fetch her Breath, and by that they knew" (46–47).
This highly sexualized scene, in which a religious leader was "laying hands"
on naked body parts of a young woman, conjuring or exorcising the devil,
imagined as the "Black man" who "resembles an Indian," into or out of her
body provoked a small stir after Calef's exposure (C. Mather, *Wonders* 75).
Cotton Mather responded to Calef's publication with a series of letters that
were all published along with Calef's account, but the stench of abuse could
not be eradicated anymore.

I read this incident as the initial cultural marking in an Anglo-American context of male racialized bodies as sexual predators.[30] The transition of evil as "the black man" from the Indigenous to the blackened bodies, possessing or molesting the bodies of European settler women that now needed to be healed by Puritan ministers, initiated a discussion that would not have happened had the apparitional tale remained within the confines of the frontier. Calef never stood up for women; rather he spoke in the name of Puritan American men and blamed Cotton Mather for letting "loose the Devils of Envy, Hatred, Pride, Cruelty, and Malice against each other; yet still disguised under the Mask of Zeal for God" (Calef 5). For Calef the fact that a member of Puritan society, albeit a woman, was affected exposed that the "Malice" was dangerous (Calef 138). It is for this reason that Calef's voice was so well heard. And while Mather could partially recover from this public exposure, the appearance of "the Black man" remained effective when accusing the innocent and excusing scenes of cruelty. As in the example of Margaret Rule, Mather assumed that these colored figurations of evil controlled the victim's mind from inside her body, confirming yet again that far-from-immaterial visitors, ghosts in Puritan America had everything to do with material bodies.

The focus on women in scenes of possession has been amply explored by the feminist historian Carol F. Karlsen, who demonstrated how standing at odds with societal expectations was likely to mark women as devil's assistants. Yet, analyzing the repeated focus on "the black man" who relates in one way or another to "the Indian" in both Mathers' oeuvres demonstrates that these scenes were often framed by satanic images of racialized male bodies marked as "Black" or "Indian" or both. Examples exposing the physicality of those ghosts are numerous and they even include public beatings, as can be seen in Calef's report: "At Examination, and at other times, 'twas usual for the Accusers to tell of the black Man, or of a Spectre, as being then on the Table, etc. The People about would strike with Swords, or sticks at those places. One Justice broke his Cane at this Exercise, and sometimes the Accusers would say, they struck the Spectre, and it is reported several of the accused were hurt and wounded thereby, though at home at the same time" (Calef 206). While the image of the devil as a "black Man" appears to have been transferred to New England from seventeenth-century British publications, it is necessary to pause at the scene of a public ritual in which the assembled men—all white settlers of European descent—were beating an imaginary "black Man" (Calef 206). The sword returns to fight the evil that now received a body. The witch trials were brought to an end in 1693, and "spectral evidence" was discredited as reliable court material; however, the national hysteria around the "Black man" who "resembles an Indian" and has the ability to possess (preferably white) female bodies had only just started (C. Mather, *Wonders* 75).[31] Tituba, the first person identified as a witch in the Salem crisis of 1692, was a woman who was known sometimes as an Indian, at other times as an African or half-African slave. Elaine G. Breslaw argued that Tituba was brought from the South American mainland to Barbados as a child. Conversely, Peter Hoffer argued that Tituba was African, a Yoruba.[32] The devil in Cotton Mather's writing oscillates between women's African and Indigenous American bodies, which might explain the difficulty in determining a fixed identity of the victims.

The Puritan Invisible World was one of the central concepts at the time that linked material and immaterial dimensions through an intricate web of signs, auguries, omens, and portents. In his *The Wonders of the Invisible World,* Cotton Mather offers the exegetic practice as the primary purpose of the Invisible World, a source of restoration as well as obligation: "I will venture to say, thus much; that we are *Safe,* when we make just as much *Use* of all Advice from the Invisible World, as God sends it for. It is a *Safe* Principle, That when God Almighty permits any Spirits from the Unseen Regions, to visit us with Surprizing Informations, then there is something to be *Enquired* after; we are then to *Enquire* of one Another, *What Cause is there for such Things?* The Peculiar Government of God, over the Unbodied Intelligences, is a sufficient Foundation for this Principle" (*Wonders* 23–24). This Invisible World was visible to Puritan settlers, not only in natural phenomena but also in figurations of the "*Black man* that resembles an Indian" and scars on young women's bodies. These, in turn, needed to be produced in order for the Invisible World to be established. Positioning ghosts and spirits as part of a national fantasy in prerevolutionary America places apparitional concepts away from questions of belief and disbelief. Instead, ghosts appear in rather profane and earthly functions embedded within increasingly secular narratives. The analysis of Increase Mather's *An Essay for the Recording of Illustrious Providences* traces this spectral transformation. A presence that grabs the reader with an "invisible hand" slowly allows for sporadic yet progressively clearer glimpses at the spectral body. Nothing less than a public renegotiation of evil within the field of the supernatural, this constellation in colonial America must be understood in its quality as a forum for negotiating race and gender. Far from a concern of belief or disbelief in "apparitions," the field of the supernatural became a space to construct identities in pronouncedly material ways. Cotton Mather expressed this sentiment himself in stating that during his own lifetime, the Invisible

World was "becoming Incarnate" and that the devil was now walking the earth in New England "more *sensibly* and more *visible*" (*Wonders* 36). While being part of the European debate on ghosts, New England contradicted the notion of a decline in magic in the face of materialist rationality, by combining science and religion in its defense of satanic possession. With its unabating appetite for ghost stories, Puritan New England also prefigured various literary and cultural trends. Examples of popular ghost stories in the early United States affirm the success of the Puritan resignification and per-sonification of evil in Black and Indigenous bodies. As will become obvious in the following chapters, some of the images established by both Mathers, particularly the "black man that resembles an Indian" and is the devil, will reappear verbatim in the writings of one of the most famous ghost-story authors in the United States, Washington Irving, and in modified forms in the writings of other canonical writers of the early republic.

∾ 2

Counter-Enlightenment
Ghosts and Morality

> Are we not Spirits, that are shaped into a body, into an
> Appearance; and that fade away again into Air and Invisibility?
> [...] Oh, Heaven, it is mysterious, it is awful to consider that we
> not only carry a future Ghost within us; but are, in very deed,
> Ghosts.
> —Carlyle, *Sartor Resartus*

Terry Castle convincingly argued in *The Female Thermometer* that "the uncanny absorption of ghosts and apparitions into the world of thought" in the mid-eighteenth century was a "momentous event in the history of Western consciousness" (171). One cannot overestimate this shift in mediation's significance as the current discourse on virtual reality. What Castle did not take into consideration in her excellent study is the implied racial hierarchies and the related production of race. The same topic has been omitted by scholars such as Hartmut and Gernot Böhme, who have demonstrated how and why "the other side of reason" was just as instrumental as reason itself in shaping what came to be called the Enlightenment in Europe.[1] Their research has been revised by more recent scholars demonstrating a strong coexistence of not only unreason but also of what Isaiah Berlin came to call "counter-Enlightenment"—a general, shared suspicion of rationality (19).[2] Most prominently, Donna V. Jones has exposed the racial dimension of the counter-Enlightenment. In her study *The Racial Discourses of Life Philosophy*, Jones demonstrates ways in which philosophical discourses that resist rational understanding joined European racism and produced racialized self-formations.

In this chapter, I demonstrate how a growing number of writers and philosophers on both sides of the Atlantic began to understand ghosts: in their ability to escape the dualism of reason and its other when presented as figments of imagination. The persistence of varied speculation on ghosts, despite visible debunking efforts by Enlightenment scholars and laypeople alike, sparked a lively public transatlantic debate within which ghosts found an entry into European moral theory. I focus particularly on the philosopher Immanuel Kant's engagement in this discourse, and his thesis that seeing ghosts connects not only the living with the dead but also all the living with each other. I argue that texts such as Kant's hypothetical theory of ghosts as mediums initiated an intellectual exchange in Germany and subsequently the United States, which, in turn, put a spectral presence, or in Kant's language "secret power," at the center of subjectivity theory in literature and culture on both sides of the Atlantic. I demonstrate how Kant's theory of ghosts is at the foundation of his still-influential theory of personhood based on a "moral state" that is organized around supposed capacities for reason. Kant's text had a direct impact on influential German romantic writers such as Christoph Martin Wieland, Friedrich Schiller, and Cajetan Tschink and indirectly on some of the most influential writers of the early republic, as is exemplified in my analysis of Charles Brockden Brown's writing. Cloaked in acknowledged philosophical models, figurations of ghosts became a powerful narrative element that settler colonial writers put in the service of affirming existing racial hierarchies. It is thus necessary to go back to European moral theory to understand antebellum ghost stories.

Ghosts as a Phenomenon

As ghosts retreated further into the human mind, their presence solidified as an aspect of human interiority. A poem published under the title "The Apparition" and signed in encrypted form with "J—L M—R—E" in 1735 spells out the often-promoted early eighteenth-century writers' certainty that ghosts are a product of the imagination. In this poem, the author states that "locomotive powers are falsely giv'n / To Spirit, which exists alone in thought." Throughout the eighteenth century, an ever-increasing number of writers engaged in either reversing this assumption or confirming it. Analyzing newspaper articles and pamphlets published in England and New England, one can trace the evolution from a few scattered pieces ridiculing or questioning the belief in ghosts and apparitions from the first part of the century to the rise of proper treatises and theories about them just a few decades later.[3] One reason for this change in attitude is the topicalization: ghosts shifted from being a novelty in scholarly discussions to becoming common and functionalized in the public discourse. Discussed as a phenomenon, ghosts ceased to be reduced to an occurrence. As a consequence, many subsequent scholars and journalists embarked on a quest to analyze the presence of apparitional figures within what would today be considered sociological, anthropological, or philosophical contexts. Edward Cave, the influential printer and publisher of one of the first US American journals, *The Gentleman's Magazine,* commonly known as Sylvanus Urban, Gent., wrote as early as 1732, in his article "Of Ghosts, Daemons, and Spectres": "If our Reason sets us above these low and vulgar Appearances, yet when we read of the Ghost of Sir George Villers, of the Piper of Hammell, the Daemon of Moscow, or the German Colonel, mention'd by Ponti, and see the Names of Clarendon, Boyle, &c. to these Accounts, we find Reasons for our Credulity, 'till at last we are convinc'd by a whole Conclave of Ghosts met in the works of Glanvill and Moreton" ("Universal Spectator"). Ghosts increasingly became part of transatlantic intellectual debates on reason. The German writer and theologian Georg Wilhelm Wegner succinctly highlighted this sentiment in his *Philosophische Abhandlung von Gespenstern (Philosophical Treatise on Ghosts)* from 1757. In the opening paragraph, he pondered the question of why ghosts reappeared in public discourse in the mid-eighteenth century after a period of "calmness": "It seems that they have recovered their old powers, and they are coming back to spook around in spite of all the work that scholars have done to dispose of them" (9). While Wegner confirmed a changing attitude towards ghosts in the mid-eighteenth century, he failed to recognize that their return was in no small degree the work of scholars like himself. Paradoxically, the numerous debunkers of ghosts in the eighteenth century faced resistance in Enlightenment scholarship that advocated an open-minded exploration of spectral matters and called for a scientific interest susceptible to description and explanation. Wegner himself left the domain of illusions and began to situate ghosts in terms of human communication.

The return of ghosts in the mid-eighteenth century led numerous scholars to discuss ghost-seeing as a human trait, if specifically a dangerous one. Only two decades after Wegner, Voltaire solidified this view in his *Philosophical Dictionary* of 1764: "THE superstitious man is to the rogue what the slave is to the tyrant. Further, the superstitious man is governed by the fanatic and becomes fanatic" (138). Voltaire's influential writings sealed the status of superstition as a project for the Enlightenment, inaugurating a lively debate about seeing ghosts and polarizing scholars along the lines of, on the one hand, those who presented ghosts as antagonists that can be used to illuminate the "dark sciences" with rationalism and, on the other hand, those who understood seeing ghosts as a notable social trait in need of examination or a creative narrative strategy. Either way, the Age of Reason found a worthy antagonist necessary for its self-proliferation.

Voltaire's attack on superstition only served to energize the arguments of those who supported the proposal that ghosts had a righteous place among the living. The following argument from the *London Magazine; or, Gentleman's Monthly Intelligencer* that appeared in the article titled "Of Ghosts and Apparitions" became a common presence in leading journals on both sides of the Atlantic: "Nothing is more natural to the mind of man than superstition, which sees everything double, and raises substance from non-entities. [. . .] We must be strangely delighted with ghosts and chimeras, when we thus take a tour out of nature to see them; and so fond are we of their company, that we frequently make them return us the visit in our homes and bed-chambers." Pondering the obvious persistence of a ghost discourse within secular, nonsuperstitious sociocultural environments discloses the rhetorical power of ghostly figurations. While the prominent US American politician and social reformer Benjamin Rush in his writings on human senses still engaged in discussions about the impossibility of physical perceptions of "spectres and apparitions" (361), Benjamin Franklin, one of the leading intellectuals of his times, had already joined a transatlantic discussion on scientific and moral aspects of spiritualism.[4] Franklin was engaged in a committee that was to determine the scientific quality of mesmerism, a belief that a ghostly magnetic fluid pervaded the body and could be redirected by a healer to cure deceases. Respectively, rather than rehashing ghostly sightings with the purpose of proving or disproving their existence, an increasing number of writers and philosophers began to wonder: how can we account for the effectiveness of ghostly figurations in storytelling, if the readers do not believe in them? The answer comes from one of the most unlikely sources.

In 1766, only two years had passed since Horace Walpole placed ghosts on the literary map with what came to be known as the first gothic novel, *The Castle of Otranto*. That year, one of the most vehement proponents of reason—the German philosopher Immanuel Kant—decided that he too should engage with the other side of reason. His aim was to accommodate "the insistent importunity of friends, both known and unknown," by dedicating a whole treatise to analyzing ghosts (*Dreams* 306).[5] By publishing *Dreams of a Spirit-Seer,* an anonymously published hypothetical treatise of ghosts, Kant entered the ongoing discussion on spectrality, and ultimately enfranchised ghosts from their religious context by asking: "What exactly is this thing which, under the name of spirit, people claim to understand so well" (*Dreams* 307)? Kant himself went on to become a rather notorious revenant, haunting modern scholarship with his theories of the human mind; his theory of spirits, however, in which he connected apparitional sightings with morality, have not provoked a comparable amount of interest in contemporary scholarship. Instead, academic contributions on ghosts and spectrality commonly cite Jacques Derrida's *Spectres de Marx* from 1993 as the driving force behind the scholarly turn towards ghost studies. According to Colin Davis, Derrida is supposed to have rehabilitated "ghosts as a respectable subject of enquiry" in literary circles, as his study "spawned a minor academic industry" (8–10).[6] Arguably, Kant's hypothetical treatise had a similar impact in the late eighteenth century. Interpretations of Kant's only text on ghosts, which, on the one hand, claimed that Kant tried to dismiss metaphysics altogether or that he, on the other hand, repudiated his early precritical philosophy, continue to hold the scholarship on this text in a contentious space.[7]

For my purposes, *Dreams of a Spirit-Seer* is significant in its relation to Kant's later critical writings on morality. This connection ultimately exposes ways in which a still-influential moral theory was shaped in relation to spectrality. I will flesh out the connection between a general sense of morality and the conjuration of spirits, using telling echoes of Kant's precritical writings on spirit-seeing within his later critical work on moral philosophy. This will demonstrate not only the relation between moral theory and the supernatural in the late eighteenth century but also the Eurocentrism of a theory presented as universal. This particular relation between spectrality and morality, in turn, informs my reading of the first generation of what today is considered canonical early American writers. Philosophy on knowledge, morals, and the self in the late eighteenth century commonly merged with issues of politics, aesthetics, and economics. Most philosophers and writers at the time began their theoretical inquiry with moral or political questions and consequently found themselves quickly faced with questions of phenomenology and epistemology. Ghosts became significant concepts for discussions of perception and the senses at that time, and as such they also entered the newly initiated discussions on morality and subjectivity. In the context of the United States this discussion framed the colonial project as a literary topic in the writings of the first generation of newly nationalized US American writers.

Immanuel Kant's "One Great Republic"

Within the secure framework of an anonymously published treatise, Kant managed to produce a rational theory of ghosts. This is in no small part due to his focus on the ghost-seer, which he already highlighted in the title:

Träume eines Geistersehers, erläutert durch Träume der Metaphysik (1766, first translated by Emanuel F. Goerwitz as *Dreams of a Spirit-Seer, Elucidated by Dreams of Metaphysics* in 1899). This publication marks a culmination of the steady retreat of the ghost into the human mind in scholarly discussions and literature alike. Kant's interest in ghosts was sparked by the publication of Emmanuel Swedenborg's *Arcana Cœlestia* in 1756. A Swedish scientist and Christian mystic with a strong interest in cosmology and human sensory perception, Swedenborg (1688–1772) was well known for his belief that he was surrounded by evil spirits. Rather neglected by the scientific community at the time, he seemed to be the least likely candidate for an engagement with the advocate of reason, a title that Kant made for himself. And yet, the German philosopher was said to be one of the first people to acquire a copy,[8] only to follow his purchase with a scalding review in the form of his *Dreams of a Spirit-Seer* in 1766. Kant stated that the dedication of his time to "spirits" was due to a wish to "expose" this "arch-spirit-seer of all spirit-seers" (*Dreams* 341) and to show the world Swedenborg's rightful place among "fantastical visionaries" (*Dreams* 335). With unusually bitter scorn and cynical wit, Kant accused the "hero," whose name he Germanified to "Schwedenberg," of being nothing but "the arch-visionary of all visionaries" (*Dreams* 341). Swedenborg, nonetheless, became a significant influence for numerous writers of the romantic period. Far from an obscure reference, he remained extremely influential, most prominently for Louisa May Alcott, William Blake, Honoré de Balzac, Charles Baudelaire, Samuel Taylor Coleridge, Johan Wolgang von Goethe, and Ralph Waldo Emerson. And even Kant's irritation was rather an anxiety of influence. The sarcastic tone in the text, as current research demonstrates, is due to the continued correlation between Kant's own work and Swedenborg's writings, which must have been disturbing to Kant.[9] As has been pointed out, most notably by Gottlieb Florschütz, even the expression the "Realm of Ends" (Reich der Zwecke), traditionally referred to as the "Kingdom of Ends," is a concept first developed by "the arch-spirit-seer," Swedenborg, under the very same name;[10] meanwhile, a central element in Kant's moral philosophy, the "Kingdom of Ends," is the spirit-world in Swedenborg's *Arcana Cœlestia*.

Kant's interest in ghosts was thus much more than a simple act of repudiation. Even if covered with a veil of disqualification, the spirit theory in *Dreams of a Spirit-Seer* found a direct entry into his later theory of morality, which, all the way into the twenty-first century, remains his most quoted work. The parallels between Kant's own oeuvre, namely between his precritical work on spirits (which he borrowed from the mystic Swedenborg) and the work of his critical phase (which covertly employed the language of spectrality), remain strangely unexplored until today. As I demonstrate in what follows, even if disavowed and ridiculed immediately upon publication, Kant's work on spirits continued to appear in his purportedly least ghostly elaboration, his work on morality.[11]

Moses Mendelssohn pointed out already in his 1767 review of *Dreams of a Spirit-Seer* that Kant's context of spirit-seeing was, in fact, used for questioning metaphysics in general (quoted in Kant, *Kant on Swedenborg* 231). As such, *Dreams of a Spirit-Seer* departs from a simple debunking effort and reveals important initial stages in the architecture of modern subjectivity, which does not depart from mysticism but rather incorporates it. In his admission that he did not know what spirits (*Geister*) are, Kant demonstrated how it is possible to understand what it is not possible to know (*Dreams* 307).

Safely cloaked in a hypothetical theory, Kant proposed a definition of spirits as immaterial beings that have reason, "beings, therefore, which lack the quality of impenetrability" and which "will never constitute a solid whole, no matter how many of them are united together. Simple beings of this kind are called immaterial beings, and if they are possessed of reason, they are called spirits" (*Dreams* 309). Spirits are, thus, immaterial beings that possess reason. This theorem did not imply that apparitions engage the domain of the possible; rather, while spirits cannot be "understood," they can be "recognized" (*Dreams* 310). This working definition highlights the essential role of the one still living in the body, who appears already in the title as the actual object of inquiry—the one who can *see* or rather *recognize* the spirit. Furthermore, this line of thinking points towards the Enlightenment's distinction between reason and understanding, which only half a century later will become central to leading romantic writers on both sides of the Atlantic. The differentiation between a rationalizing from the senses, or understanding, and higher intuitions, or reason, was at the center of US transcendentalism. It was famously introduced in the United States by James Marsh in his "Preliminary Essay," which served as an introduction to the US American 1829 edition of Coleridge's *Aids to Reflection*. Coleridge's text is basically an introduction to Kant's philosophy, which through various filters appears at the center of US American Romanticism.

Yet, as I will demonstrate in what follows, rationalizing from the senses as opposed to reason in this early text by Kant drew a demarcation line between those who possess reason and those who do not. Positioning his theory somewhere between Swedenborg's and Hobbes' ideas, Kant presented the spirit topic as a metaphysical question—metaphysics at the time being widely understood as the science of the limitations of human reason. Kant's spirit theory, therefore, was an anthropocentric meditation circling around questions of human cognition. Similar attempts at defining ghosts within an Enlightenment framework had been made before, albeit to a lesser extent. For example, the aforementioned German scholar Wegner offered what he claimed to be a "true definition" of ghosts, before Kant: "A ghost is therefore a spiritual substance, which appears in an adopted body and can be seen, felt or heard in it." Both Wegner and Kant focused on how ghosts were perceived rather than on the behavior of the ghosts, which interested previous scholars. Kant, however, takes the discussion a step further by analyzing how the presence of spirits structures the lives of the living by creating communities, thereby adding a relational level to the discussion.

Both Kant and Wegner established that the spirit needs a material form if it is to be perceived by the living. This unity of spirit and material form constitutes a new entity and calls for a different designation: the spirit, if perceived by the living, is a ghost. Unlike a spirit, a ghost only exists and can be explored in relation to the ghost-seer. This distinction between a materialized form and the immaterial presence is central and calls for separate laws, which Kant divides in pneumatic and organic laws. The peculiar laws of ghostly operations, which are hypothetically presented as external to the human being, are described as "pneumatic":[12] "I am connected with beings of my own kind through the mediation of corporeal laws, but I can in no wise establish from what is given to me whether, in addition, I am not also connected, or could not ever be connected, with such beings, in accordance with other laws, which I shall call pneumatic laws, and be so independently of the mediation of matter" (*Dreams* 357). Here one can already see the seed for Kant's later moral theory, as one is connected to one's "own kind" not only through corporeal laws but also through laws not perceivable to human cognition. Immaterial beings are of a self-subsisting nature; joined together, they constitute the immaterial world, which remains imperceptible to the living (*Dreams* 317).

However, pneumatic operations could instrumentalize bodies in the material world; in this case, Kant specified that they would then have to be considered "organic" (*Dreams* 317). In other words, spirit combined with matter produces organic laws. Setting an example for ghost studies in the future, Kant differentiated between the world of material absence (pneumatic) and immaterial presence (organic). This differentiation between a perceived immateriality and an absent materiality will remain important until current ghost theories, such as in the possibly most influential one, the theory of hauntology offered by Jacques Derrida. In *Specters of Marx,* Derrida differentiates between specters and spirits: "the specter is a paradoxical incorporation, the becoming-body, a certain phenomenal and carnal form of the spirit" (6).

Because humans enjoy an earthly spiritual existence within a somatic presence, they are connected to both worlds. Thus, the living are already semi-spirits, or semi-ghosts. Insofar as the "soul" of a person is united with a body to form a "personal unity," it senses only the material, while it receives "influences" from the immaterial world (*Dreams* 319). Kant delineated the separation between the two worlds and gathered the collectivity of immaterial beings under the phrase "the immaterial world" or *mundus intelligibilis* (*Dreams* 317). This immaterial world, when situated within the human soul, can merge with a physical presence to form a "person": "As a result, it would now happen that man's soul already *in this life* and according to its *moral state* has to occupy its place among the spirit-substances of the universe, just as, in accordance with the laws of motion, the various types of matter in space adopt an order, consonant with their corporeal powers, relatively to each other" (*Dreams* 323; emphasis added). In other words, the living are partially spirits within a "moral state." Only in relation "to each other" can a human become a "person." In *Dreams of a Spirit-Seer,* Kant therefore develops an early relational theory of personhood based on a subscription to a moral state. This relation, in turn, connects the living to their "own kind."

Upon death, the union with the body ceases to exist, and "the community in which it at all times stands with spirit-natures would continue to exist on its own; and that community would perforce reveal itself to the consciousness of the human soul in the form of a clear intuition [*Anschauung*]" (*Dreams* 319). During life, both the material and the spiritual presence are united in the human body. After death, the material shell is lost, but the spiritual presence continues to exist as intuition. Why does this intuition often look like a human when perceived by a "spirit-seer"? Kant offered a seemingly simple conclusion to this immaterial materialism: because it is the living who conjure up the pneumatic spirits, they come in thinkable forms. Constrained by the limits of imagination and language, these spirits with a body—namely ghosts—inevitably appear to resemble humans. Ghosts appear in human form because otherwise they would defy interpretation.

With this rational Kantian explanation of ghosts, I want to now return to Swedenborg, who in his writings doubts the ability of "Europeans" to connect with this "spirit"-ual self, so meticulously analyzed by Kant. According to Swedenborg's correspondence theory, even if the spiritual world is part of the natural world, it cannot be experienced by everyone; it is a world known to the "genius of the Asiatic" and "the Africans" rather than the European intellectual. Ideas that come by "influx" are "lost among the learned in the Christian world" (Swedenborg, "Athanasian Creed" 39). Pitting non-European spirituality against European rational thinking, Swedenborg confirms Achille Mbembe's proposition that "theoretical and practical recognition of the body and flesh of 'the stranger' as flesh and body just like mine, the idea of a common human nature, a humanity shared with others, long posed, and still poses, a problem for Western consciousness" (Mbembe, *On the Postcolony* 2). In *The Spiritual Diary*, Swedenborg locates in the "interior of Africa" those "who communicate with the angels of heaven" whereas "the communication is not by speech from angels but through interior perception" (no. 5946). Furthermore, "Africans excel all other Gentiles in clearness of interior judgement." For Swedenborg, the "interior" of Africa is an imagined real utopia that features as a promised land not yet found. As a site of colonial projection, an interior African kingdom features people more aligned with their spiritual self, who would educate Europeans corrupted "by perverted reasoning" in spiritual matters ("Athanasian Creed" 65). Making a sharp distinction between European rationality and non-European sensuality that he calls "interior wisdom" (65), Swedenborg confirmed the already existing Enlightenment demarcation line drawn between senses and reason as a racial distinction and affirmed the progressive view of Europe at the time as an international benefactor extending the rights of man to Africa. The material effects of this colonial fantasy are visible in the work of Swedenborg's followers. The chemist Carl Bernhard Wadström, a prominent Swedenborgian abolitionist, even developed a detailed plan on how to conduct "the establishment of regular Colonies on the extensive Coast of that hitherto illfated Continent [. . .] for the purpose of rendering thousands of Families happy, by transplanting them on those delightful shores" ("Plan for a Free Community" 44).

Kant never addresses Swedenborg's ideas about "Africans" in his review, but he does conclude his hypothetical treatise with a curious theory of "one great republic" in which only those of "one's own kind" receive the influxes from the dead and the living necessary for the "moral state" that would lead to personhood (328). Both Swedenborg and Kant center their theories on "influxes" from the "immaterial world." Swedenborg promoted a view of "influx" potentially available to all rational beings but only accessible to some Europeans, like him, and to all "Africans." Kant restricts the interaction with the immaterial world to those who inscribe themselves into "one great republic" through their "moral state" and are therefore connected to "one's own kind" (*Dreams* 328). Swedenborg's vision of a New Jerusalem unfolding in Africa, therefore, would make no sense in Kant's spirit theory, which remains firmly grounded in Europe. Instead of a colony in Africa where the "interior Africans" would enlighten the settler Europeans, Kant imagined "one great republic" restricted to those who subscribed to the moral state through a connection with the "immaterial world" right there where they lived, in this case in the middle of Germany. The romanticized and racialized vision of a superior spirituality of "Africans" that Swedenborg and some of his followers promoted is replaced by an exclusive theory of personhood.

Kant's personal struggle with Swedenborg could be brushed aside as an amusing episode in the philosopher's troubled life, had he not moved on to apply a large part of the terminology developed in the hypothetical treatise to his influential theories of morality. Almost two decades after dismissing his enquiry by acknowledging to his readers that he "does not know" if "there are spirits" or even more "what the word '*spirit*' means" (*Dreams* 307), Kant once again began to think about the collectivity of immaterial beings gathered under the phrase "the immaterial world or *mundus intelligibilis*," this time specifically in the context of morality. This central concept that designates the spirit-world in *Dreams of a Spirit-Seer* reappears in *Grundlegung zur Metaphysik der Sitten* (*Groundwork of the Metaphysics of Morals*, 1785) with a significant adjustment: it is now "a world of rational beings (*mundus intelligibilis*)" (87).[13] During Kant's famous incubation phase,[14] his theory of the spirit world had transformed into the intelligible world and ghostliness translated into morality. Kant reactivated the vocabulary he had developed in the context of spectrality within the realm of morality. His precritical "immaterial world," however, does not reappear in his critical work as the irrational; instead, in his critical work the immaterial world is the rational world or *mundus intelligibilis*. Given that Kant's *Groundwork of the Metaphysics of Morals* was intended for a general readership untrained in the history of moral philosophy, we can assume that with this publication, Kant aimed to provide a solid theory of morality that through spiritual influxes organically binds those who belong to "one great republic."

In Kant's spirit theory, the living receive "influences"—or more accurately in Johnson and Magee's translation, "influxes" (Kant, *Kant on*

Swedenborg 60)—from the spirits of the dead and the spirits of the living, and this is what guides their behavior towards others. This "speculation" addresses relations that involve the living and the dead (Kant, *Dreams* 324). Taking his reader by the hand, Kant offered a hypothetical understanding of the ghostliness of those who qualify as a "person." This required a connection between the spiritual existence and the somatic presence. In an attempt to trace this nexus, Kant began with impulses external to the human being that must therefore have originated in the immaterial world. It is these "drives" (*Triebe*) and the "secret power" (*geheime Macht*) that Kant kept returning to in his later work. In *Dreams,* it reads:

> A *secret power* forces us to direct our will towards the well-being of others or regulate it in accordance with the will of another, although this often happens contrary to our will and in strong opposition to our selfish inclination. The focal point at which the lines which indicate the direction of our drives converge, is therefore not merely to be found within us; there are, in addition, other forces which move us and which are to be found in the will of others outside ourselves. This is the source from which the moral impulses take their rise. (*Dreams* 322; emphasis added)

In *Groundwork of the Metaphysics of Morals,* this becomes: "for we like to flatter ourselves by falsely attributing to ourselves a nobler motive, whereas in fact we can never, even by the most strenuous self-examination, get entirely behind our *covert incentives,* since, when moral worth is at issue, what counts is not actions, which one sees, but those inner principles of actions that one does not see" (61–62; emphasis added). Both "secret powers" generated from the spiritual world and "covert incentives" that originate in the unknown are explained as a manipulative subconscious power that radiates from the will of the other, dead or alive. All rational beings are members of a single moral community, yet rational beings vary in their capacities for agency and capability to access reason. When Kant proposes that Indigenous Americans are "incapable of any culture" (*On the Use of Teleological Principles* 211), therefore, according to his moral philosophy, that should not only be understood as a repetition of the dominant ideas of his time but rather a structural view of racial hierarchies that grounds his theories. In another text, Kant writes: "The production of the aptitude of a rational being for any ends in general (thus those of his freedom) is culture" (*Critique of the Power of Judgement* 299). Without culture, no reason; without reason, no freedom.

To conclude, Kant developed a theory of spiritual influxes that create exclusive communities through subscription to a common moral state and thus grant personhood. This theory centered on the conflict between the wish to please ourselves and the longing for approval from "a reciprocal connection and community with each other, even without the mediation of corporeal things" (*Dreams* 317). Kant concluded that this presence is a "secret power"—an impulse that leads to actions often done unwillingly, and in conflict with our selfish inclination, as these are powers moving us in wills other than our own. This implies that humans are dependent upon the rule of the general will (*Regel des allgemeinen Willens*): "As a result, we recognise that, in our most secret motives, we are dependent upon the *rule of the general will*. It is this rule which confers upon the world of all thinking beings its *moral unity* and invests it with a systematic constitution, drawn up in accordance with purely spiritual laws. We sense within ourselves a constraining of our will to harmonise with the general will" (*Dreams* 322). The moral unity in Kant's theory functions according to his early hypothetical "pneumatic laws" among one's "own kind." It is not difficult to see the direct connection from this precritical theory to Kant's central philosophical concept, the categorical imperative.

Kant concluded his treatise on ghosts by generously allowing the reader to condemn all "spirit-seers" from then on as "candidates for the asylum" instead of thinking of them as "semi-citizens of the other world" (*Dreams* 335). But he did so only after developing a complete theory of spirits who become partial citizens—a private person who is a member of a state or nation. Why entertain this idea to begin with? If the study of spirit-seeing seemed idle and superfluous, why, even if only hypothetically, evoke spirits that together with "semi-citizens" share the space of "one great republic," thus creating a sense of morality, or as Kant wrote in his native tongue, "das sittliche Gefühl"? His application of political vocabulary (republic, citizens) to spiritual matters underlines his insistence on reading personhood as a subscription to a moral state. In this way, Kant's spirit-theory-turned-moral-philosophy paved the way for romantic nationalism in its promotion of a spiritual connection to one's own kind through moral unity. This exclusionary mechanism of belonging, which depends on impulses not accessible to individual cognition but spread among the "thinking community," emphasizes both this author's racism and universalism.

Morality, in Kant's tone-setting studies, is the domain of the European. While all humans, in Kant's understanding of the word, have the same potential, they realize it differently. It is statements like the following one that leave no space for doubt as to Kant's classification methods: "Humanity has its highest degree of perfection in the white race" (*Physical Geography*

576). European antagonists are people who are "black from head to toe" and therefore in Kant's own vocabulary "stupid" (*Observations* 61). Or, equally aggressively: "The Negros of Africa have by nature no feeling that rises above the ridiculous" (*Observations* 58). Statements like this might be a direct response to Swedenborg's proposal, which is racist in its own way.

My purpose of reproducing these blatant chauvinistic statements in a twenty-first-century publication is to highlight that these "observations" cannot be separated from Kant's moral theories, which continue to influence even current scholarship. All above-mentioned discriminatory statements were made in the context of Kant's still-influential theory of the beautiful and the sublime. In fact, they are embedded in a section in which Kant seeks to approximate a definition of beauty by discussing "the relationship between the sexes" or rather how men treat women in various parts of the world, exposing the multiple levels of supremacist subjectivity at the base of his theories. Kant's findings include the proposal that in "the Orient," "a woman is always in prison," and in "the lands of the blacks [. . .] the female sex [is] in the deepest slavery" (*Observations* 60). Far from simply rehearsing views dominant in Germany of the late eighteenth century, Kant grounds his theories in hierarchies that are constitutive to his influential scholarship, be it of the sublime and the beautiful or his architecture of morality.

Given the fact that current human rights discourses at least to some degree still rely on Kant's moral philosophy, I want to ask how these meaning-making elements shape Kant's understanding of community-building processes. Kant's racist statements have received a considerable amount of attention in recent scholarship. Charles W. Mills' "Kant's *Untermenschen*" and Theodore Vial's book *Modern Religion, Modern Race* are two thorough studies of the construction of race in Kant's work. Adding to this existing scholarship, I would like to propose the centrality of intuition to the European colonization of the mind, whereas Kant's theory of intuition is based in his theory of spirits. The provisional summary of Kant's "Part First: Which Is Dogmatic," presented above, already demonstrates how a working definition of the immaterial presence, when united with a human body, can be joined into an exclusive theory of human "intuition" that is understood to be an organizing element in building exclusive communities. It is exactly this conceptualization of intuition that became central to romantic writers in Europe and in the United States who understood themselves to be either working with, or influenced by, transcendentalist theories. Kant's spiritual connection to "one's own kind" therefore continued to shape transatlantic literature deep into the twentieth century.

As has been pointed out by Vial in his important study of the entanglement between race and religion, Kant was a monogenist. Opposing the view of numerous scholars of his time, Kant believed that all humans are of one species. Yet, as Vial already explained, in this philosopher's scholarship, some humans possess more reason than others. In Kant's philosophy, *human* refers to all members of the same species, but this does not warrant all members to be capable of personhood to the same degree. On the contrary, as is recognizable already in his *Dreams of a Spirit-Seer,* only those connected to "one's own kind" through a "moral state" are capable of reaching personhood. Swedenborg's racial and racist division between intuitive "Africans" and sadly rational "Europeans" who "think only exteriorly, and receive truths in the memory" ("Athanasian Creed") is revised in *Dreams of a Spirit-Seer* in a concept of intuition that saved European spirituality without leaving the European, organic, exclusive "community of thinking beings."

Along the lines of Mills' and Vial's claim that Kant's precritical comments on non-Europeans continue to shape his moral vision in the critical philosophy, my study demonstrates that the division runs along the lines of those capable of sensing "influxes" and those who are not, a taxonomy most pronouncedly promoted in Swedenborg's writings, if only in a reversed form. While, in his critical writings, Kant never reverts back to his theory of "one great republic," he does emphasize that only those capable of reason (*mit Vernunft begabte Wesen*) can subscribe to the moral state, which implies the existence of those who have no access to such membership. The German word *begabt* means apt, gifted, or talented and is not a misnomer in this theory. While the human species is biologically considered to be a unity, it is reason that features prominently as the dividing line in this philosopher's taxonomies, which survive even the existence of a somatic presence. Death is not an interruption of this supremacist ethical web of spectral communication; rather, Kant concluded that death is but a continuation of our (moral) existence and, consequently, the post-mortal immaterial world is not exempt from, but included in, this earthly community of thinking beings and white supremacist fantasies.

Staying beyond his stated intention, Kant solidified the figure of the ghost as an integral part of the realm of the living, presenting it as a form of disembodied morality. Relocating spirits from outside the body into the mind, Kant delineated the confines of "another world" right within this one, thus marking ghost theory as an early source of not only psychology but also European romantic nationalism. Whether or not Kant was himself a ghost-seer, his treatment of the subject at the very least laid fertile ground for mapping out a European theory of European morality that can claim universality in spite of its explicit exclusion of all non-Europeans. The therein-proposed conceptualization of personhood demonstrates that moral universalism, as inherited from German Idealism, relies on racial hierarchy based supposedly in the capacity for reason. With this long exposition on Kant's instrumentalization of spectral vocabulary for purposes of constructing a supremacist theory of morality that addresses the unconscious nature of communities, three takeaways can be gleaned: first, Kant drew from a late Enlightenment recognition of the promise borne by the study of spectrality, which was increasingly understood to be a vehicle towards understanding what was presented as human cognition and, particularly, questions pertaining morality; second, this acknowledgment laid the groundwork for early Romanticism in the late Enlightenment; and third, it is particularly within this philosophical discourse that writers of the time found the resources that would later merge into what came to be called the gothic genre, as will be demonstrated in the next chapter.

Literature and Magic Philosophy

Approved by one of the most fervent advocates of reason himself, ghost-seeing sprinkled with romantic nationalism could safely return not only to philosophical soirées and literary salons but also the writings of Enlightenment intellectuals eager to explore the workings of the human mind and related questions concerning relational aspects. In such an intellectual environment, it was only a matter of time until fiction writers discovered the power of spectrality and ghostly figurations as a literary tool, asserting its effectiveness even outside of the classic ghost story or gothic novel frameworks. Prompted by Kant's publication, lively discussions about the applicability of ghostly figurations in literature began to spread in Germany in the late eighteenth century, whereas many departed from Kant's critical stance. Gotthold Ephraim Lessing, for example, wrote in support of ghosts as an artistic element just one year after Kant's publication. In 1767 he wrote in his highly influential *Hamburgische Dramaturgie* (*Hamburg Dramaturgy*): "And does poetry not provide many examples in which a genius defies all our philosophies, and things that we sneer at in cold reason manage to appear frightening to our imagination" (Lessing 65). He continued encouraging writers to explore the power of ghostly figurations: "But the lack of belief in ghosts according to this understanding cannot and should

not keep the dramatic poet from using them. The seed of belief lies in all
of us, and most of all in those for whom he primarily writes" (Lessing 66).
Exposing the powerful poetics of the ghost and defending it against "cold
reason," Lessing called for an acknowledgment of the perspectives of the
ghost and the ghost-seer as effective narrative tools. Various German writers
such as Christoph Martin Wieland, Friedrich Schiller, and Cajetan Tschink
followed Kant's and Lessing's lead.

According to the German studies scholar John McCarthy, the writer and
philosopher Christoph Martin Wieland was by far the most translated German author in North America before 1790.[15] On remembering his visits
to Berlin, John Quincy Adams corroborated the leading role in literature
Wieland played not only in the US but also in his native Germany. Thomas
Jefferson, too, deemed Wieland important enough to order his collected
works for the University of Virginia (Kurth-Voigt, "Reception of *Wieland*"
97–98). The fact that leading politicians promoted this writer's work demonstrates his influential standing in the United States. Wieland retained
an interest in ghosts and spectrality throughout his writing career. In 1781,
he published an essay in which he analyzed ghosts, intermediary beings
between the human and the divine, salamanders or fire spirits, air spirits
or sylphs, goblins, gnomes, mermaids, guardian spirits, and teasers. The
first version of the essay was published in *Teutscher Merkur* under the title
"Betrachtung über den Standpunkt, worin wir uns in Absicht auf
Erzählungen und Nachrichten von Geistererscheinungen befinden"
(Reflections on our current stance towards tales and information about
ghosts). This title clearly demonstrates the Enlightenment thinker's scholarly interest in understanding the fascination with ghosts apart from questions of belief or disbelief. The article was republished in 1796 to great
acclaim with the new title "Über den Hang der Menschen an Magie und
Geistererscheinungen zu glauben" ("On the Human Tendency to Believe
in Magic and Ghosts").[16] Wieland, however departs from his predecessor
Kant, only alluding to "a certain philosopher who dedicated a whole study
to ghosts" (Wieland 78), by insisting that rather than creating "one great
republic," the world of spirits was the world of ideas and images that *all*
the living help to form. Driven by Enlightenment proposals and invested
in correcting Kant's theory, Wieland suggested a cosmopolitan approach
to ghosts, advising his readers that no matter how urgently people tried to
exclude spectrality from their lives, ghosts would always find a place "in our
imagination and in our hearts" (67). Confirming a common need, Wieland
asked: "Why would a ghost surprise anyone, philosophy in its pythagorean,

platonic, or Alexandrian realization has always included the return as well as the existence of spirits" (70). Promoting the idea that thinking about the provenance of ghosts and the settings preferred by apparitions might be a reasonable, enlightened way of thinking about human nature, this influential author separated ghosts from occultism and proposed a more prosaic and embracing view: "Yes, even the philosophers, while denying the truth about the incidents that ghost-seers use as the reasoning for their belief, even the philosopher feels suddenly tricked by his fantasy. His conclusions are seldom convincing enough to suppress the instinctual tendency toward the supernatural, which he shares more or less with the unlearned—the secret desire to be convinced to the contrary by means of undeniable facts" (68). Opposing Kant's exclusionary theory, Wieland indexes Enlightenment's favorite antagonists—the ignorant, the unlearned, the primitive—in close proximity to the sophisticated scholar via ghosts. Refusing to rank human ability for reason, Wieland also defends the study of ghosts against the common view that only uneducated people would succumb to such a silly activity. Only a short time later, Edmund Burke writes: "Superstition is the religion of feeble minds; and they must be tolerated in an intermixture of it in some trifling or some enthusiastic shape or other, else you will deprive weak minds of a resource found necessary to the strongest" (234). The power game over who is reasonable and who is superstitious received a renewed energy after Kant's demarcation of the immaterial world within the realm of reason. Wieland tirelessly went on promoting a pronouncedly transnational concept of ghost-seeing. Assembling unusually long lists of spectral creatures, he underscored how well-versed his contemporaries were with something that in the scholarship of his time was presented as inexistent. Pointing out the transcultural and ahistorical quality of ghost stories, he concluded: "A tradition, as old as humanity or at least a few centuries older than philosophy, produced a form of general belief and an agreement among all nations about these things" (56). Explicitly departing from Kant's community-building theory of spirit-seeing, Wieland proposed a theory of the ghost as a connecting element "among all nations."

Given Wieland's popularity, it is most likely that this text was circulated in revolutionary America and its content discussed in articles about Wieland in local journals. It is worth revisiting the basic arguments relevant to the Enlightenment transatlantic ghost discourse, because Wieland's essay contains some of the key ideas concerning spectrality in relation to late Enlightenment discussions of humanity at that time. In this lexicon of eighteenth-century spectrality, Wieland carefully repeated the need to recognize the position of supernatural concepts within the process of reasoning, the rejection of which, according to his text, could have serious consequences for nothing less than humanity. Similar to Hobbes but transitioning into a secular context, he proposed that understanding the *human* affection for ghosts was necessary, because otherwise, "Isis' priests, magicians, fakirs, bonzes, mystagogues, oneirocritics, masters, spies and thyrspakurns, treasure seekers, and exorcists" would take control over this intrinsic human trait, which was open for misuse and abuse (85). Repeatedly employing lists as a narrative tool, Wieland argued that instead of focusing on individual cases of ghostly apparitions, the omnipresence of ghosts should be acknowledged. In doing so, he hoped to expose the power of the ghost and ways in which it affects the whole "poor humankind" (85). Wieland thus called for a theory of reason that included its own unreasonable elements apart from Kant's "one great republic." Poets, priests, and a "large number of philosophers" were called upon as advocates of "this romantic way of doing philosophy," which Wieland termed "magic philosophy" (70). Those who understood magic philosophy were in possession of a power that could nothing less but shift the human closer to divine, and that was "the greatest possible ennoblement of mankind" (71). Wieland described "magic philosophy" as "a key that can open the door to an invisible spiritual world. The visible world relates to the invisible one in the same way that letters relate to words—and words to ideas, of which they are only signs, or like a dead image to a living person" (71). This call to inspect spectral matters as a sign from an enlightened standpoint would be responded to a good decade later in what is often referred to as the first US American gothic novel. Charles Brockden Brown's *Wieland; or, The Transformation, an American Tale* (1798) even promotes the name of this German writer in its title. But before I can move on to Brown, it is necessary to introduce one more text that will help delineate the role of spectrality for the establishment of national US American literature, a truly ghostly field.

The ultimate expression of an acknowledgment of ghosts as powerful rhetorical and literary tools can be found in one of the Enlightenment's most notorious texts, Constantin François de Chassebœuf, Comte de Volney's *Les ruines; ou, Meditations sur les revolutions des empires*, a text that was to leave a significant mark in the former colonies.[17] Here the ghost is presented as the voice of reason. Volney's *Ruines*, first published in 1791, was admired and consequently translated in several English editions, one of which, even if only partially, by Thomas Jefferson under the title *A New*

Translation of Volney's Ruins; or, Meditations on the Revolution of Empires.
The last four chapters were subsequently translated by the prominent poet
and diplomat Joel Barlow.[18] This text, which was not only influential in the
United States but also throughout Europe, opens with a narrator wandering
through the ancient ruins of Palmyra, Lebanon. There, he stumbles upon
a ghost that takes him into outer space and presents to him a vision of all
the people of the world rejecting religion in favor of "the principles
of individual happiness and of public prosperity" (130). For what Priestman called a "key text of revolutionary atheism," one might be surprised to
find that the narration was largely taken on by a ghost (Priestman 22). Seen
in the context of the time, however, it is clear that Volney's choice was no
coincidence. With the ghost as the voice of reason, Volney manages to construct un unbiased transnational enlightened vision. Indeed, with the fash-
ioning of the modern Self in the late eighteenth century came an awareness
of perspective.[19] Introducing a ghost in a text enabled a unique opportunity
for narratives to address matters of central concern from a superior vantage point without involving the speaker directly in worldly controversies.
The reader's inability to attach a gender mark to the ghost added to the
unique narrative situation. It, she, he, or they had an advantage of speaking simultaneously as an external and internal focalizer unaffected by
constraints such as gender, nation, or even humanity. Existing outside of
the bonds of chronological time, a ghost could easily act as a corrective
from the past or a warning from the future, as Volney's ghost most succinctly exemplified.

The first English translation of *Ruins* in 1792 was an instant success. Robert Irwin remarked: "everybody read this book. It was a bestseller and talk
of the salons, spas and, gaming rooms" (135). Even Frankenstein's creature,
yet another ghost,[20] in Mary Shelley's famous novel published a short time
later in 1818, received his first lessons on mankind from Volney's *Ruins*—it
is the text that Felix De Lacey read to Sophia to teach her French. Hiding
from the two, the creature overheard their conversations and learned how
to communicate and express a sense of Self based on Volney's vocabulary.
Thomas Jefferson jeopardized his presidential candidacy by anonymously translating *Ruins,* which is at least partially a ghost story, and which
at the time was often considered a pagan text. Abraham Lincoln later went
on to praise the text (Herndon 102), while Walt Whitman even claimed to
have been raised on *Ruins* (Whitman 445).

The power of *Ruins* lies to a large degree in its narrative technique,
which makes use of an ontologically empty space: the apparition. The text

opens with an "invocation," as the introductory chapter is titled, with the words "Hail, solitary ruins, holy sepulchers and silent walls! you I invoke, to you I address my prayer" (ix). After the narrator introduces his laments and shares his traveling coordinates, the reader is presented with a chapter titled "The Apparition" (15). There he addresses the silent remains of a once-blossoming city. His address appears to have summoned a ghost: "I thought I saw an apparition, pale, clothed in large and flowing robes, such as specters are painted rising from their tombs" (15). As Wieland claimed, readers of any cultural background would be able to interpret this image, the effect of which is arresting, urgent, and personal—and, due to Enlightenment interference, also secular. After establishing such a powerful setting by the entrance of the apparition alone, the rest of the chapter gives voice to the spectral presence. The ghost is enraged about the human tendency to blame mankind's misery on divinity or fate instead of taking responsibility for their own active engagement in creating their destiny. Volney, thus, reversed Glanvill's call for more engagement with spectral matters and Hobbes' warning against it by putting the ghost in the service of human autonomy instead of religion. The speech calls for a change in attitude on various levels. The apparition reveals to the narrator that "man vainly ascribes his misfortunes to obscure and imaginary agents" while actually being "governed by *natural laws*" (42). Paradoxically, it takes an imaginary agent for humanity to face this problem. To progress, humanity needs to understand the power of imagination: "Let man then know these laws! let him comprehend the nature of the beings that surround him, and also his own nature" (43). Understanding the power of imagination equals understanding what it means to be human, which, in turn, leads to a more just society. In the chapter titled "Exposition," the narrator receives an opportunity to respond, taking over the lead only to support the apparition's claim: "the justness of thy discourse restores confidence to my soul" (24). As if in response to the prior chapter, the speaker concludes with what the apparition had already proposed and what amounted to his initial thoughts as he ventured out into the ruins to begin with. The ghost, in this example, provides access to one's "own nature" (43). Subjectivity is multivocal, dissolved in a community of speaking voices, some of which are spectral. Now that the power of the ghost as a narrator had been recognized and established within the realms of reason among intellectual circles on both sides of the Atlantic, the door to the invisible world was pushed wide open for writers to enter.

Free Philosophy in the Revolutionary United States

While exploring ghosts within what Glanvill termed "free philosophy" and Wieland described as "magic philosophy" was well established throughout Europe at the end of the eighteenth century, ghosts had a more difficult time in the revolutionary US. Still scarred from the Salem witch trials, the country's intellectual circles chose a more cautious approach, towards a view of ghost-seeing as a human trait. Long articles debunking ghost stories continued to dominate important newspaper editorials in the new republic at a time when they were long diminished within the public sphere in Europe. An exemplary case can be found in a much-reprinted article from 1792 titled "The Morristown Ghost Delineated," published under the penname "Philanthropist." The article detailed a case of fraud through pretended spectral agency. Resonating with Wieland's warning, the journalist aimed to expose how a rural town, "the county of Morris, in the state of New-Jersey, in the year 1788," retained its Puritan belief in witchcraft. Its inhabitants presented easy targets to deceivers skilled in the art of the pretended conjuring of spirits. The writer concludes with a warning about the power of the irrational: "I am confident that there are many such kinds of impositions transacted by particular persons, and many illiterate and vulgar readily believe that they have power that have long slept dormant in the earth: But let reason be our guide, and we shall soon exclaim against such capricious declarations." Unlike Wieland, this author gives the advice to his readers to forget about ghosts rather than study them. Like numerous US scholars and journalists at the time, Philanthropist proposed learning and science as a cure for such "followers of imaginary hobgoblins." The report failed, however, to account for the continued existence of ghost-seers. Nor did the author question the apparatus of reason in its ability to combat ghost-seeing.

The US American author, deist, and publisher Elihu Palmer expressed this sentiment most succinctly in his journal launched in 1803, *Prospect; or, View of the Moral World*. Palmer explained his wish to discuss questions of morality, and he did so by warning his readers in each issue about the dangers of irrationality, which he deemed to be "a commanding influence over human sensation" ("Superstitious Terrors"). The first issue of his journal goes as far as proposing that teaching the Bible is a dangerous activity. In particular, he contests the trust in dreams and visions as promoted by Christian theology. For example, Palmer questions the idea that Joseph, who is warned by God in a dream to escape with Mary and the "divine infant" into Egypt, would actually follow up on this "most uncertain" thing:

"This bible system of religion however has set the whole world a dreaming from the day of the prophets down to the present time" ("Your Old Men" 28). In Palmer's view, encouraging people to rely on dreams, visions, and "reason proscribed by superstition" is contradictory to "the general improvement of the world" ("Reason Proscribed by Superstition"). It is for this reason that he launched his journal to begin with, as he explains in the letter to the public in the first issue (Palmer, "To the Public"). Palmer announces that the underlying topic of his journal—the exploration of "the nature and character" of "moral principles" and the ways in which those "regulate the conduct of intelligent beings"—is closely related to superstition. In one of the issues, he even claims that "the flagrant crimes, the horrid murders and widespread devastation" in the past have "resulted from superstition claiming social intercourse with celestial powers" ("To the Public"). It is again Brown's novel *Wieland* that will pick up on exactly this topic.

Palmer's aggressive stance towards superstition set the tone in the United States. With the publication of *Principles of Nature* in 1801, he was quickly acknowledged as the author of "one of the most influential philosophical treatises not only of Deism" (Hamilton 389). After losing his eyesight due to the yellow fever pandemic in Philadelphia in 1793, Palmer decided to dedicate all his time to preaching and writing, becoming one of the most fervent and famous Deists of his time. However, his central focus throughout his career remained the attack on fanaticism and superstition that he considered to be at the heart of Christian teachings of his time. Interestingly, like Volney, he even used ghosts to convey his point. Palmer promoted the work of John Rannie, one of the most famous early ventriloquist and phantasmagoria showmen to travel New England. Phantasmagoria shows were theatrical performances with "magic lanterns" that projected ghostly images or macabre subjects onto a wall in order to frighten the audience.[21] A simple apparatus consisting of a concave mirror and a light source, such as a candle, sufficed to produce the desired effect. The following is an advertisement for a phantasmagoria show staged in the City Hotel in New York in 1803:

> PHANTASMAGORIA, or, wonderful display of Optical Illusions. Which introduces the Phantoms, or Apparitions of the Dead of Absent, in way more completely illusive, than has ever yet been witnessed, as the objects freely originate in the air, and unfold themselves under various forms and sizes, such as imagination alone has hitherto painted them, occasionally assuming a figure and most perfect resemblance of the heroes and other distinguished characters of past and present times. This Spectrology professes to expose the

practices of artful imposters and exorcists, and to open the eyes of those who still halter an absurd belief in *Ghosts* or *Disembodied Spirits*. (Anonymous, "Advertisement" 3)

The advertisement distinguishes between "Spectrology," the art of constructing ghosts, and the belief in ghosts. Palmer hoped that a study of the apparatus that produces spectral imagery might lead to a more informed understanding of ghosts. It is for this reason that he promoted Rannie's show in his journal, comparing Rannie's efforts to enlighten the masses favorably with the efforts of Copernicus and Archimedes. An announcement in Palmer's 1804 journal introduces the show with the sentence: "The age of superstition has not yet passed!" It goes on to praise Rannie's ability to exterminate "the very dregs of fanaticism." The author of the article also offers a warning to Rannie, assuming that he might be "avoided and detested by the remnants of the disciples of illiberality" (Anonymous, "Rannie's Exhibition"). It is therefore liberality, or the acceptance of different types of beliefs, that Palmer was hoping to defend.

Yet, Rannie continued to be celebrated as a conjuror rather than as a showman. And philosophical discussions relating to questions of perception in New England around 1800 remain married to the supernatural, which in turn increasingly becomes a blueprint for discussing moral issues. Palmer was not successful. Although the phantasmagoria performances were disclosed as illusion, as they were often intended as a demonstration of the fallibility of human perception, they eventually produced the opposite effect, proving and exposing the human desire for enchantment. Pamphlets and daily newspapers repeatedly addressed this conundrum:

> Such are the Forms Phantasmagoria shows,
> And such the dread which round about us glows,
> As when the weary limbs repose in sleep,
> What wild fantastic forms their vigils keep,
> Men, Devils, Angels, unconnected train,
> Compose the motley visions of the brain. (Lemoine)[22]

Terry Castle expressed this sentiment most fittingly: "One knew ghosts did not exist, yet one saw them anyway, without knowing precisely how" ("Phantasmagoria" 30). Indeed, providing an image for what before was not visible promoted ghost-seeing to new and unexpected realms, as phantasmagoria showmen and ventriloquists who pretended to channel the dead appeared in New York and Philadelphia. As a consequence, theories of sight in relation to imagination as expressed in spectrality became a notable topic once again.

Public intellectuals like Palmer and his supporter Thomas Paine as well as most journalists at the time were rather reluctant to acknowledge the popularity of ghosts in the newly inaugurated United States, and yet, they could not stop the spread of the traveling magicians and ghost shows that populated public squares in all major cities. In fact, as Terry Castle and Marina Warner have demonstrated most convincingly, the dialectics of Enlightenment is perhaps best expressed by the popular phantasmagoria shows that spread throughout Europe and New England in the 1790s. In Philadelphia, where Palmer lived for a while, they became a staple of public life. In this way, once again, as in Volney's *Ruins,* ghosts could return to public life by way of the Enlightenment, even in the writings of the most dedicated debunkers, such as Palmer. Instead of exposing the deceit, these Enlightenment ghosts bring to light ways in which imagination shapes human relation. It is for this reason that the first professional US American writer, Charles Brockden Brown, centered the first US American gothic novel at the intersection of ghosts and morality, as I demonstrate in the following chapter.

3

The Voice of Conscience
Settler Colonial Ghost Whisperers

> So talk we of graves and goblins. But, what have ghosts to do
> with graves?
> —Nathaniel Hawthorne, "Graves and Goblins"

Christopher Castiglia argued that the eighteenth-century discourse on the
human mind led to the development of what he termed the "interior state,"
within which in nineteenth-century United States "the interior became a
micro-version of the social." According to Castiglia, the "inside" simply
"became a reflection (and increasingly a displacement) of the ideological
conflicts of the social world" (*Interior States* 3). This work confirms what
Judith Butler had pointed out in her work on subjection: "It is a significant theoretical mistake to take the 'internality' of the psychic world for
granted" (*Gender Trouble* xvi). Following these important interventions
into theories of modern subjectivity, I look into the colonial framing of
the construction of "internality" through spectrality. Retracing ways in
which the ghost came to move from the outside and the social to the private
or the inside of the human mind in early United States reveals a colonial
shift from spectrality to morality.

A writer whose work most strongly exemplifies this point is Charles
Brockden Brown. Firmly situated within the above described transatlantic
context, Brown's oeuvre exemplifies the late eighteenth-century literary effort to challenge the Enlightenment proposal of the sovereignty of reason
and the evidence of the senses as the primary motivation for action. Not
only *Wieland; or, The Transformation, an American Tale* (1798),[1] commonly acknowledged as the first US American gothic novel to reach international acclaim, but even more so the later published prequel, *Memoirs of
Carwin, the Biloquist* (1803–5), are invested in using spectrology to address
a nation in peril. Centering on ghostly voices, both of these publications
circumscribe the supernatural as a space of knowledge production. In what
follows, I demonstrate that Brown, in fact, joined the growing discourse

that perceptibly expressed a need to discuss the irrational not as the other side of reason but as a dangerous source of knowledge itself. I particularly demonstrate Brown's indebtedness to the ghost discourse led by Kant, Lessing, Schiller, Wieland, Volney, and Palmer that I have already introduced. Doing so highlights the colonial framing of Brown's investment and the settler colonial origin of the original document of the American gothic or US American literature in general.

Brown fostered a life-long interest in German philosophy and literature, which is expressed in his focus on reprinting mostly German sources in his role as a publisher and editor (Warfel 357). Particularly his appreciation of Wieland's work cannot be overlooked—the main protagonist in Brown's novel is a fictional cousin of "the modern poet of the same name" who "may be considered as the founder of the German Theatre" (*Three Gothic* 6). Historically, Gotthold Ephraim Lessing, rather than Wieland, would be considered the father of German theater. The fact that the narrator in Brown's novel provides Wieland with this title only confirms Brown's admiration for this writer. In addition, *Die Geschichte des Agathon* (1766), translated as *The History of Agathon* in 1773 by John Richardson of York, Wieland's most famous novel, is a bildungsroman that focuses on the costs of enthusiasm and thus demonstrates some telling congruences with Brown's *Wieland*. Yet, a proper contextualization of Brown's work within the German romantic debate at the turn of the eighteenth century is still missing.[2] What's more, relying on Henry Warfel's criticism, Edward Cahill asserts that "Brown's German influence appears to be more one of literary models than philosophical traditions" (63). Liselotte E. Kurth-Voigt pointed out the obvious correspondences between Brown's *Wieland* and C. M. Wieland's *Private History of Peregrinus Proteus, the Philosopher* (1791, English translation 1796) in mystical experiences, visions, hearing of voices and finally death in fire ("Reception of *Wieland*" 120). This chapter presents a hypothesis that Brown explored a theory of morality through the genre of fiction in relation to the German discourse on spectrology and indirectly in relation to theories introduced by the German philosopher Immanuel Kant. The work of Brown aligns with several of the ideas proposed by Kant in *Dreams of a Spirit-Seer* (1766) and in his much more influential *Groundwork of the Metaphysics of Morals* (1785); specifically, the use of spectrality and its conjunction with questions of morality binds the two writers. Drawing from the philosophical debate in German literary texts that were influenced by Kant's theories, Brown addressed morality through spectrality in a specifically US American settler colonial context.

Charles Brockden Brown on Apparitions

Like all the writers discussed so far, Brown had a philosophical interest in ghosts, or rather in what at the time was often referred to as "spectrology"— a term that addressed "the science of study of specters" ("Spectrology"). In 1799 he founded a periodical that he called *The Monthly Magazine and American Review.* The first issue, published in April of that year, features a cover story with the title "On Apparitions. In a Letter from a Country Gentleman to his Friend in Town," signed with the initials F. R.[3] The authorship of the text is not indisputably confirmed. The fact that this is the first proper article in the first issue of a periodical Brown founded in 1799 confirms at the least that he thought the piece important.[4]

   The article opens with a rhetorical question: "Pray, Sir, what is your opinion respecting the power which the living may obtain over the dead?" Resembling Kant's spirits, which are part of life, the author turned the common question around in highlighting ways in which the living shape relationships among themselves by adjusting the past to their own purposes via ghosts. The dead do not haunt the living; rather, the living have powers over the dead. Brown's well-recorded interest in the dangers emanating from sense deception[5] involved in performing witchcraft and conjuration was in no small degree influenced by the teachings of Elihu Palmer but also by two German authors who managed to redefine the ghost-story at the time and adapt it to Enlightenment purposes: Friedrich Schiller and Cajetan Tschink. Both writers were introduced to the US American audience by the publisher John Bull, who made sure that their enlightened gothic texts were accessible to the US American readers in his serial installments of novels and fragments in his magazine the *New-York Weekly Magazine or Miscellaneous Repository.* Even if the journal existed only from July 1795 to June 1797, Bull managed to publish translations of both texts that became canonical: Friedrich Schiller's *The Ghost-Seer; or, Apparitionist: An Interesting Fragment, Found among the Papers of Count O** (in this journal first published as *The Apparitionist*) and Cajetan Tschink's *The Victim of Magical Delusion.*[6] Brown read and admired both Schiller and Tschink and the writing style that along with Ann Radcliffe's writing set a new standard for ghost stories. Radcliffe, Schiller, and Tschink along with numerous epigones made use of the type of gothic plot that relies on necromancy and spiritualism with the exclusive purpose of merging science and philosophy with literary speculation. Never leaving the confines of science, they used the supernatural to explore the mysterious workings of the human mind.

The German titles of Tschink's original text, *Geschichte eines Geistersehers* (History of a Spirit-Seer), as well as Schiller's title, *Der Geisterseher* (*The Ghost-Seer*, later *The Spirit-Seer*) already indicate their indebtedness to Kant's *Dreams of a Spirit-Seer*. Both intertwine aesthetics and ethics in the act of ghost-seeing in order to explore psychological manipulation and, in the end, propose that a morally intact society can only be established if affect and the senses are taken into consideration. In a letter to Christian Gottfried Körner, Schiller explicitly confirms being influenced by Kant: "I talked about the Ghost-Seer and how this essay had attained a certain celebrity. The matter pleased him [Herder] and we further embarked upon it. He has his own fertile ideas in this, too, and leans toward the assumption of a mutual interaction of spirits according to unknown laws. . . . A vivid thought of mine could awaken a similar one in somebody close to me etc." (*Schillers Werke* 124–25). As in Kant's theory, in Schiller's work, ghosts do not signify the return of the dead but rather the activation of somebody else's thought in the mind of another, whereas this person might be either dead or alive. As a secular version of the Puritan devil who controls the mind of those possessed, these ghosts rely on the activation of the will of another in the mind of the ghost-seer.

Schiller's writings were much discussed in the revolutionary United States. Even before publishing *The Ghost-Seer*, in his most famous and in the early republic extremely popular text, *Die Räuber* (1781, translated as *The Robbers, A Tragedy* by Alexander Fraser Tytler in 1792), Schiller already had convincingly argued that epistemic uncertainty is elemental to terror and thus needs to be studied. Schiller was therefore already established as a popular writer in the former colonies by the time *The Ghost-Seer* was translated. Both Schiller and Tschink reached great acclaim on both sides of the Atlantic shortly upon publication of their ghost stories, and with their corresponding texts turned spectrality into a literary trope that could be instrumentalized for purposes of grounding democratic politics by placing the instability of the human mind and uncertainty at the center of attention.

Much more than simply a part of this tradition, the text "On Apparition" reads like a condensed variation on Schiller's *The Ghost-Seer*, which was not only serialized by *New-York Weekly Magazine* in 1795 but also widely excerpted elsewhere in the late eighteenth-century periodical press.[7] Schiller's ghost-seer is identified in the English subtitle as an "apparitionist," a designation that effectively collapses into one the acts of seeing and producing an apparition. Consequently, particular attention was paid to the physicality of the necromancer and the affective transfer with the audience. Harking back to the conjuring tricks performed by "the Armenian" described in Friedrich Schiller's *The Ghost-Seer,* the author of "On Apparitions" carefully observers the efforts undertaken by an alleged conjurer of ghosts referenced only as "the Hungarian": "His eye was bent down and was immovably fixed for more than fifteen minutes. His tranquility of features gradually gave place to emotion. The muscles of his face were observed to grow tremulous. This agitation became vehement, and extended to every muscle of his body. His hands were clasped forcibly together, and he breathed with difficulty." (n.p.). Detailed descriptions of the conjuror's features are prominent in both texts, as if to suggest that the apparition was spreading through each individual body first before being projected out (literally on the wall).[8] Details about audience's reactions also focused on the physicality of the performance.

In "On Apparitions," the narrator highlights this focus on an externalized interiority as a new aspect of conjuring that relies on the power of the mind rather than on rituals. The narrator explains this transformation from performance to a psychological force: "Instead of an intellectual operation, they [the audience] expected the farce of incantation, mystic characters, traced with charcoal, and high-sounding jargon" (n.p.). Rather than with a spectacle, the audience is confronted with a scene of meditation and mediation. This conscious embodiment of the spirit by the medium, rather than a possession, exemplifies the literal interiorizing of ghosts at the turn of the nineteenth century. It also shifts the power of the ghost to the power of the host.

Much more than a sighting, ghosts emerge upon careful contemplation and introspection as a material projection of those who are able to recognize the realm beyond reality. The medium advanced into the center of attention, rather than the ghost; the performance becomes the phenomena. Consequently, the author of this short article demonstrated more of an interest in the performative aspects, the moments of connection with the audience, and the spectators' desire for enchantment than in the actual apparition. Adapting ghost stories to the demands of the times entails a careful construction of a powerful performance with psychological consequences for both the presenter and the audience. In such circumstances, confirming the existence of the apparition is beyond the point: "The credulous believed, the skeptical doubted, but all ran with speed to the fountains of intelligence, to the houses of those who were said to have been present when the necromancer waved his ivory wand, and *spirits of the dead obeyed his call.* Rumor carried the miracle farther than the confutation would ever reach" (emphasis added).

This pronounced attention paid to senses, perception, and the effects of imagination, rather than the appearance of a ghost, is a novel addition to the genre.[9] The spirits of the dead do not simply appear, they obey a call. The terror created by the act of conjuration does not emanate from a ghost but from the audience's fascination with what the ghost inevitably signifies: the unknown lurking within one's own mind. Rather than awaiting an answer, the audience studies the ghost-seer and participates in this search for a definition that will determine the shape of the ghost. A mixture of fear and attraction is described in a sublime tension between the audience and "the apparitionist" that ultimately seems unbearable. The text ends fittingly with the banishment of the alarming ghost-seer: "The Hungarian, for fear of being mobbed and hooted at for holding commerce with the devil, was compelled to leave the city." The reader, however, is left with questions about mediation, susceptibility, and manipulation.

"On Apparitions" is much more than a lead story that engages in the late eighteenth-century debate on sense and perception, imposture, and the dangers involved in spectral performances by means of exploring the confines of the gothic. Deviating from a simple debunking effort by an author concerned with the impact that the belief in ghosts might have on the credulous population, the text for the largest part focuses on the power of the will of another. The narrator, a "country gentleman," continues to wonder about "the will of him to whom they appeared" and the idea "that voices may be made to salute my ear, and image to hover in my sight, at the will of another" (F. R.). Like Kant's concept of "secret powers," "On Apparitions" implies that a ghost story does not necessarily need a ghost, nor does a ghost-seer depend upon the appearance of a ghost. Rather, the presence of the ghost manifests in the will of another guiding the actions of the receptor. The focus of attention in this essay is the moment of connection between "the apparitionist" and the audience, locating the power of the ghost in the host. The ghost-seer is literally a medium that binds the wills of those dead and alive. Brown draws from this discussion in his fiction, where the reader is confronted with the power of the spectral to conduct the lives of the living. It is this type of performative spectrology that, influenced by the writings of Wieland and Schiller who in turn were influenced by Kant, would lead to Charles Brockden Brown's inauguration of the American gothic.[10]

Brown's choice to feature "On Apparitions" prominently as the opening piece in the first issue of his periodical demonstrates the importance of the narrative perspective that explored the unknown as a site of reason, suggesting that reason as a reliable "guide" was much more perilous than the workings of any of the many charlatans populating the main squares of New York and Philadelphia at the time. Reason, if perceived to be relational, relies on the will of the other. As such it can appear to be supernatural. If subjectivity is understood to be intrapsychic, as it is in Kant's theory, all members of thinking communities are subject to being remotely controlled by the will of another. It is only within this relation that one can understand Brown's instrumentalization of spectrality for questions of morality in his novels. Although there is no evidence that Brown read Immanuel Kant's work before publishing his novels, as a founder and major contributor to early American periodicals, he must have read at least the various articles published on Kant's philosophy in British and local periodicals.

As early as 1796, a reader wrote a letter to the editor of the *Monthly Magazine or British Register* asking for more English translations of this "very intelligent German writer" whom "the majority of your curious readers are, doubtless, acquainted with" (Beddoes 265). The reader-author continued by offering a long list of reasons why Kant's writing should be made accessible to English-speaking readers, mainly concentrating on this philosopher's "examination of our intellectual faculties" (Beddoes 265). His call met various followers, demonstrating that already by the late eighteenth century, Kant's was a known name in the United States. The *Monthly Review* printed a thorough introduction to Kant's philosophy as early as 1798 with a focus on his distinction between appearances and "things by and in themselves" (Anonymous, "Kantian Philosophy" 151) as well as an even longer introductory essay in 1799 by A. F. M. Willich. Kant's essay "Zum ewigen Frieden" (Project to perpetual peace) had already been summarized and interpreted in the same newspaper in 1796 (Anonymous, "Kant's Project"); passages of it were reprinted from Friedrich Nitsch's *A General and Introductory View of Kant's Principles* in the *New-York Magazine or Literary Repository* in 1796 (Anonymous, "Explanation and Vindication").[11] An original reaction to the materialism of John Locke and the Scottish school of common sense, Kant's transcendentalism represented "an offensive and defensive measure against conservative resistance" in the new republic, and thus promised reform to those dissatisfied with the early policies of the so-called founding fathers (Hochfield 10). Brown was perhaps the most prominent writer at the time who sought to express his dissatisfaction with his government's domestic policies. As the first US American professional writer immersed in transatlantic literary, philosophical, and cultural exchanges, he was certainly familiar with Kant's main ideas.

There is also evidence that Brown maintained an interest in the philosopher's life long before Kant became a household name throughout US American literary salons. From 1803 to 1807, Brown served as editor and chief contributor to the *Literary Magazine and American Register*. In May 1805, the journal printed an article titled "Memoirs of Immanuel Kant," which praised "Kant's intellectual qualifications."[12] While the article contains some peculiar observations concerning Kant's physique, including his "large head" mounted on a delicate body "covered with so little flesh, that his clothes could never be made to fit, but by artificial means," which makes Brown's authorship rather unlikely, the anonymous author tellingly expresses his admiration for the philosopher's "extraordinary faculty of retaining words, and representing absent things to himself" ("Memoirs").[13] That certainly would have sparked Brown's interest. The author praised Kant's ability to recognize the imperfection of humans: "He discovered, therefore, so easily, the incongruities of other men's sentiments, and traced, with unspeakable precision, their errors to the true source" ("Memoirs"). Given Brown's life-long interest in "the man of errors" (*Three Gothic* 230), it is hard not to assume that he was, if not influenced by, then at least sympathetic to Kant's theories. At a crucial moment in Brown's first novel, *Wieland*, Carwin explains addressing Theodore Wieland: "Man of errors! Cease to cherish thy delusion; not heaven or hell, but thy senses have misled thee to commit these acts. Shake off thy phrenzy, and ascend into rational and human. Be lunatic no longer" (*Three Gothic* 230). Finding the true source for the incongruities and human errors is at the center of this novel. Both Kant and Brown drew some of their ideas and theories about morality in relation to senses and perception from the same sources and sentiments accessible in late eighteenth-century Europe and the newly inaugurated United States.[14] It is thus possible to conclude that Kant's moral theory via the spectral and German ghost-seer novels had a significant influence on the founding of the American Gothic.

Fiction as a Space between Affect and History

In an "Advertisement" published in the first edition of *Wieland* on September 3, 1798, Brown himself interpreted the novel as no less than an "illustration of some important branches of the moral constitution of man" (*Three Gothic* 3). By the time he published his fourth novel, *Edgar Huntly; or, Memoirs of a Sleep-Walker*, in 1799, Brown was already calling himself a "moral painter" (*Three Gothic* 641). In fact, at the center of all his hastily constructed novels[15] are protagonists immersed in problematic situations that function as a setting to question their moral capabilities. In his essay "Walstein's School of History," Brown specifically spells out this desire to analyze morality "by exhibiting a virtuous being in opposite conditions"—in other words, by depicting fictional individuals in situ rather than tackling the "uncertainty of history" (335). In this essay published in the *Monthly Magazine and American Review* in August 1799, the narrator, Krants, presents revolutionary ideas developed by a fictional German history professor who proposed that history relies on appearances rather than on so-called historical facts. Krants is no Kant; but the correspondence in both their theories and their names is obvious. The narrator in Brown's article compares the work of the historian to the work of a physician: "I am apt to think, that the moral reasoner may discover principles equally universal in their application, and giving birth to similar coincidence and harmony among characters and events" ("Walstein" 335). As demonstrated in this and other texts, Brown believed fiction rather than history to be the proper genre for education. It is this concern that urged the writer to send his first novel, *Wieland,* along with a personal letter, to Thomas Jefferson three months after its publication. Jefferson most likely never took the time to read the book that would have presented him with the spectacular death of a father followed by the unaccountable madness of his son, who strangled his wife and four children, attempted to kill and possibly rape his sister, and finally committed suicide. Theodor Wieland, the main protagonist, claimed to have heard voices that commanded him to murder his family, which he obeyed. Structured as a series of letters written by Theodor's sister Clara to an unidentified addressee, *Wieland* is based on a true murder case that happened in upstate New York.[16] The novel thus explores a classic gothic theme: the altered mind. Does the unconscious mind function independently of a person's will?

"Walstein's School of History" is an important text for understanding the ways in which Brown interlaced questions of spectrality with morality in *Wieland* in order to explore the unconscious. In this essay, the narrator writes: "Actions and motives cannot be truly described. We can only make approaches to the truth" ("Walstein" 336). This revolutionary theory of history proposes that a historian's "deeper insight into human nature," acquired by paying attention to human motivation rather than historical facts, will necessarily result in greater factual "arrangement, and a deeper concern in the progress and issue of the story" ("Walstein" 338). Convinced of its political character, while fearing indifference or contempt from a man "engrossed" by his "public office," Brown endorsed in his letter to Jefferson the social importance of fiction and explained persuasively, "if I had not this belief, I should unavoidably be silent" (Brown, *Collected* 445). Fiction is therefore understood as a ground to play out possible historical scenarios. It is the belief described in "Walstein"—that fiction rather than history can provide access to understanding human motivation for certain actions and thus also provide the foundation for a more just politics—that led Brown to construct a complex novel in which he merged Enlightenment theories and the art of conjuration with ideas about democracy and state formation, all with the aim to develop a theory of morality. To understand the murder case in upstate New York, therefore, it would have been necessary to take a step away from the fact that the murderer was a religious fanatic, as this, in the end, cannot provide an explanation. Instead, a deeper understanding of his environment and the workings of human senses and perception can lead to a better understanding of his motivation. Acknowledging the fiction of history, in turn, enables a more informed conception of state politics. In the letter that was delivered to the then vice president of the United States on December 15, 1798, Brown expressed his hope that the narrative would be "capable of affording pleasure" (*Collected* 445). Alas, Jefferson shared neither Brown's belief in the imperative link between fiction and politics nor his conviction regarding the connection between a local murder and the policies of the new republic; he replied a month later, rather cordially, with the promise to find time for this "work of imagination" in the future.[17] Perhaps as a consequence, Brown, indeed, turned silent. He abandoned his career as a fiction writer only three years later and dedicated all his attention to political journalism instead.

Yet, it is in his literature and particularly in his treatment of spectrality that his politics comes to the fore the strongest. To avoid any confusion: no ghost appears in Brown's *Wieland*. But as demonstrated in this study so far, the ghost story at the time when Brown was writing his novel has shifted its attention from the apparition to the apparitionist. The entrance of a ghost marks the erasure of subjective certainty. Immediately exposed to philosophical discussions relating to spectrology and ghosts in his literary and private circles, Brown drew from Enlightenment theory and phantasmagoria charlatanry alike. Beset with professional frustration and struggling to establish writing as a vocation in the new country, he published his first novel instrumentalizing intellectual debates on ghosts to explore sensationalist psychology but primarily driven by a desire to expose the deficiencies of rationalist philosophy to provide a grounding for organizing society. In

doing so, he marked the contours of the US American gothic by delineat-
ing a form of spectral relationality reminiscent of Kant's moral theory in
Dreams of a Spirit-Seer. It is thus necessary to delve into this much-studied
text one more time in order to expose the tension between spectrality and
morality, which in turn will highlight the central function that ghosts
have held in the colonial project of US American literature since its early
beginnings.

Transgenerational Phantoms

Wieland is written in epistolary form from the perspective of
Clara Wieland, the sole survivor of the family tragedy. Since her brother
is dead by the time Clara writes the letters, readers are forced to assess the
reliability of her account. This becomes increasingly complex as Clara wonders repeatedly if spectral agents might have caused her brother's horrific
behavior (Brown, *Three Gothic* 167). The novel revolves around attempts to
determine the source of the voices that at times are produced by a ventriloquist named Carwin but in crucial moments cannot be explained. Clara
further exposes her unreliability: "What but ambiguities, abruptness, and
dark transitions can be expected from the historian who is, at the same
time, the sufferer of these disasters" (*Three Gothic* 137). At the center of
the novel is the insufficiency of reason to enable both Theodor Wieland to
understand his own actions and Clara to make sense of them. To express
this conundrum, Brown uses a peculiar narrative technique: it is through
Clara's ideas about ghosts or "spectral agents" that the reader gets involved
in assessing Wieland's situation. Just as a historian is always situated in the
present and cannot but rely on ghosts from the past to construct a story for
future generations, Clara herself repeatedly insists that she has no access to
the truth she seeks to convey.

In *Wieland,* Brown constructed a complex web in which irrational
elements of rational structures kept resurfacing within seemingly supernatural frameworks that never left the confines of reality. Brown's specific
technique of weaving the supernatural into the natural to retrace the ways
in which the culture of the early republic had wrongly shaped ideas of progress and knowledge was situated within the specifically US American Enlightenment's attempt to use reason as a tool to control the "wilderness"
encountered in the New World. In 1765, long before Immanuel Kant famously answered the question "What is Enlightenment?" John Adams had
already called upon his fellow citizens to "let us dare to read, think, speak

and write. [. . .] Let us read and recollect and impress upon our souls the views and ends of our own more immediate forefathers, in exchanging their native country for a dreary, inhospitable wilderness" (Adams 123, 128). Brown took Adams at his word and wrote a novel about a settler colonial subject: a white man of European descent, a property owner, who spent his life "in Schuylkill, within a few miles of the city," exclusively reading, thinking, speaking, and writing—the consequence of which was insanity, murder, and suicide (Brown, *Three Gothic* 9). The causal relation between Wieland's isolation, his education, and his murdering of his family continues to keep critics and scholars guessing even today. Evidently hoping to communicate a message to the whole nation with his novel, Brown chose a symbolic addressee to send it to, namely the father of American republicanism, Thomas Jefferson.[18] So, what was the message that the first professional US American writer so insistently tried to convey with the help of spectral agents and from the perspective of a survivor?

I suggest that Brown was following two famous predecessors and ghost-story writers, Shakespeare and Horace Walpole. In such good company, he sought the help of ghosts to address paternal guidance gone awry. Shakespeare's *Hamlet,* one of the most famous ghost stories, and Walpole's *The Castle of Otranto,* widely acknowledged to be the first gothic novel, are both texts that are structured by a masculine economy passed from one generation to the next. Brown's *Wieland* follows these famous examples and tells a story about a son troubled by the mental heritage left by his father, a topic carefully introduced in the first part of the novel. And like the two more famous authors before him, Brown topicalizes transmission by means of spectrality.[19] As in Kant's and Schiller's theories, the ghost signifies a transference. Before the unhappy Wieland children were able to inaugurate their own story, their father "contracted a habit of morose and gloomy reflection. He could not accurately define what was wanting to his happiness" (Brown, *Three Gothic* 7). Introducing depression to the US American reader before this illness even had a name, *Wieland* revolved around a depressed father who embarked upon a religious self-help quest and traveled to the New World, where he hoped to find somebody who might be willing to listen:[20] "The North-American Indians naturally presented themselves as the first objects for this species of benevolence [. . . H]e converted his little fortune into money, and embarked for Philadelphia" (*Three Gothic* 9). The father attempted to tame and control a diffuse body of people the narrator simply calls "Indians." Seen from the perspective of this distraught immigrant, all of the large Indigenous population featured as his mental projection, the Other, a sign of hope and a means of escape. D. H. Lawrence once claimed that even the Pilgrim Fathers turned "America" into a refuge as they "came so gruesomely over the black sea" (5).[21] Brown insists on this view of "America" as a refuge for the European settler, by meticulously describing the troubled situation Wieland senior finds himself in before embarking on his trip from Germany. However, the transferential constellation between missionary and victim that Wieland senior had hoped to establish in the New World proves untenable: "Here his fears were revived, and a nearer survey of savage manners once more shook his resolution" (*Three Gothic* 9). The colonial desire held by this European "father" to transform the Native inhabitants almost reads like a farce: "Terrified at first by the perils and hardships to which the life of a missionary is exposed," he returns to Philadelphia to build a great estate using slave labor instead (*Three Gothic* 9). Proving conflicting with father Wieland's needs, the missionary quest was quickly abandoned and the initial mission was effortlessly replaced by slavery.

The seeming solution to father's problems is summed up in two short sentences: he found his "true" vocation, moved to a new continent, became a missionary, abandoned this vocation, and started a farm. "He passed fourteen years in a thrifty and laborious manner" building a great estate thanks to "cheap land" and "the service of African slaves," which, as the narrator insistently reminds her readers, "were then in general use" (*Three Gothic* 9–10). The "cheap land" around Philadelphia is presented as empty, whereas the presence of the Indigenous population was alluded to only once as, a perceptible sound of war somewhere at "a distance" (*Three Gothic* 25). Without reflecting on these details, the narrative follows the father in his effort to build a temple, with the help of slaves, to which he could retreat in the darkness of the night to construct "his own" enlightened and free religion (*Three Gothic* 11). The presence of enslaved Africans is not mentioned again. The solipsistic narcissism of this solitary religious project is exposed in the conclusion: "His own system was embraced not, accurately speaking, because it was the best, but because it had been expressly prescribed to him" (*Three Gothic* 11). The failed American missionary celebrated individualism and his own exclusive religious freedom in a house built by the enslaved on "cheap land" where he embraced the solitude of this endeavor.

A German settler who attempted to Christianize "Indians" deems this task too complicated and decides to let enslaved people build a temple for his own individual religion instead. This is how the first widely read and discussed US American novel circumscribes the European arrival in the

"New World." In carefully arranging the topics of religious freedom and individuality for the price of civility and community, the forceful exclusion of a vast natural environment including its inhabitants through majestic architectural seclusion and a depressed European exile acquiring wealth through slavery, Brown set a standard for American literature to come.

Although the two resources that enabled the life of the immigrant Wieland—Indigenous land and slave labor—are the very elements that define *Wieland* as an American gothic novel, they are seldom discussed in detail in the abundant scholarship that exists on the novel. In fact, it took over two hundred years until Lisa M. Vetere, motived by questions relating to the Anthropocene, considered the role of land in this gothic novel, in her reading published in 2022. Writing about the "villa, Mettingen, on the 'suburban' outskirts of Philadelphia," Vetere exposes the very material afterlife of the "plantations" along the banks of the Schuylkill, which is what the suburban mansions surrounded with pleasure gardens were called even at the time when the novel was written (119).[22]

The hypocrisy inscribed in the early American idea of freedom in the face of the enslavement of African people and the displacement of the Indigenous population is subsumed under the myth of paternal protection, which in this novel at first is enveloped in silence, then surrounded by voices that cannot be accounted for, and eventually ends in murder. The particular aesthetic Brown developed to convey his message can be best described as ghostly. Wieland senior's morbid behavior ended in a scene that reminds of medieval images of infernal punishment by putrefaction while alive. Just like his increasingly "gloomy" depression, which merged into "insupportable anxiety" when "his brain was scorched to cinders," his exit is shrouded in mystery (*Three Gothic* 13).[23] As if possessed, Wieland Sr. left the family in a spectacular scene that was marked by "piercing shrieks [. . .] uttered without intermission," without any explanation as to the cause of his horrific demise. His body was torn by "fever and delirium terminated in lethargic slumber," and all along, "insupportable exhalations and crawling putrefaction had driven from his chamber and the house everyone whom their duty did not detain" (*Three Gothic* 17). The scene recalls descriptions of demonic possession and exorcism.[24]

Clara repeatedly wonders in her testimonial narrative how the psychic condition and disturbing death of this German immigrant and religious fanatic might have affected the subsequent generation. Both her brother and her father died mysteriously: one claimed to have heard voices that commanded him to kill his family and finally commit suicide, while the other spontaneously combusted.[25] Clara, both the patient and the analyst, underlines the connection between the death of her father and the death of her brother when revealing her torment from sensing the terror transferred from one generation to the other. Facing her brother's demise, she asks: "Was it the infraction of a similar command that brought so horrible a penalty upon my father?" (*Three Gothic* 62). She considers the possibility of herself being affected by the same predicament: "What was my security against influences equally terrific and equally irresistible?" (166). The vertiginous character-development, tamed only by the death of the father and the suicide of his son, supports her as a possible object of transference.

As has been pointed out in a footnote by Charles Brockden Brown himself, Theodore Wieland's condition is based on the descriptions of *mania mutabilis* by Erasmus Darwin in *Zoönomia; or, The Laws of Organic Life (1794–1796)* (Brown, *Three Gothic* 165). Brown's close friend Elihu Hubbard Smith had a strong interest in Erasmus Darwin's work, and he had published an American edition of the first volume of Darwin's *Zoönomia* in New York in 1796. It is thus certain that Brown also took a cue from Darwin's ideas about evolution and heredity, which, in turn, are widely acknowledged as having influenced Jean-Baptiste Lamarck's theory of inherited characteristics from one generation to the next. The literary device Brown develops to express this transgenerational transference is the son's hearing of unaccounted-for voices that are experienced as ghostly.

Following the trace of ghostliness in this text reveals a striking parallel between the plot in *Wieland* and the psychological theory of the "transgenerational phantom": "a formation of the unconscious that has never been conscious—and for good reason. It passes [. . .] from the parent's unconscious into the child's" (Torok and Abraham 173). The theory was developed by Nicolas Abraham and Maria Torok in Paris in the 1970s to account for unseen and unheard transgressions of family members that could provoke trauma-related symptoms. Importantly, just like in *Wieland,* Abraham and Torok use the language of spectrality to describe this pathology: "The phantom is therefore also a metapsychological fact, what haunts are not the dead, but the gaps left within us by the secrets of others" (171). There is another parallel between Abraham and Torok's instrumentalization of the language of spectrality and Brown's own. The two psychologists rely on the concept of ghosts to depart from Freudian theories of the return of the repressed. Instead, they propose that the "phantom" is a heterocryptic "ghost" that returns from the unconscious of another and not one's own (171).[26] As such, the "transgenerational phantom" could not be analyzed in reference to the psychic life of the subject, nor could it be explained in terms of repression or phantasms, as the pathology is understood to be a radically alien presence that comes closer to possession than transference (173). Consequently, they termed this presence a "ghost" or a "phantom." The illness or breakdown which this phantom causes in some circumstances differs significantly from common psychological disorders, because the symptoms that are manifesting in the body of the patient are understood to be somebody else's. What these ghosts are describing is a reaction to somebody else's memory. In other words, the patient is moved by the will of another.

The intimate relation between spectrality and psychology is already in-scribed in the Greek word ψυχή (*psyche*), which refers to "life" in the sense of "breath" and derives from the verb ψύχω (*psycho*, "to blow"). Given that *psyche* refers to the act of blowing breath into something, thus animating something that prior to this activity was considered not alive, it is not a sur-prise to discover that derived meanings include "spirit," "soul," "ghost," and ultimately "self" in the sense of "conscious personality" ("psyche"). Ghosts have thus even in the Western tradition often marked a transgenerational intersubjectivity. Drawing from this context, as Abraham and Torok did, Brown traced a psycho-spectral constellation from the depression of the father to the son, with the help of the narrative structure of a ghost story. In Brown's example, the scene was an isolated building in a rural setting; the typical gothic castle was replaced with a temple built by enslaved people in the midst of a "wilderness" cleansed from its original inhabitants. This setting connects the father and the son and marks the state of affairs in the new republic. This intrusive structure also provides the setting for the deaths of both Wieland fathers: "Backward, it was hidden from distant view by the rock, and in front, it was screened from all examination, by creeping plants, and the branches of cedars. What recess could be more propitious to secrecy?" (*Three Gothic* 89).[27] Ceremoniously set at the same spot con-ducive to secrecy, the temple is renovated by the next generation into a neo-classical summerhouse and turned into an Enlightenment stereotype—a place to think, discuss, and celebrate. In spite of the transformation from the oppressive system of religion to the freedom of education and moral philosophy that this site marks, both father and son face the same tragic end.

The doom lurking in Clara's exclamation is striking: "The future, like the present, was serene. Time was *supposed to* have only new delights in store" (Brown, *Three Gothic* 21; emphasis added). Turning the music ever louder, the next generation already appears doomed, and the reader is ready for a gothic turn of the event. Just like the elder Wieland, who previously withdrew into the isolation of the "temple" to conduct his studies of the French Protestant group the Albigenses, Theodore Wieland begins to dedicate his time to the solitary study of the philosopher Marcus Cicero.[28] The subsequent generation replaces religion with philosophy yet remains equally oblivious as to how to justify their presence in the world. Theodore Wieland's decision in particular could be construed as delusional, but there is method to his ostensible madness.

Neither the father nor the son in *Wieland* reflect upon the colonial setting that they were a part of. Brown went to great lengths to describe their efforts to push aside any thoughts about the location of their home. Even in the face of war, the Wieland offspring were lulled into safety, exposing their ignorant bliss: "The Indians were repulsed on the one side, and Canada was conquered on the other. Revolutions and battles, however calamitous to those who occupied the scene, contributed in some sort to our happiness, by agitating our minds with curiosity, and furnishing causes of patriotic exultation" (*Three Gothic* 25). This almost sarcastic description exposes the early republic's indifference to violence and injustice, but it also resolves the current generation of any responsibility. Brown proposed a theory of intrapsychic communication that calls for inspecting communities rather than individuals.[29] Neither actively participating in shaping their history nor offering a humanist reflection, the young people living in isolation in Schuylkill in the midst of war appear as the victims of a government that abandoned them. The naivete and innocence of the Wieland children turns them into peons on the dark board of political chess.

Abraham and Torok offer a methodology that can advance Brown's scholarship. Their concept of "the phantom" represents an obstacle to what Freud called the process of "working-through"—a sense of which can be recognized in all of Brown's writings: protagonists oblivious to a problem and confused by it are eventually subsumed by it. The phantom in Abraham and Torok's theory leads to an "incorporation" of what they call "the stranger" or "the secret" or "the ghost." It creates "a crypt" inside the body that entombs it. In their theory, the ghost prevents a working-through of a particular trauma (125–32).[30] Clara's musings about Wieland's condition leave no doubt about the psychological connection between the father and the son: "There was an obvious resemblance between him and my father in their conceptions of the importance of certain topics, and in the light in which the vicissitudes of human life were accustomed to be viewed" (*Three Gothic* 21).[31] Opening the discussion to spiritual influxes (in a philosophical reading with Kant) or transgenerational phantoms (in a psychoanalytic reading with Abraham and Torok), Brown introduced the idea of ghosts: "That conscious beings, dissimilar from human, but moral and voluntary agents as we are, somewhere exist, can scarcely be denied. That their aid may be employed to benign or malignant purposes, cannot be disapproved" (*Three Gothic* 167). As Brown himself warned his readers in the advertisement of the first edition of *Wieland,* the incidents, "perhaps, approach as nearly to the nature of miracles as can be done by that which is not truly miraculous" (*Three Gothic* 3). In a parallel manner, Abraham and Torok explain: "Finally, it [the intrapsychic secret] gives rise to endless repetition and, more often than not, eludes rationalization" (175). Theodore Wieland thus carries the ghost, his father's secret, which prevents him from "working-through" his family trauma.

Using the concept of ghosts in an attempt to provide a moral theory for the newly initiated nation, Brown introduced psychological transference long before the birth of psychology in the United States.[32] *Wieland* exposes the troubles of two settler generations without engaging the perspective of those who are affected by the lives of these characters, the previous in-habitants that are strangely absent and the abducted Africans that make a cameo appearance. As Toni Morrison most succinctly demonstrated: early American literature of the American gothic tells the story of the inaugura-tion of a nation through silence.[33] While the African American characters are silenced, the presence of the Indigenous population is framed as absence.

Silence and absence always have the potential to materialize through spectral agents. This, however, is well known not only to those who have no voice but also to those who speak for those who are silenced. Given Brown's interest in the role of the state within subject formation, as well as the central placement of the transgenerational phantom in *Wieland,* it can be argued that Brown constructed Wieland's murders to demonstrate how the forceful exclusion of dealing with extreme forms of violence such as slavery and dispossession in the young republic affects the psyche of the newly inaugurated citizens. However, the problem is displaced to the lives of the previous generation. Dominated by his father's unscrupulous life and his spectacular death, and his own education in moral theory, Theodore turned into a murderer, driven by the intrapsychic ghost. Elevated to a state level, the phantom secret—that is, the trauma that has been passed over from the father to the son without the son's involvement—raises questions about accountability. The ghost as a secret passed by the previous generation relieves the next generation of any responsibility. As an inverted Hamlet figure, Theodore Wieland is presented as a product of laborious and lonely studies of ethical philosophy, but, unlike the famous Prince, he acts. The novel insists that Theodore's decision to extinguish his family grew out of a state of clarity. Clara's surprise reveals his determination: "Did my ears truly report these sounds? He knew himself to have been betrayed to the murder of his wife and children, to have been the victim of infernal artifice; yet he found consolation in the rectitude of his motives. He was not devoid of sorrow, for this was written on his countenance, but his soul was tranquil and sublime" (*Three Gothic* 167). Theodore Wieland establishes his fatherly role within the colonial American community as a murderer. He took over a household established by a failed missionary and enslaver on land formerly owned by displaced people currently at war with the state-supported army. He concealed the secret of this inheritance in acts of virtue and a strong sense of justice, until the two collapsed in a voice that called for absolute self-destruction. Interpreted in this way, Theodore Wieland appears more like a victim than a perpetrator.

Future recipients of Wieland's secret would have been his children. As Clara reported, it was in the temple that her "brother's children received the rudiments of their education" (Brown *Three Gothic* 22). Discontinuing the transference in death continues the violence. Richard Slotkin's famous thesis, that violence has a fundamental significance for the creation of US American mythogenesis as a moment of rebirth, does not apply to this novel. In *Wieland,* violence holds no promise of regeneration.[34] The violence is directed not against characters marked as the Other but against the self, crushing Emerson's call for self-reliance before it was even conceptualized. In passing the secret on to his family, Theodore betrays the ethical convictions that are so carefully woven into his character at the beginning of the novel. His sole occupation was pondering on questions of morality; in fact, this became his only "duty" (*Three Gothic* 208). Torn by this sense of duty, he chooses a future divorced from the hierarchical order established by his father, claiming agency in the act of murder. He communicates the devastating emotional consequences of the entombed secret passed on by the (founding) father(s), in the murder of his family. Wieland's murder presents an act of insanity in a state of rationalization and marks the violence of rational thinking in a free democracy built on slavery and dispossession. Stripped of any moral responsibility, the children of the upcoming revolution appear infantile and vain. Pulling back to study problems of social interaction and communal life in ancient history while living next to a current war, Theodore returns to this scene as a murderer. His act of murder was communication by way of extermination, violence without regeneration.

Biloquism and Intersubjectivity

It is tempting to leave this much-interpreted novel at the psychological reading as a transgenerational haunting through the return of a family's repressed secret to subsequent generations, were it not for the entrance of a "stranger," a curious figure by the adopted name of "CARWIN" who is introduced as a ventriloquist (Brown *Three Gothic* 49).[35] Brown's negotiation also uses the registers of spectrality, but in more subtle ways. Rather than producing a ghostly abject to visibly mark an alternate subject position, the early gothic is carefully producing race through hierarchies of presence. This material affirmation is often expressed vocally. The exclusivity of the settler perspective is justified in the present absence of alternatives. To construct a model within which the subaltern cannot speak, Brown uses the absent voice. Ventriloquism is perfectly suited for this colonial fantasy, as it erases the body of another while incorporating its presence. Ghosts are an aid to such silencing methods, as they emphasize incorporation rather than abjectification. To explain this colonial agenda in early American literature, it will be necessary to take a closer look at how the ghostliness of the disembodied voice structures the novel. To do so, I will need to introduce yet another text by Brown.

Carwin in Brown's *Wieland* remains the most famous ventriloquist in US American literature. Yet, prior to publishing *Wieland,* Brown had already worked on the character of a mysterious vocal artist under the same name in *Memoirs of Carwin, the Biloquist*—an unfinished prequel to the novel that was serialized only much later, between 1803 and 1805, in the *Literary Magazine*.[36] Initially intended as part of *Wieland,* the fragment on Carwin seems to have developed into a story on its own. On September 4, 1798, just before finishing and publishing *Wieland,* Charles Brockden Brown writes to William Dunlap about having already written the fragment on Carwin and about his plan to expand it into a book-length publication: "I have written something of the history of Carwin which I will send. I have desisted for the present from the prosecution of this plan & betook myself to another which I mean to extend to the size of Wieland, & to finish by the end of this month, provided no yellow fever interpose to disconcert my schemes" (Brown, *Collected* 417). The wish to dedicate a separate novel to Carwin manifests the importance of this character to Brown's literary agenda.

It is within *Memoirs of Carwin* that Brown develops his focus on intersubjectivity via spectrality. The text opens with an outcast son who runs after his father's cow into a forest to escape the paternal grip. There he imagines himself surrounded by "goblins and specters" while "solitude and darkness" embrace him (Brown, *Wieland and Memoirs* 185). The haunted forest is an "object of the most violent apprehensions," so Carwin decides to distract himself by "hallowing as loud as organs of unusual compass and vigour would enable" him: "I uttered the words which chanced to occur to me and repeated in the shrill tones of a Mohock savage . . . 'Cow! cow! come home! home!'" (185). This scene is a crude example of the author replacing European castles with North American wilderness, and the feudal ghost with the "savage Indian," as promised by Brown himself. In the oft-quoted preface to his novel, *Edgar Huntly; or, Memoirs of a Sleep-Walker* (1799), Brown determines that in the new US American novel, "the incidents of Indian hostility, and the perils of the western wilderness" are to replace the rather European "puerile superstition and exploded manners; Gothic castles and chimeras" (*Three Gothic* 641–42). Most critics have followed the influential scholar Leslie Fiedler, who supported Brown's idea that "Indian hostility" could replace ancient family homes and dynasties as a building block for a nationalized genre. Dominant definitions of the US American gothic continue to juxtapose the collapsing state power structures in the European gothic novels with the New World formation of hegemonic constellations in the wilderness as a specifically American trait. Yet, *Memoirs of Carwin* points at a more thorough engagement with the Mohawk population.

As an original document of the American Gothic, *Wieland* located multivalency at the heart of this genre. It did so through the concept of the voice. And indeed, in *Gothic Utterance: Voice, Speech and Death in the American Gothic,* Jimmy Packham writes: "At the heart of America's gothic tradition is the horror of the voice" (Introduction). His prime example is Carwin in Brown's *Wieland*. This motif, however, can only be understood in relation to *Memoirs of Carwin*. Spectralized, the voice speaking in the tone of a native character belonging to the Mohawk people of the Iroquois Confederacy is interiorized by the European settler character. In *Iroquois Culture, History, and Prehistory,* Elisabeth Tooker writes about the League of the Iroquois in the colonies as a sovereign political model and demonstrates that, counter to prior scholarship, this confederacy rested on distinctly Iroquois principles. As such, this confederacy held a great source of fascination for European settlers of the early republic. Much more than simple fascination, this scene marks fantasies of outright replacement. Upon hearing his words repeating "in a different quarter," Carwin is first startled and then realizes that he is hearing his own echo reverberating "in the shrill tones of a Mohock savage" (Brown, *Wieland and Memoirs* 185). The eidolic setting in the haunted forest was rationalized through an explanation that was just as unusual as an apparition. The explained supernatural here relies on the spectralization of the Indigenous population, which, in turn, relies on the setting in the seemingly haunted forest.

The forest animated by the spirits of the Indigenous dead is central to antebellum literature in general and the US American ghost story in particular. Here, the voice of the Mohawk American is produced by the European settler, which makes them both, the absent Mohawk and the present settler, echo as one in the forest. The forest is therefore fundamental to establishing this settler colonial motif. What initially seems to be a haunted forest is rationalized in the next step as a space filled with the estranged voice of the self. Carwin proceeds in a scientific manner and slowly learns the art of ventriloquism: "From speculation I proceeded to experiment. The idea of a distant voice, like my own, was intimately present to my fancy" (187). It is this "distant voice," so much like his own, that keeps Carwin's mind occupied (185). In this scene, the closeted ventriloquist, who is about to learn of his ability to "accommodate [his] voice to all the varieties of distance and direction" (187), surprises himself by speaking in the voice of a Mohawk. He ran away from the oppressive "primitivism" of his father towards freedom, which is symbolized by the forest. In this ecogothic setting, the intradiegetic narrator of *Memoirs* highlights the centrality of the voice himself: "A little reflection was sufficient to shew that this was no more than an echo of an extraordinary kind" (186). Emphasizing the particular nature of the echo, the narrator instrumentalized the voice of the Mohawk for his path to freedom.

Among the few scholars who analyze *Memoirs of Carwin,* only David Kazanjian argues for the importance of the Indigenous voice in the text and proposes that "Carwin's judgement in the rocky passage allegorizes the very assimilation policy being directed against Iroquois at the turn of the nineteenth century, drawing specifically on colonial discourses about Mohawks" (157).[37] Adding to Kazanjian's interpretation, I'd like to highlight the importance of the spectral element and ways in which it enables this colonial narrative project. Just as Carwin is not in control of "the tone" by which he is spoken (rather than in which he speaks), the European settlers were not impervious to the cultural influences of the Mohawks. If one is to assume that Carwin is the same character in both *Wieland* and *Memoirs,* his newly acquired art of ventriloquism receives an important twist in *Wieland*—there, Carwin cannot help but "use his art:" "A thousand times had I vowed never again to employ the dangerous talent which I possessed; but such was the force of habit and the influence of present convenience, that I used this method" (Brown, *Three Gothic* 185).[38] Ultimately, he employs his artistry a last time to protect the novel's narrator, Clara, from being murdered and potentially raped by her brother. Thus, rather than developing into a villain, Carwin emerges as the sole character who speaks (as a ventriloquist) in the name of justice. Intertwining the cadences of a Mohawk with the son of a Pennsylvanian farmer of European descent vouches for a morally superior position. Speaking as one in the curious character of Carwin prevents yet another atrocious murder in the Wieland family. This forced unification of the Indigenous voice with the voice of the European settler, produced under the signum of the absence of the former and the presence of the latter, produces a colonial setting in which the Mohawk is not simply replaced but rather incorporated by the European settlers. The incorporation of the ghost, described in universal terms by Abraham and Torok, yet again receives a very material racialized context.

Carwin's status as an unfortunate, confused and knowledge-thirsty migrant US American complicates an interpretation of him as a self-involved settler colonial subject or simply villain.[39] Brown juxtaposes Carwin with his brother, who was driven by fear of punishment; Carwin is driven by curiosity. His interest in ghosts provides him with the desired insight into humanity: "My senses were perpetually alive to novelty, my fancy teemed with visions of the future, and my attention fastened upon everything mysterious or unknown" (Brown, *Wieland and Memoirs* 183). Carwin realizes that the "mysterious or unknown" voice comes from inside, merging the enlightened solipsism of the subject—a Kantian return to the "Self" as a law-giving member—with the realm of "otherworldly" possession, or the voice (will) of the other. While the colonial structure turns the figure of the Mohawk in this text into an incorporated presence prevented from materializing, the voicing is a colonial multivalent subjectivity that can simultaneously erase the voice of the Indigenous character and function as an acknowledgment of the dependency of the new citizens on the voice of the prior inhabitants. This narrative structure marks an erasure of the presence of the Indigenous inhabitants in a literal incorporation of their voice. Similar to Swedenborg's colonial fantasies of enlightening the European with "African" spirituality, the European settler Carwin is enlightened by the Mohawk unearthliness. Whether this inner voice is interpreted as possession, divine annunciation, a transethnic phantom, or an oracular utterance, in spite of its anatomic explanation, Carwin is the active participant, and the Mohawk voice an instrument in his act of freedom. As such, a spectral presence with no agency is created that remains perceptible until the end of the text.

Early instances of ventriloquism were interpreted as the voice of the dead in one's belly. In an early study entitled *Anatomical History on the Organs of Voice and Hearing* (1601), Julius Casserius explained ventriloquism as a diabolical activity.[40] Joseph Glanvill wrote in *Saducismus Triumphatus*: "For *Ventriloquy,* or speaking from the bottom of the Belly, 'tis a thing I think as strange as witchcraft, nor can it, I believe, be performed in any distinctness of articulate sounds, without such assistance of the Spirits, that spoke out of the *Demoniacks*" (258). Brown's narrative is an example of both the literary trope introduced by Puritan scholars, of spectralizing and of demonizing the Indigenous population, and a form of taming the demon within. By merging science with superstition and religion with secularism, the fragment *Memoirs of Carwin, the Biloquist* denies the existence of monoethnic subjectivities, but only under the erasure of the Indigenous voice.

Borrowing from Francis Jenning's study of the myth circulated among settler colonials of an Iroquois empire, Kazanjian explores the specific attraction to representations of Mohawks by white settlers of the late eighteenth century (153). Philip Deloria further demonstrates the simultaneous desire and repulsion visible in the widespread impersonation of "Indians" by white Americans throughout the nineteenth and twentieth centuries.[41] The "hobby-Indians" claimed to capture "the spirit" of what it meant to be Native to the United States (Deloria 128–29). Freedom is central to this costume party: "When the colonials dressed as Indians, they sent the signal of total rebellion. To associate with 'savages' (the natives) was the sign that the colonists would go to the last measure to obtain their freedom" (Deloria 181).[42] Carwin's enlightened effort in the forest, marked by the tones of a "Mohock savage," adds a new dimension to the colonial project of replacing "the Indian." His version can be interpreted neither as the act of a "hobby Indian" nor as the typical romanticization of the motives of warriors among the Mohawk people most famously exemplified in James Fenimore Cooper's *The Last of the Mohicans*.[43] Working within the delicacy of ghostliness, his is a much more subtle form of enfranchising the settler population. The colonial incorporation of the disembodied presence of the Native American character within the body of the European immigrant produces knowledge of a discomforting kind. And, it is not only Carwin who is sensitive to this discomfort—everyone around him is affected by it, creating an atmosphere of uneasiness. In *Wieland,* Carwin is a Euro-American migrant who is wandering around dressed "in the manners of a clown," and while he himself is confused, he is an object to be both dreaded and adored by others (Brown, *Three Gothic* 184). "The subject was extraordinary," exclaimed Clara (*Three Gothic* 63). Presented by Clara as a villain in the opening pages, Carwin quickly turns fainthearted and submissive: "Carwin, irresolute, striving in vain for utterance, his complexion pallid as death, his knees beating one against another, slowly obeyed the mandate and withdrew" (164). Clara's depiction of Carwin reveals an unease that keeps her simultaneously attracted to and revolted by this unfortunate character.

Rather than an assimilationist, Carwin, indeed, is a biloquist. Brown introduced this neologism for a type of nonsupernatural possession that points at the conditioning of meaning by the wills of others. Similar to Kant's origins of moral theory in the language of spectrality, Brown detected in the aesthetics of ghostliness a way to address seemingly universal moral issues in the early republic under the erasure of those who have always been internally excluded.[44] As in Kant's conjecture in *Dreams of a Spirit-Seer,* the immaterial presence (the voice of another) is located within the body of the living. This voice of another (spirit) puts the living in hierarchical relation to others, both living and dead. Carwin's coming-of-age experience in the forest is the result of him putting himself in relation to the presence of the Mohawk. Theodore Wieland rejected this relationship and transformed into a murderer. Carwin survived. The spectral "tone" stresses "the torments of dubbing," yet, at the same time, it enables a literal incorporation of the Native population and thus signifies survival.[45] While this unsettling heteroglossia calls for expression, it can only ever be ventriloquized in the early republic, where the presence of the Indigenous population is relegated to absence.

The last two decades of the eighteenth century saw various developments in theories of the human voice. In 1780, the Royal Academy of Science in St. Petersburg even offered a prize for a machine that could reproduce vowels. The assignment was supposed to explain the physical property of the human voice (Dolar 7). Leigh Eric Schmidt in *Hearing Things: Religion, Illusion, and the American Enlightenment* explains that ventriloquism served an important role in Enlightenment thinking, since it turned spiritual voices into "a rational entertainment and perceptual fallacy" (9). The character of Carwin exemplifies this conjecture and proves Brown was familiar with these discussions. His decision to reduce ventriloquism to its quality of double-voicedness connects the voice of the Indigenous population with the voice of the estranged settler character. In calling this form of ventriloquism "biloquism," Brown introduced a specific form of nonsupernatural agency that addresses a colonial twoness that relies on the erasure of the Indigenous body. Biloquism in *Wieland* is an exploration of the unsettling undefined inner space within which Brown created an American gothic version of a voice that articulates the silence of the Other within oneself.

Neither first- nor third-person, ventriloquism in *Carwin, the Biloquist* is a multiple narrative perspective. Whether one follows Ernst Jentsch and Sigmund Freud and calls the effect of ventriloquism in *Carwin, the Biloquist* uncanny, or rather Tzvetan Todorov and marks it is as fantastic because of the continued oscillation between the explained and the unexplained, either outcome is the result of the spectral presence of the Mohawk voice, a disembodied presence that comes as close to the ghostly as possible without leaving the confines of reality.[46] The choice of an Indigenous nation that always had a strong presence and a *loud* voice and the offering of an image of that voice pushing through the body of the settler invites the reader to engage with the idea of a specific other within. This spectral multiple narrative perspective determines the American gothic throughout the antebellum period and coalesces into a recognizable narrative element that has marked the gothic mode in the United States into the present.

When Fred Russell, the "father of modern ventriloquism," was asked shortly before his death to recall the beginnings of his artistic career, he recalled the early advice of his father to "keep his mouth shut," the upshot of which is expressed in his conclusion: "So I became a ventriloquist" (Vox 90). The art of speaking somewhere else, with somebody else's voice, is honed as a consequence of feeling under transgenerational duress. Carwin also begins to practice his art of talking with a voice that appeared to belong to someone else, in a response to the pressure his father exerted on him. The US American literary aesthetic was formed by a paternal multivalency that in relation to the concept of possession and hauntedness exposed the urgency of recognition. The colonial image of the literal incorporation of the Indigenous voice within the body of the white male settler marked a productive unease at the heart of the nation. A voice within is at first suppressed by the violent father; it eventually emerges through the body of the son. *Wieland* and *Memoirs* propose that positioning the voice of the "Other" within the "Self" as a law-giving member as theorized by Kant is of uttermost importance in constructing a functioning society.

Other than Kant, who excluded all non-Europeans from the realm of law-giving members of a community of thinking beings in his ghost theory, Brown's spectralizing and incorporating voices is a colonial project that enabled settler characters to transform from villains into confused and sympathetic migrants.

Brown's insistence on conveying a moral message via ghosts with his "work of imagination" did not go unheard. *Wieland* remains one of the most interpreted literary texts of the early US American period.[47] Even today, the continuous flow of scholarly engagements with Brown's work demonstrates, at the very least, that his writing addressed a central concern of the early republic, and one that perhaps reaches into our current times.[48] Most sympathetic scholars praised *Wieland* as the novel that kicked off the gothic literary genre in the United States;[49] indeed, the specific construction of a gothic mood continues to make Brown's writing relevant to new generations of scholars. Yet, while the gothic in Brown's novel has certainly been acknowledged by most critics, to date, the central spectral elements have not been sufficiently addressed. This is most likely due to the often wrong conception of a ghost story as narrative that centers on the return of the dead in life. Ghosts stories have always structured the lives of the living rather than accounted for the dead. The voices that Wieland heard are presented as those of ghosts by his sister, the narrator. And Carwin himself reflects on the ghostly voices that he produced. In their introduction to the recently published *The Routledge Handbook to the Ghost Story,* Scott Brewster and Luke Thurston praised the ghost story of the late nineteenth century as a medium "for redefining the boundaries of literary culture and giving it a wholly new affective intensity" (Brewster and Thurston 4). Brown's novel deserves to be counted among the texts that led to this new affective power concentrated within the field of spectrality. In fact, its inclusion might change the way ghost stories are perceived in popular culture even today.

~ 4

The Politics of Absence
Race, Land, and Ecogothic Ghosts

> In the Great American Indian novel, when it is finally written,
> all of the white people will be Indians
> and all of the Indians will be ghosts.
>   —Sherman Alexie, "How to Write the Great American
>   Indian Novel"

By the turn of the nineteenth century, ghosts were an accepted and popular literary element deployed not necessarily to provide insight into the Beyond but to offer a more thorough knowledge of the workings and the trappings of the human mind. When in 1816 Mary Shelley, Percy Bysshe Shelley, Lord Byron, and John Polidori gathered around the fireplace in the Swiss Villa Diodati and decided to each write a ghost story, they were thus responding to a literary impulse.[1] In Germany, the writer E. T. A. Hoffmann, also known as "Gespenster-Hoffmann" (Hoffmann the Ghost), was ardently working on providing literary material for Sigmund Freud's later theory of the uncanny. In France, Jacques Cazotte established spectral lovers as a respected narrative element and initiated a whole literary movement that wrote ghost stories focusing on the devil in the shape of a woman. In the United States at the turn of the nineteenth century, Washington Irving was considered the most prominent ghost-story writer. His popular tales of the supernatural often take place in a natural setting that in his narratives is regularly described as haunted by Indigenous spirits such as "an old squaw spirit" in "Rip van Winkle" (Irving, *Sketch Book* 785) or "an old Indian chief" in "The Legend of Sleepy Hollow" (*Sketch Book* 1059), to name only the most famous ones.[2] The central role of Indigenous motifs in Irving's ghost stories is underlined by how artist Arthur Reckham titled his illustrations of a 1916 edition of Irving's "Rip Van Winkel": "Long Stories of Ghosts, Witches and Indians, illustration from Rip van Winkle by Washington Irving 1783–1859." With the entrance of Irving's tales of the supernatural into the transatlantic literary scene, the convergence

96

of ghosts and Indigenous characters was firmly established as US American popular culture.

Borrowing from Puritan writing, Charles Brockden Brown's treatment of the gothic, and the European fascination with spectrality, Irving sought to promote a specifically US American ghost-story model. He succeeded to the extent that his writing was acknowledged in Europe, and he set the standard for future ghost stories produced in his country that through Irving received a pronouncedly colonial framing. Irving's repeated installation of neglected historians, who coincidentally manage to leave a mark in the annals of history by discovering stories about ghosts, follows a specific pattern. Mute African American ghost-storytellers framed by fictitious historical narratives that relate their biographies reappear in all publications following: *A History of New York* (1809), *The Sketch Book of Geoffrey Crayon, Gent.* (1819), *Bracebridge Hall* (1822), and *Tales of a Traveller* (1824). The conjecture of history with spectrality in the form of the "negro" character telling (ghost) stories about "Indians" that are being collected and retold by Dutch historians so far has not been recognized as a topos in Irving's writing.[3] By exposing and interpreting this point of convergence, I will demonstrate how Washington Irving set a standard colonial framework for US American ghost stories.[4]

Gespenster-Irving and His Silent African American Ghost-Storytellers

In Washington Irving's first book-length publication, *A History of New-York, from the Beginning of the World to the End of the Dutch Dynasty, by Diedrich Knickerbocker* (1809), the narrator attempts to describe "a typical domestic situation" in the postrevolutionary United States.[5] A "happy regulated family" of Dutch origin is introduced: the father smoking a pipe, the mother knitting stockings, and "the young folks would crowd around the hearth, listening with breathless attention to some old crone of a negro, who was the oracle of the family,—and who, perched like a raven in a corner of the chimney, would croak forth for a long winter afternoon, a string of incredible stories about New England witches—grisly ghosts—horses without heads—and hairbreadth scapes and bloody encounters among the Indians" (Irving *History* 479).[6] Following the standard set by Increase Mather with his *An Essay for the Recording of Illustrious Providences* in the seventeenth century, here witches and ghosts join "hairbreadth scapes and bloody encounters among Indians." In this scene, an old woman marked as African American is mediating "incredible stories" about apparitional creatures and the Indigenous population, while the mother knitting stockings, the warmth of a fireplace, and the intimacy conveyed by a first-person narrator are intertwined in an effort to produce what is offered as a "typical" image of harmony and felicity in the United States shortly after the country's acquisition of independence. "Negro," "Indian," "ghosts," and "witches" are assembled in a spectral room of their own and staged as a source of wonder and amusement for the ordered, "regulated family" of European descent. This narrative setting was already carefully assembled in Puritan colonial America in the form of an apparitional tale and presented by Increase Mather as Natural History, therefore paradoxically naturalizing the supernatural and along the way constructing what Michel Foucault called a "subrace" for the purpose of affirming racial hierarchy (83). The same narrative structure now reappears as a literary source of joy and pastime.

The narrative tension is generated through the enigma surrounding the storyteller. Her outsider position and animistic description creates the anticipation that she will provide insight into clandestine and occulted spheres of knowledge. The reader assumes that she is in possession of secret information, parts of which she is now willing to share. The reader herself has an interest in retaining the alienation of the storyteller, as this distance grants suspension and initiation into otherwise inaccessible spheres of knowledge. To an Anglo-Saxon audience in 1809, the character of a (formerly) enslaved person must have appeared highly suitable for this task, as the imagined distance in experience, habits, and culture in comparison to a "typical" Euro-American family is considerable. For this purpose, the storyteller appears dehumanized. Animalized, she is "perched like a raven," and rather than speaking, she "croaks." Presented as an "oracle of the family," she is positioned halfway between regulated happiness and threatening mysteries; she is presented less as a storyteller than a medium, less human than nonhuman.

Charles Brockden Brown had already educated the US readership as to the importance of mediums—those who claim to be able to see or hear ghosts. In his novel *Wieland,* ghost-seeing became a spectacle of mediumship that calls for an inspection of the performance and the reception rather than a discussion about the appearance of the ghost. Irving's mediums are equally important, even if they are carefully nestled within numerous layers that occlude their centrality. The ghosts are equally irrelevant. The scene depicted above is framed by an introduction in which a landlord, Seth Handaside, recalls a story about a ghost-storyteller, which he claims to have read in the papers of the fictitious historian Diedrich Knickerbocker (Irving, *History* 370). Knickerbocker, whose character combines logocentric authority with village gossip, is also introduced as an unacknowledged oracle: "Indeed he was an oracle among the neighbors, who would collect around him to hear him talk of an afternoon, as he smoked his pipe on the bench before the door" (374). It is thus through the historian's tales that the occluded stories narrated by the first "oracle" receive their first public exposure, turning Knickerbocker into an insightful philosopher with access to the unknown. The historian is simply collecting stories about ghosts and therefore not in danger of being subject to superstitious beliefs. It is within this colonial framing that the historian replaces what has been presented as the Native Informant. What in the colonial period was "the Black Man" that needed to be narrativized and exorcized is transformed in Irving's narratives into a racialized spectral informant whose stories need to be preserved by the European settler. Rather than an antagonist, the non-European narrator knowledgeable in the occult spectralizes himself within European ghost stories. Never fully there, this narrator is only present for the settler colonial historian to take over.

The locally famous yet generally unacknowledged historian Knickerbocker and the African American ghost-storyteller return with more alternative histories in Irving's later publications. In *The Sketch Book of Geoffrey Crayon, Gent.,* published serially between 1819 and 1820, it is markedly Knickerbocker, an "old gentleman of New York," whose informed perspective is trusted, as he is "very curious in the Dutch history of the province, and the manners of the descendants from its primitive settlers" (*Sketch Book* 767). Invested primarily in fieldwork, Knickerbocker is commonly seen strolling around in the neighborhood collecting tales among "common people" (475). The manuscript he finds holds otherwise inaccessible information that official annals of the American past might have excluded. Jeffrey Insko argued that Irving constructs a metahistorical discourse with his hobby historians in order to create a national past, and this argument has been repeated numerous times. Yet, where does this imagined past place racialized people, and what type of subjectivity is produced during this process? To answer this question, I will focus on less famous and little-discussed tales by Irving rather than his most analyzed tales "The Legend of Sleepy Hollow" and "Rip van Winkle," but my final conclusions apply to these famous tales as well. My focus on rather neglected tales will demonstrate that Irving's colonial framing of spectral matters was structural rather than restricted to individual examples.

A recollection of undocumented history is also the topic of Irving's collection *Bracebridge Hall* (1822), written during his stay in England. The
collection was awaited by critics and readers, with excitement on both
sides of the Atlantic, as it was to solidify Irving's leading role in the (new)
world of American literature that he had acquired by publishing *The Sketch
Book*. Irving reacted to this transatlantic acclaim by focusing on what in
early nineteenth-century Europe were topics commonly understood to be
American: exploration of the frontier and the creation of a new nation.
Whereas in his earlier writings, Irving had presented European topics from
a North American perspective, he now develops a sense of foreignness by
moving away from home. That sense of estrangement paradoxically provides the basis for strong national sentiments and solidifies his role as a
leading US American writer. Reminiscent of the growing nationalism in
expat situations that has been effectively described by Benedict Anderson
in *Imagined Communities, Bracebridge Hall* puts typical postcolonial topics such as cultural definitions and identity questions at its center. Pushing
back against the European gaze, Irving provides a sense of Indigeneity for
his settler characters.[7] The fictitious author of *Bracebridge Hall*, Geoffrey
Crayon, explains this tension when opening the work with the author's address to the reader: "I was looked upon as something new and strange in literature; a kind of demi-savage, with a feather in his hand, instead of on his
head; and there was a curiosity to hear what such a being had to say about
civilized society" (7). Promoting the settler writer as subject to an ethnic
gaze and therefore erasing and replacing the Indigenous writer in this position, Irving now reacts to what he imagines to be a European view of the
United States. The established character of a historian now openly takes
on the role of a spokesperson for Indigenous issues whereas these are, as
demonstrated in my analysis of Brown's writing, in fact, settler colonial issues. An increasing number of African American characters join the settler
historian's cause by mediating between what is presented as the Indigenous
spirit world and the realism of what is called "common people" (Irving,
History 475). In this way Irving's oeuvre maps out the supernatural ghost
story with racial and ethnic colors that were already set in place in the Puritan apparitional tale and fine-tuned in Brown's tone-setting publications.
Embedded within the realism of Dutch American villages, this narrative
setting is, in turn, effectively offered as a storage space for silenced voices
and the unacknowledged past, the spokesperson for which now becomes
the non-British European male colonial settler. In a manner reminiscent
of the ministers who collected apparitional tales throughout the colonies

only to mark them with racial insignia, Irving constructs a postcolonial version of the US American ghost story that turns out to be rather colonial, with a European hobby historian who mediates between African American and Indigenous topics and European settler concerns.

A complex of interrelated tales, all published as part of *Bracebridge Hall*, exemplifies this narrative setting. The individual tales are "The Historian," "The Haunted House," "Dolph Heyliger," and "The Storm-Ship." In "The Historian," Diedrich Knickerbocker is again introduced, by his landlord, now Geoffrey Crayon, as a descendant of the Dutch families that remained in New York "after it was taken possession of by the English in 1664" (Irving, *Bracebridge* 298). Knickerbocker is thus marked as a member of an ethnic group that had to submit to the political power of the English: "The descendants of these Dutch families still remain in villages and neighbourhoods in various parts of the country, retaining, with singular obstinacy, the dresses, manners, and even language of their ancestors, and forming a very distinct and curious feature in the motley population of the state" (*Bracebridge* 298). The distinctly Euro-American but not British history of the region is recognizable in the preservation of cultural elements such as dress, language, and manners, all of which are shared by the historian who speaks from an outsider's perspective: "With the laudable hereditary feeling thus kept up among these worthy people, did Mr. Knickerbocker undertake to write a history of his native city" (298). The fact that the following tales are presented as part of yet another found manuscript demonstrates the preservation of historical memory threatened by erasure under British rule.

The title of "The Haunted House," together with its epigraph, which is taken from Shakespeare's *Winter's Tale* and promises a "sad" story of "sprites and goblins," makes the reader anticipate a gothic plot (Irving, *Bracebridge* 298). But instead of a ghost story, "The Haunted House" turns out to be Knickerbocker's own concise autobiography. Describing his former neighborhood, "the ancient city of Manhattoes [...] when [he] was a boy" (300), the historian reduces his report to one element, the "old mansion" of "the early Dutch settlers" known as "a country residence of Wilhelmus Kieft, commonly called the Testy, one of the Dutch governors of New Amsterdam" (301). A detailed description of the owner promises a historical reconstruction of the "important history of the Dutch settlers," yet this expectation is subverted, too. Carefully established facts are exposed as mere interpretations; the question of belonging is "lost in the obscurity that covers the early period of the province" (298). This topical beginning in contested ownership and belonging relegated to obscurity finds an expression in a classic gothic element: a house that seems to be producing its own agents. While the question of ownership is obscured, the current inhabitants are well known among the neighbors as well as to the narrator: "It is a fact" that the current residents are "ghosts," explains Knickerbocker (301).

Upon introducing a common gothic setting—an abandoned haunted house—the narrator follows his stream of consciousness and suddenly shifts the attention to reminiscing about "a gray-headed curmudgeon of a negro who lived hard by" and who was known to tell ghost stories (302): "The old crone lived in a hovel, in the midst of a small patch of potatoes, and Indian corn, which his master had given him on setting him free" (302). Similar to "the old crone of a negro" in *A History of New York,* this former slave is characterized solely as a ghost-storyteller: "He would come to us, with his hoe in his hand, and as we sat perched, like a row of swallows, on the rail of the fence, in the mellow twilight of a summer evening, he would tell us such fearful stories, accompanied by such awful rolling of his white eyes, that we were almost afraid of our own footsteps as we returned home afterwards in the dark" (302). The focus of this analepsis is Pompey, "the grey headed negro," constructed as a joyful source of threat, whose stories of pain and danger serve to recall the biography of the narrator. Consequently, the reader does not learn the content of the supernatural tales. Instead, the story shifts back to the present tense, and the historian Knickerbocker returns to the haunted mansion to find out about "a knot of gossip speculating on a skull which had just been turned up by a ploughshare" (301). Next, the narrator finds the skull and informs the reader: "I knew it at once to be the relic of poor Pompey," "the gray-headed negro," who "went to keep company with the ghosts he was so fond of talking about" (302). Deciding to leave the villagers to "their stories," the narrator presents himself as Pompey's solitary ally, constructing his own "story": "I took care, however, to see the bones of my old friend once more buried in a place where they were not likely to be disturbed" (302). The narrative is establishing what will become a trope in the twentieth century and what Gordon and Hernán discussed as the White Savior format within which "the messianic white self" appears as "the redeemer of the weak" who are regularly presented as "black" and "Indian" (3).

In *Bracebridge Hall,* this narrative structure is nestled within a tale that evokes familiar ghost-story elements and gothic settings but clearly breaks with the British tradition. Introduced as a classic ghost story under the patronage of Shakespeare, "The Haunted House" turns out to follow a rather unconventional plot. Instead of activating the past in the present, in "The

Haunted House" the past is erased in the present without conjuring it. Two narrative levels are interlaced in this short tale: the untold ghost stories by the now dead narrator and those ghost stories told about him. The space is haunted by an apparition that never appears; spectrality thus is put in the service of the historian's biography. As the ghost of Pompey never materializes, he is spectralized not in order to become an agent and receive a voice of his own; on the contrary, his voice is erased even in death, and his life appears only as an element of Knickerbocker's autobiography.

The anticipated ghost story functions as a vehicle that enables the historian to take the remains of the dead body to their second and final resting place. Instead of reactivating unfinished business from the past by letting it manifest itself in the present, this semi–ghost story shifts the present—the historian's present—into the past, putting the ghost to rest without giving it a chance to materialize. What seems to be Pompey's ghost story is revealed as Knickerbocker's history. Knickerbocker—who at first seems to be an extradiegetic narrator—now appears as the focalizer, and "The Haunted House" turns out to be a narrative about a Dutch historian burying the final remains of a person who was formerly enslaved.

What is presented as a polyphonic story with various narrators is actually a settler colonial autobiography of one man. Irving's ghost stories are a continuation of Charles Brockden Brown's spectral multivalence, within which the voice of the racially marked characters is absorbed and silenced. The African American auguries never get to tell their stories, not through spectral means nor through ventriloquy; nor are they verified through multiple perspectives, not even as spectral agents. Instead, they are installed in association with ghostliness itself, which constructs a distance between these characters and their audience. This, in turn, allows the reader to identify with the "regulated family," which is the audience and not the narrator. Whereas spectrality in Brown's *Wieland* and *Memoirs of Carwin* served the purpose of promoting a colonial theory of intersubjectivity at the heart of constructing a multivalent national imaginary suggesting assimilation in the early republic, Irving's spectral elements pursue the opposite objective. Siding with the audience, the reader unconventionally imagines a lack of shared values with the storyteller, who cannot be made subject to one's own standards. Vexing the role of the storyteller, Irving provides a literary fantasy for European American readers in the new republic, within which a scene of domestic bliss could include African American characters via ghost story right in the center of the circle of a "typical happy family" while simultaneously refusing their entrance. Aided by the supernatural framework, these characters are internally externalized. Brown's mental incorporation here receives a structural external pattern.

Colonization of the Spirit World

To construct his supernatural tales, Irving uses a complex concentric structure of stories nested within other stories, with the significant deviation into private libraries of neglected historians and the unveiling of questionable publishing methods. Through this simulation of a ghost story, the past is repeatedly reconstructed in the present, and Irving's historians come to the fore with their chance discoveries set apart from acknowledged mainstream annals of American history. At the center of these multiple *Rahmenerzählungen*—frames within which a narrator tells the story—is the supernatural core interlaced with fictitious historical elements and embodied by a silent African American ghost-storyteller.

The ghost story perfectly suits this structure given that multiple narrators are a standard element of the genre. Additional perspectives convey a sense of reliability within a highly unreliable plot. Paradoxically, the reliability of the narrator grows with his insecurity. The more the narrator doubts the content and the more second opinions he consults, the closer will he draw the reader into the narrative web. In this way, the reader can identify and consider his personal methods of verification. Famous examples include: a narrator who questions his own stance within a first-person point of view, as in Mark Twain's *A Ghost Story* (1870); or a narrator who engages in a tripartite framework that shifts the attention to different perspectives, for example, Henry James' delivery of the governess' story through the character of Douglas through an anonymous narrator in *The Turn of the Screw* (1898). Regardless of the manner, the further removed the storyteller is from the supernatural content, the higher the expectation of authenticity. In this way, the narrator and the audience join in constructing the unknown: the (hi)story of a ghost. Irving is playing with these genre conventions, but he deconstructs specifically the authority of those who tell the story and their relation to the audience; the connection between reader and narrator is erased by eliminating this shared perspective and repeatedly breaking the tales off exactly at the expected appearance of the spectral element. The ghost, the storyteller, and the audience are silenced; only the framework—the so-called ghost story—remains, making space for the historian's settler colonial tale.

William Hazlitt famously called Irving's writing "literary anachronisms," and Mary Weatherspoon Bowden points out in her reading of *A History of*

New York that nineteenth-century characters such as Hudson, Van Twiller, Kieft, and Stuyvesant are displaced to seventeenth-century New Amsterdam (Bowden 29). In *Bracebridge Hall,* as well as in *The Sketch Book* and *Tales of a Traveller,* the literary anachronism holds true even for spheres where "time is out of joint"—the sphere of the supernatural. Even ghosts are displaced as they are remembered by historians who prevent their materialization. "The Haunted House" entails all the classic elements the reader expects: a haunted house, a quest to identify the ghost, a ghost-seer with a personal interest who returns after a considerable period of time has elapsed, and veiled indications of a potential crime committed in the past. But the narrative is temporally reassembled in an unconventional manner that takes the agency away from the ghost, who commonly appears as the agent of history. Even the ghost-seer is stripped of agency, shifting it to the ghost-teller, distinct form to the ghost and ghost-seer. In this way, Irving rewrites the story of the American ghost as a story of the American host.

The function of installing a ghost-storyteller as a mediary without allowing the ghost to appear becomes clearer if one recalls what the appearance of a ghost historically has been able to convey. From one of the first concise treatise on ghosts, published in 1586, Pierre Le Loyer's *Quatre livres des spectres; ou, Apparitions et visions d'esprits, anges et démons se montrant sensiblement aux hommes* (*Treatise of Specters; or, Strange Sights, Visions and Apparitions*), to Jacques Derrida's 1993 *Spectres de Marx* (currently the most quoted reference in the context of spectrality), the appearance of a ghost has always oscillated between imagination and knowledge. Even long before these disparate writers sparked respective discussions about the sociopolitical importance of studying ghosts in their own times, Aristotle connected in *De anima* the appearance of what he calls a phantom to the act of acquiring knowledge by tracing the ancient Greek word *phantasia* (φαντασία) from *light* (φάος). Phantasia is the act of making visible and presenting to the eye, and stems frequently in derivatives of φαίνεω, to show, cause to appear, or bring to light. Conclusively, a phantom is not only something that is missing but also the act of bringing to light what has been missing (as is particularly recognizable in phrases such as "phantom pain" or "phantom limb"). In light of Irving's numerous narrators, who seem to be reevaluating ghost stories as important sources for alternative views on history, the nonappearance of a ghost in these stories must be understood as a colonial erasure of historical memory that was reactivated for the purpose of obliteration.

Only a very few ghosts do appear in Irving's spectral tales, and their provenance is a telling indication of the power of materialization. After burying Pompey, Knickerbocker turns to a ghost story told by John Josse Vandermoere, who promises to outdo Pompey's idiosyncrasies. The tale relates the adventures of another of Irving's familiar character types, the ne'er-do-well male character in the manner of Rip Van Winkel or Ichabod Crane. Dolph Heyliger is a "most mischievous" person with a "gamesome spirit, which is extolled in a rich man's child, but execrated in a poor man's" (Irving, *Bracebridge* 306). Prototypically, the ghost-seer is rich in spirit and poverty-stricken. In order to earn a living for himself and his mother, Dolph replaces the recently deceased assistant of a famous German doctor, Karl Lodovick Knipperhausen. This act allows him to enter the world of magic. A sorcerer-like physician, Dr. Knipperhausen consulted the stars; like Cotton Mather, cured "old women and young girls" of witchcraft; and became famous in "managing cases not laid down in the books" (*Bracebridge* 312). The doctor's study, "almost as the den of a magician," again misleadingly mimics a gothic setting. It consists of a chamber of horror, complete with "a claw-footed table," and features a corner in which "grinned a human skull," as well as "glass vessels, in which were snakes and lizards, and a human foetus preserved in spirits" (308). This setting, which is presented as alien to Dolph's nature, proves—with little spectral help—to be the key to his happiness. Secluded from social contacts except for "the wild striplings of the place, who were captivated by his open-hearted, daring manners, and the negroes, who always look upon every idle, do-nothing younger, as a kind of gentleman," Dolph is ordered by the doctor to spend a night in a newly acquired haunted house to prove it free of evil spirits and raise its market value (314).[8] His friendship with "negroes" becomes his spectral pass as an "old black cook," the narrator's "only friend in the household," ties an amulet around Dolph's neck to protect him (318). The amulet was "given her by an African conjurer, as a charm against evil spirits" (318). Swedenborg's racial divide, supported by Enlightenment scholarship such as Kant's, between those who are spiritual and those who are reasonable comes to the fore again. This charm passed from the African conjurer to the African slave is now ceremonially given over to the Dutch settler for purposes of securing property and raising its market value. Swedenborg would have been proud of Irving.

Armed with Native American friendship and African American charms, Dolph spends a night in the haunted house and survives. This time, however, the ghost does materialize. Its identity is discovered in small installments. At first there are only steps—"tramp-tramp-tramp!"—and "whatever made the sound was invisible" (157). The ghost's final appearance bears more spectacle in its choice of fashion than in its existence: "It approached along the passage; the door again swung open, as if there had been neither lock nor impediment, and a strange looking figure stalked into the room. It was an elderly man, large and robust, clothed in the old Flemish fashion. He had on a kind of cloak, with a garment under it, belted round the waist; trunk-hose, with great bunches or bows at the knees, and a pair of russet boots, very large at the top, and standing widely from his legs" (158). Dolph proves conversant in the face of the anthropomorphized apparition and remembers that all one needs to do is address it: "Whether alive or dead, this being had certainly some object in his visitation; and he recollected to have heard it said, that spirits have no power to speak until they are spoken to" (324). Following formulaic ghost-story arrangements, Dolph initiates a ceremony to which the old man's recognizably Dutch apparition proves responsive. Dolph feels encouraged to follow the lead of the ghost and boards a ship that leaves for a long sail down the Hudson River. Just like Ichabod Crane, who enjoys gossiping with the "old Dutch wives of Sleepy Hollow" and telling ghost-stories deep into the night, or Rip van Winkle, who is only mildly surprised about ghostly demands in the middle of the forest, Dolph realizes that "there was something strange and incomprehensible about the unknown, that inspired awe and checked familiarity" (325). As in William Gilmore Simms' "Grayling; or, 'Murder Will Out,'" which similarly features one of the few instances of the sighting of a ghost in antebellum literature, this ghost, significantly, is of European-American descent; it is the ghost of a former major who fought in the revolutionary war. His appearance serves a patriotic purpose even after death. Whereas the stories told by the African American character served the purpose of distancing, this ghost creates a feeling of "familiarity" and can be instrumentalized for purposes of constructing a heritage and a present in relation to the past. The ghost that materializes in front of this Dutch settler enables Dolph to construct a historical line of heritage and carve out a sense of belonging. The sphere of the supernatural allows outsider characters like Dolph to position themselves in society. The supernatural is thus instrumental in marking a space for European settler characters who confront their ghosts, by making this very positioning impossible for African American characters.

Various male protagonists in Irving's work are outsiders associated with "ghostly" spheres long before they become ghost-seers. This is indicated by the actions they take outside of the moral framework of English Protestant ideology: They socialize with women and Native American and African American characters and connect with these characters through telling ghost stories about (spectral) "Indians." At times, they even join these characters in their nonfunctional activities. Ichabod is fond of reading and dancing, for which he "was the admiration of all the negroes, who, having gathered, of all ages and sizes, from the farm and the neighbourhood, stood forming a pyramid of shining black faces at every door and window, gazing with delight at the scene, rolling their white eye balls, and showing grinning rows of ivory from ear to ear" (1077). Rip likes hiking in the forest. Tom Walker is lazy. Dolph wanders around the village. The ghost-seeing of these characters implies an exceedingly playful innocence, a separation from mainstream traditions, and a responsiveness toward the unknown that is implicitly marked as non-British. Their near-childish ingeniousness conveys a knowledge supposedly acquired through friendship with marginalized racially marked characters, a knowledge that helps them subvert the requirements of an ordered small-town community.

While this connection between settler outsiders and generic Indigenous characters persists throughout Irving's writing, it is particularly central to the plot of "Dolph Heyliger." It is in this story too that the centrality of the forest comes to the fore. One day, far from the restrictive life in the village, Dolph wanders into the forest and becomes acquainted with a society that complies with his nature. He meets a "large stout man," apparently "the principal personage, or a commander," whose "face was bronzed almost to the colour of an Indian's" (333):[9] "He wore a hunting frock, with Indian leggings, and moccasins, and a tomahawk in the broad wampum belt round his waist. As Dolph caught a distinct view of his person and features, he was struck with something that reminded him of the old man of the Haunted House" (333). Later Dolph will befriend this man who resembles an Indian but also the ghost he had seen. The explanation follows: Antony Vander Heyden turns out to be "a great friend of the Indians, and to an Indian mode of life" and a descendant of the man who appeared to Dolph as a ghost (334). With the help of Antony's spectral ancestor, Dolph finds marital bliss and, conveniently, a large sum of money hidden in the well in front of the haunted house. Keeping the legend of the ghost alive, he spends the rest of his life with exclusive access to money, the house, and the love of Antony's beautiful daughter, securing property, affirming patriarchal gender structures, white supremacy, and heteronormativity.

"To understand the various ways Americans have contested and constructed national identities, we must constantly return to the original mysteries of Indianness," writes Philipp Deloria (2). Irving's ghost stories play a significant role within these national fantasies. In this narrative,

Dolph, whose "only friends" were "the wild striplings of the place" and "negroes," joins Antony, a wealthy man who refuses the controlled life of a Puritan settlement and chooses to spend his time in the forest "playing Indian." Antony's household is described as follows:

> The room was decorated with many Indian articles, such as pipes of peace, tomahawks, scalping knives, hunting pouches, and belts of wampum; and there were various kinds of fishing tackle, and two or three fowling-pieces in the corners. [. . .] The negroes came into the room without being called, merely to look at their master, and hear of his adventures; they would stand listening at the door until he had finished a story, and then go off on a broad grin, to repeat it in the kitchen. A couple of pet negro children were playing about the floor with the dogs, and sharing with them their bread and butter. (351)

Dolph and his new friend Antony establish the appearance of a close emotional connection to anonymous African American and Indigenous characters. As such, a non-British domestic is created within the US in a concentric structure organized around a "master." Portrayed in association with Blackness, these characters are free to live out their Whiteness; "playing Indian" provides a sense of moral exculpation and cultural identity apart from the British rule.[10] The appropriation of the "Indian" lifestyle and the animalization of African American children strolling around and sharing food with dogs expresses Antony's and Dolph's humanity. What makes them human is their inclusion of non-European characters, which is perceived to be an anomaly in a society based on the exclusion of these groups. It is the non-humanity of these characters that affirms Dolph's humanity.

As yet another example of internal exclusion, the imagined friendship between settlers, the Indigenous population, and African American characters can only be constructed by way of the supernatural. Antony's appearance, which simultaneously recalls the image of an "Indian" and of a ghost, makes both "Indians" and ghosts superfluous. They are replaced with Antony. Irving constructs an intricate web of ethnically and racially marked characters, excluding them from society through a questionable inclusion for the sole purpose of carving out a space for Dutch settlers apart from the history of markedly British Puritanism. Serving the sole purpose of establishing the Dutch American protagonist's moral integrity, African American and Indigenous characters have a ghostly presence themselves, appearing only to disappear. Their secret knowledge of the ghost world is passed on to the Dutch settler, who can now live a life in moral peace and financial prosperity. The settler's peace is conveyed by his own spectral ancestry, and he is released from being haunted by either colonial or postcolonial ghosts.

The supposed friendship between the protagonists and marginalized characters serves to legitimize the wealth of Dutch settlers and to distance them from questionable governmental policies of exclusion. Using the language of the supernatural, Dutch American characters elevate themselves from their outsider status into the role of a mediator and spokesperson for disempowered inhabitants of early America. The spectral constellation demonstrates how under certain conditions, exposed interpersonal contact between socially distinct groups can be the most effective way of preserving xenophobic prejudice.[11] To conjure a ghost while preventing its materialization must be understood as an erasure of suppressed historical memories on the verge of reactivation. It prevents the exposure of something that has been perceived and marked as missing, the amputation of a phantom limb.

The Return to "Devil's Territories"

Irving constructs the many spectral gaps in his tales of the supernatural around America's Indigenous inhabitants and their relation to nature as well as the origin of wealth in slavery as a strategy to produce a usable social imaginary for the new republic. In the work of the psychoanalyst Jacques Lacan, the Imaginary is the accessible and conscious register of psychic subjectivity. The social imaginary in my context, similarly, relates to the restricted sphere of self-awareness, thus who and what citizens of the early republic imagine themselves to be and not to be. The numerous missing apparitions represent a resourceful method concerned with producing an image repertoire for the national narrative that manages to address death and destruction without negotiating it. This structure reaches its peak in Irving's next publication, *Tales of a Traveller* (1824).

The collection was not successful among critics, who lamented that Knickerbocker "grows somewhat superannuated" some critics even experienced "pure unmingled disgust" (Anonymous, "Washington Irving Review"). Yet, Irving's style had not changed much. In one of the collection's most famous tales, published under the title "The Devil and Tom Walker," Irving reactivates all of the already established and analyzed elements: the isolated and impoverished but sympathetic Dutch settler character, the superstitious African American spectral informant, spirits of Native American descent, the landscape of New England supposedly haunted by Indigenous spirits, and the appearance of the ghost of a specific settler character. In this popular tale, all these narrative elements that Irving has been carefully constructing since his very first publication coalesce into a quintessential settler colonial ghost story. What began in "The Haunted House" as a fantasy of the early republic in which a hobby historian of Dutch provenance could take the disturbed remains of former slaves to a final resting place is rounded up in "The Devil and Tom Walker." The same elements can be found in another tale published as part of the collection under the title "Adventures of the Black Fisherman," which demonstrates the colonial formula in Irving's oeuvre. But it is in "The Devil and Tom Walker" that Irving makes a direct reference to Cotton Mather's "Black Man" who generally resembled "an Indian" in *The Wonders of the Invisible World* (75). I will focus on this text.

"The Devil and Tom Walker" is a ghost story about a man who avoids punishment for the national debt of slavery and dispossession by opting for capitalism instead. In this story, greedy European settlers are punished for slavery and the dispossession of the Indigenous population by a satanic character who, just as in Mather's text, is identified as halfway between "negro" and "Indian" (Irving, *Tales of a Traveller* 657). The tale begins with Tom Walker accidentally stepping on a skull in a swamp near Boston. Looking down, he discovers "an Indian tomahawk buried deep" in the ground, an indication that the skull must be of Indigenous origin. This chance discovery of a skull is a repeatedly instrumentalized element in Irving's writing. In the supernatural tale "Adventures of the Black Fisherman," the formerly collected skulls of an African American slave and the "Indian" skull are joined by the skull of a royal Dutch settler, completing the literary collection of ethnically marked remains buried in the same ground. In this way, postcolonial America is being restructured in death under European auspices.

This skull motif is corroborated in the next scene, which establishes a causal relation between the stepping on the remains and the appearance of a "stranger," a "black man" (Irving, *Tales of a Traveller* 657). Entering the enchanted ground of New England is sufficient for conjuring a ghost; no incantations are taking place, no long and mysterious rituals are needed; Tom's stepping on "a cloven skull with an Indian tomahawk buried deep in it" alone activates the appearance of "a great black man, seated directly opposite him on a stump of a tree" (657). Always already haunted, the American forest brings together the "great black man" and the "Indian," who are yet again joined in a spectral space of their own and presented to the settler character. The narrator describes "the stranger" who appeared as a being that oscillates between supernatural and racially marked otherness: "the stranger was neither negro nor Indian. It is true, he was dressed in a rude, half Indian garb, and had a red belt or sash swathed round his body, but his face was neither black nor copper colour, but swarthy and dingy and begrimed with soot, as if he had been accustomed to toil among fires and forges" (657). Just like his European model, the American infernal agent, "the old Scratch," has no power over the individual. What can be described as a figuration of an ethnic devil invites Tom to become a slave trader, which would make him rich for the rest of his life. Tom is free to decide for or against this deal; except, Tom's freedom is limited by poverty. He refuses the offer but opts for becoming a usurer instead, or, expressed in modern terms, a broker. Refusing slavery has shifted Tom away from the role of the traditional greed-driven contractee. When "a meager miserly fellow" who "lived in a forlorn looking house, that stood alone and had an air of starvation" enters a deal with the half "negro" and half "Indian" devil (655), the collaborator can easily be seen as a victim. In this version of the legend of Faust, rewritten under the auspices of the new republic, the devil appears as a spokesperson for the victims, while the poor man's Mephistophelian contract is a question of survival. Exposing the complexities of European immigration, the Dutch settler finds moral exculpation halfway between fantasies of racial punishment and the violence of poverty in a capitalist promise of extra value. The common initial separation between victims and perpetrators that is so central to the gothic genre loses its stability in the service of establishing a functional colonial-capitalist national imaginary in the new republic.

A ghost haunting the forest is introduced only at the end of the tale, but its appearance is of central importance. In the middle of a banal fight in his office, Tom exclaims: "The devil take me, if I have made a farthing!" (Irving, *Tales* 665). Obediently, "the black fellow" appears immediately to follow Tom's wish: "The black man whisked him like a child into the saddle, gave the horse a lash, and away he galloped, with Tom on his back, in the midst of a thunderstorm" (666). Since this incident Tom was never seen again, except in the shape of a ghost on horseback, "which is doubtless the troubled spirit of the usurer" (668). Tom's ghost and the devil now haunt the same ground that still hosts the Indian remains, while "the good people of Boston shook their heads and shrugged their shoulders, but had been so much accustomed to witches and goblins and tricks of the devil in all kinds of shapes from the first settlement of the colony, that they were not so much horror struck as might have been expected" (666). The reference to the "goblins" of the "first settlements" is telling. Irving corroborates the motif of the devil in the shape of a "black man," so firmly established in the writing of Increase and Cotton Mather during the colonial period, and relates it to the looming question of how to justify the blatant dispossession of Indigenous peoples in the country. In *A History of New York* (1809), Irving's first book-length publication, the historian Diedrich Knickerbocker warns about the consequences of "taking possession of a country [...] without asking the consent of its inhabitants": "until this mighty question is totally put to rest, the worthy people of America can by no means enjoy the soil they inhabit, with clear right and title, and quiet, unsullied consciences" (Irving, *History* 412). "The Devil and Tom Walker" is a tale that provides a cultural fantasy in the function of reaching that goal. The conjunctive expression "and" in the title implies symmetry, exchangeability, and a common ground inhabited by Tom and the devil. Refusing slavery, Tom escapes his immediate death and replaces "the black man" to subsequently haunt the "Indian fort" himself (Irving, *Tales* 660). By persisting in his spectral presence, Tom has bested the devil, who collects him away from his earthly existence but cannot erase his presence in death. His haunting is his way of denying the devil's penchant for burning the perpetrators and victims. Tom, the devil's only truly formidable opponent, is not dismembered, with pieces of the body hung up in a tree for carrion birds to feast on, like the only female character in this tale.[12] Nor is he the nameless Indigenous spirit that blackened characters supposedly talk about, hobby historians write about, and "common people" like to hear about. While nameless Indigenous spirits only structure these taxonomies in settler colonial writing, Tom is a proper ghost—an agent of history and the only proper ancestor for generations to come.

With "The Devil and Tom Walker," Irving offers a model for the non-British European settler, who—in spite of slavery and genocide—retains his property rights over North American land. His haunting persists as a trace, a reminder, a voice from the past never granted to either the spectralized Indigenous characters nor to African American spectral informants. In close relation to Puritan apparitional tales, this narrative structure established African American storytellers and their untold stories about the Indigenous population as a central element in the design of the racial fabric of the early republic. With the spectral "black bailiff," "neither negro nor Indian," who acts in the interest of the ones who have been wronged, the literature of the early republic provides a national fantasy of a defensive spokesman pleading on behalf of the dispossessed without risking radical measures or even social criticism.

The Disempowered Dead and Systems of Racial Hierarchy

Rememory is a concept, famously introduced by Toni Morrison in her novel *Beloved*. It marks the process of activating collective memories that have been suppressed and can come to the fore forcefully in the appearance of a ghost. The concept is related to haunting. Haunting or a rememory can initiate a specific reevaluation of the past in the present. It can even lead to a repetition of the past in the present. The ceremonial laying of the ghost, a way for the living to carve out a space for what the ghost represents in the present, traditionally interrupts this anticipated repetition, leading to a peculiar settlement within which memorizing an event allows for pacification. The memory is not erased, but it is accepted, or rather positioned in relation to other memories. Rememory and certain types of haunting are—often painful—inscriptions of previously erased histories into the makeup of the present. Verbalizing this past event or providing images for it are elemental to this process. A ghost is appeased when spoken to. Irving's ghost stories circle around this central tension that engages in questions of national guilt, yet they evade the rememory or haunting by repeatedly reading the present into the past instead. Only ghosts of European settlers appear; only those can be appeased.

It is difficult not to read Irving's tales as examples of what Laura Murray calls the "aesthetic of dispossession" and explains as "a Euro-American sense of vulnerability with respect to Britain" (205). Tracing this tendency in Irving's work, Murray proposes that his plots have the effect of exculpating Euro-Americans from their colonizing role with respect to Indigenous Americans. This chapter demonstrates that supernatural elements and the specific form of the ghost story are essential in structuring these narratives of vindication. The fantasy of friendship between Dutch settlers and heathens (be they Natives or former slaves), which is epitomized in the mutual understanding of the spiritual world, functions simultaneously to create distance from North America's past and from the British-American present. Employing a supernatural framework, Irving constructs a space in which ethical questions can be discussed: Slavery and genocide can be rendered as a moral guilt of the British, and formative narratives foster an alternative national imaginary of acquittal.

Within narrative structures that negotiate the process of creating a new nation, African Americans (agglutinated into one group marked with the term "negro") and people indigenous to North America (agglutinated into one group marked with the term "Indian") are imagined in anonymous, spectralized supporting roles. This is contrary to the frequently made suggestion about the centrality of these characters as the national Other, as an imagined enemy that paradoxically endows national consistency. It is also an interpretation opposed to the argument put forward by Werner Sollors and Donald Pease, who contend that Indigenous spirits in American literature play an essential role because of their function as substitute ancestors. This interpretation, as demonstrated by Irving's spectral tales, needs to be complicated. As Indigenous spirits either do not materialize in Irving's narratives or receive embodied selves only in the form of the devil, they cannot be put into service as substitute ancestors.

To my knowledge, the only tale within which an Indigenous ghost receives a voice in Irving's work appears in "Traits of Indian Character," first published in *Analectic Magazine* in 1813 and a few years later published as part of *The Sketch Book*. It is the story of the sachem of Passonagessit, who in protest of the violation of his mother's grave recalls how the spirit of his mother appeared to him to warn him not to accept such an atrocity. The story was retold numerous times, dating back to William Hubbard in 1677, before Irving's and to William Apes in 1829, after Irving's retelling of the famous narrative. In all cases, the story of the restless spirit of the mother is retold almost verbatim, making an instrumentalization of the story by Irving for purposes of extending agency to Indigenous ghosts unlikely. The tale opens with the narrator calling "the character and habits of the North American savage" sublime, thus putting himself at a safe distance somewhere between fear and awe (*Sketch Book* 1002). Lamenting the bad treatment of "the Indians" by "the white man," while painting a romantic picture of the natural man roaming the "vast lakes, boundless forests, majestic rivers and trackless pains" (1002), the text recalls a historical episode from 1677, the sachem speech in William Hubbard's *A Narrative of the Troubles with the Indians in New England*. It is thus a retelling of a story retold in what was at the time a more than a century old colonialist text that was often used to promote the agenda of "Indian eloquence" (1006). Rather than making space for an Indigenous ghost, this solitary episode confirms the erasure of Indigenous presence in transforming it into the settler's past. "Traits of Indian Character" suitably ends with the narrator making space for the words of "an old warrior," but only to let himself confirm his own erasure: "a little longer, and the white man will cease to persecute us—for we shall cease to exist!" (1012).

With Irving's supernatural tales, the literature of the nineteenth century has established a national image repertoire that depicts male characters of non-European descent, and women regardless of their origin, in a spectral space of their own that can be embedded within European American national creation myths. This spectral space confines a state of internal externality that can be integrated into the larger image of a new and just nation that cannot afford to exclude issues of slavery and dispossession. "To be haunted," writes Avery Gordon, "is to be tied to historical and social effects" (190). It is thus essential to identify who is haunted and who is haunting in the new republic. The ground of New England in Irving's writing is described initially as haunted by Indigenous spirits: "it was asserted that the savages held incantations here and made sacrifices to the evil spirit" (Irving, *Tales* 657). Yet instead of materializing, these spirits are replaced— tale by tale—with ghosts of Dutch settlers. These tales of the supernatural are narratives that excuse the takeover of Indigenous land by white settlers. Irving's ghost stories are a vehicle for the production of a purified nationalized imaginary that serves the purpose of creating the appearance of a democracy that can remain intact in spite of slavery and dispossession. "There is no subjugation so perfect as that which keeps the appearance of freedom, for in that way one captures volition itself," writes Jean-Jacques Rousseau in *Émile* (119). Irving's treatment of the supernatural indicates a similar didactic stance. A highly effective simulation of freedom is obtained in establishing a supernatural setting introduced through perfectly integrated male outcasts of European descent who surround themselves with the dispossessed: African American men and children, always already dead Indigenous people, and European American women.[13] In spite of the accusatory tone and the seemingly gothic style that promises to expose systematic oppressors and involve the reader by provoking sympathy for the victim, the agents are never exposed and remain anonymously numbered among the wealthy. The act of retribution is sealed off under the exclusion of the story of the victims. In this way, readers in the early republic could enter the supernatural framework in order to identify with sympathetic young Dutch settlers who are friends of "negroes" and lead "Indian lifestyles" without departing from white normativity and racial stereotypes of blackened people in racially subservient positions. The insistence on the founding of wealth through slavery on violently appropriated land is consequently transferred to someone else somewhere else. The scholarship on this writer's work is complicit with this project, as Irving, apart from two publications, remains celebrated: In 1970 Kenneth T. Reed published an article entitled "Washington Irving and the Negro" wherein he demonstrates that Washington Irving not only avoided slavery as a topic but also kept returning to "the negro" and promoting stereotypes "illustrating the black man as a happy, lazy, superstitious, altogether ridiculous animal" (43). Almost fifty years later, in 2017, Jason Richards returns to this topic in his study *Imitation Nation: Red, White, and Blackface in Early and Antebellum U.S. Literature* demonstrating that Irving, in fact, draws on "the nascent communities of blackface culture" to "Americanize his writing" (65).

Constructing an alibi by presenting the victims of European colonialism exclusively as frolicking friends in order to avoid an ethical call for action parallels one of the most telling laws passed in the new republic. The simultaneous insistence on free speech and quiescence is exposed in the so-called gag rule passed in the US House of Representatives in 1836, prime time for Irving's so-called ghost stories: "*Resolved,* That all petitions, memorials, resolutions, propositions, or papers, relating in any way, or to any extent whatsoever, to the subject of slavery, or the abolition of slavery, shall, without being either printed or referred, be laid on the table, and that no further action whatever shall be had thereon" ("Register of Debates"). Talk of slavery was regarded to be an intrusion, an obstacle to be avoided for patriotic reasons; President Jackson even denounced it as "ultimately undemocratic" (Holmes 19).[14] Abraham Lincoln wrote about the most avoided topic during the formative period: "You must not say anything about it in the free states, *because it is not there.* You must not say anything about it in the slave states, *because it is there.* You must not say anything about it in the pulpit, because that is religion and has nothing to do with it. You must not say anything about it in politics, *because that will disturb the security of 'my place.'* There is no place to talk about it as being a wrong, although you say yourself it *is* a wrong" (Lincoln 809). "The security of 'my place'" in the early republic openly and publicly depends on silencing a "wrong." While ghosts theoretically have the potential to articulate this silence, they can also be muted. In this way, literature exemplified in Irving's oeuvre found a way to be silent while speaking, creating a "public secret" strong enough to become a building block for a nation.

In light of the founding politics of taciturnity, American ghost stories would have had the facility to function as an ethical corrective. Ridiculing the authority of one leading voice, the onion structure of ghost stories promotes alternative views, luring even the reader or listener into an act of continual verification. Moreover, the gothic formula, with its multiple perspectives often delineated through the same protagonist, indicates the insufficiency of human faculties to produce consistency. This image of complexity that calls for a synthesis by the reader is opposed to a politics based on leading voices and paternal figures. Irving's stories, just like their Puritan predecessors, however, are veiling while revealing—they provide a secure forum for European settlers to dissociate themselves from the national debt even in death.

The power of the fantastic tale as an alternative source of information seeking public exposure is never sufficiently employed, which is why most of Irving's tales of the supernatural remain fragmentary. The skull that Tom steps on "was a dreary memento of the fierce struggle that had taken place in this last foothold of the Indian warriors" (Irving, *Tales* 657). This significant fictional termination of the wars with the Indigenous nations in Irving's writing suggests that the present is a time of recovery. Displacing a current problem, such as the question of freedom for all in the new republic, to a discussion among "the pious fathers" shifts the question of responsibility into the past and away from the new republic and its own founding. Acknowledging the existence of slavery and genocide in one's own country, the protagonists are carving out a space that would exempt them from the responsibility for the same. Irving's consistent exclusion of the Indigenous perspective and the perspective of the formerly enslaved required the spectral framework within which these voices could appear only to be erased without materializing. These narratives simulate a mutual symbolic order. The anachronistic settings point at a time before death and destruction, a time "before the red man have been exterminated by you white savages" (*Tales* 659). The vocative case defers the accusation temporally and spatially onto an imaginary other. Traveling through enchanted forests and stepping on haunted grounds, which leads to a discovery of skulls that belong to the Indigenous population and enslaved African people, is dislocated to Puritan New England in spite of the very imminent presence of the War of 1812, the second Barbary War, illegal slave trade, and the First Seminole War in 1818. The haunted house in Irving's narratives is presented as a museum of American history that one can walk through but not *work through*.

Establishing narratives based on European models and decorated with spectralized Native American and African American semi-lives marks the realm of the supernatural as a secure place for a critique without political consequence. The insistence on rural and domestic spheres naturalizes the supernatural within the fantasy of an independent country that has by now learned how to deal with its shortcomings by creating a spectral "one great republic" for "one's own kind" (Kant *Dreams* 328). The supernatural, appropriated and obstructed by realism, is constructed as a subversive power that subverts the affected. If the appearance of a ghost, the agent of haunting, commonly initiates a process of remembering, repeating, and conclusively working through (as in Shakespeare and Freud), Irving's ghost stories can be understood neither as retribution narratives nor as a forum for exposing missing voices of the marginalized. Irving's introduction of the celebrated free-willing counter-Protestant male American of European descent to the ghost world is an act of appropriation. Only within spectrality could a simulation of a close relation or friendship with nonnamed characters identified only as "negroes" and "Indians" be enacted. This fantasy facilitates a free-spirited and morally justified European American male identity shortly after the revolution. The ghost-story framework is central to this fantasy, traces of which are to determine American literature and culture all the way into our own ghost-ridden twenty-first century.

5

The Voice of Nature
The Invisible World and the Great Spirit

And, lost each human trace, surrendering up
Thine individual being, shalt thou go
To mix forever with the elements,
To be a brother to the insensible rock
And to the sluggish clod, which the rude swain
Turns with his share, and treads upon. The oak
Shall send his roots abroad, and pierce thy mold.
—William Cullen Bryant, *Thanatopsis*

The exploitation of topics with an Indigenous focus was at its peak in the 1820s. This is exemplified most succinctly by James Fenimore Cooper's Leatherstocking Tales, which offered up images of white hypermasculinized characters established against the background of idealized and sentimentalized representations of "Indians" as noble savages or bloodthirsty warriors who together roam the forest. Sarah Rivett interpreted this trope as an attempt to "inscribe a usable indigenous past into the nation's make-up" ("Indigenous" 239). Cooper's stereotypical characters were revealed as colonial fantasies in much of the scholarship throughout the twentieth century, yet they have left long-lasting effects. "'Clothes upon sticks': James Fenimore Cooper and the Flat Frontier" by Sandra Tomc is a revealing study about the many satires that Cooper's Leatherstocking novels provoked in the second half of the nineteenth century already. The article demonstrates how racial stereotypes produced in these texts could, in fact, be remodeled even while they were ridiculed in the decades after the Civil War. In the previous chapter, I demonstrated how Washington Irving was already working on generating a myth for early nationalism that integrates settler colonial Indigeneity in his internationally acclaimed ghost stories. Irving's tales consolidated in the Puritan apparitional tales introduced compounds of the ghost, the witch, the (satanic) "black man," and "the Indian," who all dwell together in the forest and can be interpreted by settler colonial characters.

In Cooper's and Irving's narratives, the frontier romance and the gothic fuse together into a central national genre of the postrevolutionary literary period, ultimately contributing to an enforcement of the colonizing divide. Stressing the centrality of the frontier to early American literature, Carol Margaret Davison writes in "American Gothic Passages": "the Frontier Gothic illuminated American psycho-geographies, casting a long shadow from Brown to Cooper, Neal, Bird, Hawthorne and beyond" (277). As I will demonstrate in this chapter, the forest as a restricted location where reason does not reign was central in establishing this image repertoire of settler colonial supremacy.

Perhaps because parodying or appropriating Indigenous practices was so firmly established in the United States by the 1820s, a growing resistance to the agenda-setting guided by Cooper and Irving led to significant counternarratives, all of which reached great popularity at the time. Since much has been written about the role of Cooper's narratives in the context of settler-Indigenous relations, and Irving's writing was explored in the previous chapter, I will now take a closer look at these counternarratives that put the presence of the Indigenous population at the center. This chapter demonstrates that even novels that sought to produce alternative visions, in the end, did not construct a viable national imaginary to counteract the colonial racial divide. What follows is an analysis of novels that pronouncedly sought to either correct dominant or to provide alternative visions of the depictions of the forest as a dark and enchanted wilderness established by the Puritans and solidified in the 1820s popular Frontier Gothic. Texts analyzed in this chapter focus on a European settler character who leaves the settlement for a life in the forest, a trope already introduced in what is most likely the first US American gothic novel, *St. Herbert—A Tale* (1796), published under the penname Anna. And just like in *St. Herbert,* all texts discussed in this chapter include a renegotiation of the Puritan Invisible World in narrative constructions of spectralized forests. But before John Neal's *Logan* (1822) and Nathaniel Hawthorne's "Roger Malvin's Burial" (1831) can be analyzed, the spectralization of the Indigenous population in the poetry of Philip Freneau needs to be sketched out, as his poetry provides the blueprint against which the latter two writers were constructing their own conceptualizations of forests.

The "Force of Nature" in Philip Freneau's Poetry

The codification of the "wilderness" as a space of terror was a carefully constructed narrative strategy. In his famous 1670 jeremiad, in which he called upon all his followers "to excite and stir us all up to attend and prosecute our Errand into the Wilderness," Samuel Danforth praised the wilderness as a "woody, retired and solitary place" where even Jesus went for contemplation ("Brief Recognition"). Depictions of "wilderness" were thus central to positioning Europeans within what was termed "the New World" from the time the first settlers arrived on shores of the North American continent. Only some twenty years later, in Cotton Mather's *The Wonders of the Invisible World,* does the same wilderness become a place where "New-Englanders," who are "People of God settled in those, which were once the *Devil's* Territories" (20). The seemingly effortless transformation from an environment worthy of Jesus to devil's territories exemplifies how nature that is presented as wild or hostile is directly implicated in the modern world's violence and oppression. Paul Outka explains how natural experience became racialized within the modernist discourse: "The civilized/ white versus savage/wild binary was replicated mile by westward mile, a sort of factory that consumed the wild and the native at one end, and extruded gender, the pastoral, and whiteness on the other" (33). To scrutinize nature inevitably means to scrutinize stories of racial oppression, segregation, and exploitation. Hannah Arendt, in *The Origins of Totalitarianism,* specifies this cultural construction and goes as far as locating the invention of race in hostile nature: "At any rate, races in this sense were found only in regions where nature was particularly hostile. What made them [savages] different from other human beings was not at all the color of their skin but the fact that they behaved like a part of nature, that they treated nature as their undisputed master, [...]. They were, as it were, 'natural' human beings who lacked the specifically human character, the specifically human reality, so that when European men massacred them, they somehow were not aware that they had committed murder" (192). Arendt's telling extrapolation exemplifies not only the exclusion of certain humans from humanity by way of nature but also ways in which the construction of nature as estranged and antagonistic was implicated in the invention of race. Relegated into the background of European man, both nonhuman nature and the natural human become a site of ravaging and extermination.

In US American literature, the nonhuman nature that includes certain humans comes to the fore most explicitly in the trope of the so-called

Vanishing Indian.[1] Deeply embedded within a tradition dramatically initiated in Puritan texts that demonized the Indigenous population in their
habitat, wilderness was recast by revolutionary American writers in a more
tamed version as a space where first nations "retreat" to "die" supposedly of
their own accord. This is unequivocally expressed in the poem "On the Emigration to America and Peopling the Western Country" by Philip Freneau,
published in 1784. In this poem, the prototypical "unsocial Indian" simply
retreats into ever-darker forests, never to be seen again. In much of his poetry, Freneau promoted visions of American forests as "the Indian burying ground," where ghosts appear in "many a barbarous form," relegating
the presence of the Indigenous population to "the ancients of these lands"
(Freneau, "Indian Burying Ground"). The centrality of Freneau's work for
establishing the cultural imaginary in the early republic is expressed in a
statement by Thomas Jefferson, who credited Freneau, through his literary
output, with having "saved our constitution which was galloping fast into
monarchy."[2] Freneau's poems, therefore, were influential enough to contrib-
ute to the image repertoire necessary for the creation of a nation; and they
did so via the myth of a dying or dead Indigenous person. Bergland convincingly demonstrates in her study *The National Uncanny: Indian Ghosts
and American Subjects* that a method of "ghosting" Indigenous characters
by presenting them as always already dead in literature and culture was an
important element within practices of cultural erasure (5). Short-lived Indigenous characters repeatedly not only vanish but dematerialize in their
white antagonists' imagination as ghosts. Far from threatening, these ghosts
are rather accommodating. Drucilla Wall expresses the notion of replacing
real Indigenous people with virtual ones most succinctly: "the dominant
culture wishes the difficult and complex Native to disappear so that the
constructed, controlled, and purely simulated Indian can conceal Indian
people rather than reveal them" (103). Ghosts served these processes of
personal simulation perfectly; rather than disposed of or murdered, the
Indigenous peoples could be imagined as a present absence.

Freneau's poetry already exposes the ways in which spectrality is implicated in what would become the dominant trope of vanishing, as his poetry
regularly exhibits figurations of ghosts to assert the erasure of Indigenous
cultures in the United States. Freneau's famous poem "The Indian Burying
Ground" went through numerous reprints between 1787 and 1829 (Smeall
258). In all its variations, the poem most notoriously reduced *all* Indigenous
people(s) in the colonies to future ghosts, lamenting their death before
it was even occasioned. Referencing postmortem Indigenous characters

became a topos in Freneau's oeuvre. Another striking example can be found in the poem "The Indian Student; or, The Force of Nature" (1787), in which an Indigenous student abandons his scholarly career in order to die in the forest due to the titular "force of nature" (Freneau, "Indian Student"). Spectralization has been acknowledged most succinctly in Bergland's study as a colonial strategy of replacing the Indigenous population with Europeans. In her study, she writes that all representations of "Native Americans" by European settler writers rely on the language of ghostliness: "They [authors of Anglo-Saxon descent] call Indians demons, apparitions, shapes, specters, phantoms, or ghosts. They insist that Indians are able to appear and disappear suddenly and mysteriously, and also that they are ultimately doomed to vanish" (Bergland 10). Much less discussed, however, is the fact that the supposed disappearance of the Native population is paradoxically grounded in the material presence of natural elements. In one of the first editions of Freneau's famous poem, published in 1787 under the title "Lines Occasioned by a Visit to an Old Indian Burying Ground," one will find "a lofty rock" that remains and "an aged elm" that "aspires." Furthermore, the memory of the "activity" of the "hunter" and the "deer" in this poem evokes images of the forest, even if in the end they are revealed to be shadows and illusions. As the supposedly disappearing material bodies are replaced with specific representations of nature, the Indigenous characters in these texts are not only spectral but imagined to be absorbed into the forest. In "The Dying Indian; or, The Last Words of Shalum," the "Indian" narrator put forward by Freneau even exclaims:

> I, too, must be a fleeting ghost—no more—
> None—none but shadows to those mansions go:
> I leave my woods—I leave the Huron shore—
> For emptier groves below!

What the ghosted "Indian" leaves behind is the forest. The poem continues:

> Ye charming solitudes,
> Ye tall ascending woods,
> Ye glassy lakes and prattling streams,
> . . . .
> Adieu to all!
> . . . .
> Adieu the mountain's lofty swell,

Adieu, thou little verdant hill,
And seas, and stars, and skies—farewell,
For some remoter sphere!

Through Freneau's poetry, the "unsocial Indian" who inevitably retreats into "darker forests" to peacefully die received significant exposure and political prominence in the revolutionary United States (Freneau, "On the emigration"), paving the way for the literary trope of the Vanishing Indian that quickly achieved national significance.

Central to this national agenda-setting is the forest. Jean O'Brien explains the role of nature and tradition within relations between Indigenous peoples and settlers in her poignant study *Firsting and Lasting: Writing Indians Out of Existence in New England*: "The master narrative of New England was that it had made a stark break with the past, replacing 'uncivilized' peoples whose histories and cultures they represented as illogically rooted in nature, tradition and superstition, whereas New Englanders symbolized the 'civilized' order of culture, science and reason" (xxi). Progressive US American ideas of modernity and modernization were thus constructed in relation to Indigenous antagonists, who were presented as natural, traditional, and superstitious. Yet, these acts of othering and antagonism are much more complicated than a simple binarism. In *This Violent Empire,* Carroll Smith-Rosenberg demonstrates the ways in which the constitution of the Others provided the early republic "with an inner cohesion" that it lacked (52).[3] Her description of the New York Tammany Society's multiple receptions of the Creek delegation by white settler officials in "full Indian costume" in 1790 offers one of the strongest scholarly images to convincingly exemplify how othering often works under the premise of inclusive erasure rather than exclusion or antagonism. To this end, Smith-Rosenberg describes the centrality of mimicking of an Indian lifestyle to the establishment and survival of a distinctly settler colonial body politic. Recalling images of European middle-aged men with painted faces dancing in grotesque postures and chanting in garbled voices, Smith-Rosenberg concludes: "In parodying native practices, the odd assortment of 'braves' and 'sachems' who welcomed the Creek delegation were declaring that European Americans had indeed replaced Native Americans as rulers of American lands" (196). O'Brien's and Smith-Rosenberg's studies manifest that not only replacing but becoming the Indigenous bodies was fundamental to early American cultural myths seeking to excuse the occupation of North American territories. Adding to these studies, I demonstrate ways in which the spectralization of the forest played an elemental part in establishing these fantasies of settler colonials as the patrons of a supposedly expired Indigenous population.

Particularly trees and stones, which already occupied a prominent place in Freneau's poetry as markers of allegedly disappearing—for the most part unnamed—"Indians," are repeatedly employed to index ghosted bodies. In this way, the forest is transformed into a gothic space by way of its infusion with Indigenous remains. The dead, significantly, do not come back to haunt the living but rather in transfigurations that appear more ornamental than eerie. The seventeenth-century image of "American Indians" as "Devil-worshipers" performing their "sorceries" in the forest was thus replaced within the project of the Vanishing Indian by the unmarked grave of the noble warrior (Lovejoy 611–12).[4] Without a grave, the spirit could potentially inscribe itself anywhere in the forest.

In a reaffirmation of the trope of the wilderness as a ghostly Indigenous space, initiated in Puritan writings of the seventeenth and eighteenth centuries, the spectral forest found even greater exposure in the postrevolutionary period in Freneau's writing. Subsequently, Washington Irving turned this now recognizably national trope into stories that could be exported and thus become *American* in a transatlantic context. What once was presented as "devil's territories" was therefore gradually transformed in newly nationalized settler imaginaries into "charming solitudes" and "tall ascending woods," populated by the spirits of the Indigenous dead, that consequently remained empty and available for European immigrants to move in (Freneau, "Dying Indian"). Yet, just mourning the supposedly absent Native population was not enough for a settler imaginary to take hold. Eventually, those very spirits in the same "woods" could be replaced, as is exemplified in Irving's most popular tale, "The Legend of Sleepy Hollow," by "the dominant spirit, [. . .] the ghost of a Hessian trooper" (*Sketch Book* 1059), or by the ancestors of the "original Dutch settlers," such as the ghost of "Antony Vander Heyden" in Irving's "Dolph Heyliger" (*Bracebridge* 334). The affect of superiority and heritage rights conveyed by the European ghosts within the genre of the frontier gothic mark a colonial project that extends into the Invisible World of the newly independent nation.

"Super Natural" Ghosts in John Neal's *Logan*

The idea of "humans living amidst the wilderness is one that is seen either as the most natural, or the most unnatural thing in the world," writes

Elizabeth Parker in her study of gothic representations of forests (214). On the one hand, the forest can be interpreted as a place of origin, where the *return* to nature would imply a nourishing effect; on the other hand, it can be understood as a regression into a state long overcome, which implies fearful, unpredictable, uncontrollable, and dangerous circumstances. According to Parker, "if we deem civilisation seriously flawed, or even evil then the forest becomes an idealised alternative to it. [. . .] Conversely, if we read civilisation—and progress—in essentially positive terms, then the forest is demonised. It becomes a deep, dark, and degenerative space" (215). In the following examples, it will become obvious that the intersection of nature and ghosts in the early republic destabilizes this clear-cut taxonomy. In fact, a criticism of "civilization" through dedicated periods spent in the (spectral) forest might be one of the most common ways of establishing an even more superior position in terms of cultural hierarchy or a "civilization" ranking. Furthermore, the reordering of temporality and spatiality in the movement beyond life (ghosts) and beyond human (rocks and trees) manifests cultural representations of forests that are neither threatening nor nourishing. Instead, envisioned as an unexplored territory where nature is animated by human spirits, spectral forests in antebellum literature become rehabilitation parks for settler characters to cleanse their colonial conscience. This deep ecological engagement between human and nature was rather effective as a colonial measure.

John Neal's two-volume novel, *Logan, a Family History* (1822), is one of the strongest examples of spectralized natural environments in early American literature. The novel remains one of the strangest and, perhaps as a consequence, one of the most poorly interpreted novels of the early republic despite having been widely read at the time of its publication.[5] It is loosely structured around the historical person of the same name, the Haudenosaunee chief whose family was murdered by vengeful settlers on the Ohio river in 1773.[6] By the time Neal wrote his novel, the prominent diplomat and leader Logan had already become a national myth due in large degree to Thomas Jefferson's mention in his widely read *Notes on the State of Virginia* (1781/1785). There, Logan is famously featured as an example of a great North American orator, in company of George Washington as a great warrior, Benjamin Franklin as a great physicist, and David Rittenhouse as a great astronomer (Jefferson, *Notes* 69). Placing an Indigenous leader next to such widely acknowledged statesmen and scientists—even marking him by his name and lineage—must be and has been understood as a political act. Logan, in his famous speech given in response to the massacre of his family, presented himself as the last of his people with no possibility of being mourned, thus implicitly inviting the settler community to pay their due to his wronged family. Speaking to citizens of a community organized around the public secret of genocide, Logan could provide a space for the new republic to mourn the deaths of the wronged Indigenous population and by doing so relieve themselves of a looming identification as perpetrators. In "The Necropolitics of New World Nativism," Jillian Sayre compares ways in which beneficiaries of colonial violence "rewrite themselves as native patriots through rituals of mourning" and comes to the conclusion that in both cases a national feeling is crafted out of the ritual of lamenting irremediable loss (713).

The massacre of the innocent described in Logan's lament was quickly augmented to a national tragedy much discussed in contemporary scholarship. Jonathan Elmer describes the importance of this ritual: "Unable to mourn or be mourned, Logan becomes, in a sense, immortal; or, alternatively, we might see his fate as an inassimilable event manifesting itself in traumatic repetitions" ("Melancholy" 153). Logan, in his role as the last man, became a national symbolic figure who could secure a presentable past based on the image of a neatly constructed public mortuary. As Jean O'Brien demonstrates most convincingly, mourning Logan's tragedy created a mythology that helped settler colonials to break away from an undesirable history and install themselves as the pillars of modernity. Most importantly, Logan's question still echoes throughout numerous classrooms in the United States: "Who is there to mourn for Logan?—Not one!"[7] Unified in the act of mourning, the white settler colonial nation responds as one and perpetuates the colonial divide into the future.

John Neal's novel complicates this necropolitical conjecture with a fictional response to the national Logan myth as early as 1822. The subtitle, *A Family History,* indicates an attempt to reinterpret, if not correct, the extinction narrative that this national legend inevitably invoked even in the 1820s.[8] Neal unmistakably introduces the topos of the Vanishing Indian in the opening pages: "The family of Logan, 'The Mingo Chief,' is now extinct." The text immediately proceeds to the legend: "The sun of their glory hath set in darkness. [. . .] Who has not heard of Logan? Who cannot recount the deeds of his generation?" (1:6). Yet, immediately after establishing Logan as a mythical figure of national concern, the actual Logan bursts this image in the form of a gothic character of excess and transgression, challenging, in particular, the concept of the material disappearance of bodies marked as "Indian" (1:16). This rupture of the public mortuary by way of reanimation of a not-dead figure marks the instability of the division between death and life in the early republic.

Logan, in this version, is a paradoxical construct represented from the perspective of settler colonial characters as a ghostly appearance of hyperphysicality. The perspective of the governor in particular demonstrates this point. When Logan first enters the scene, the governor describes him as "a hot and smoking war-horse" and a "being" that provoked "doubt and horror" (1:6), "a phantom" (1:12), and "literally and truly a devil" (1:4). Reminiscent of Puritan depictions of Indigenous people that oscillate between materiality and immateriality in their satanic appearance, the governor sees in Logan a presence somewhere between an iron man and an apparition at their first encounter: "The Indian stood before him like an apparition. His attitude (it is worth describing—for it was very peculiar) was not entirely natural, nor perhaps entirely unstudied. He stood motionless and appalling; the bleak, barren, and iron aspect of a man, from head to foot strong and sinewed with desperation, and hardened in the blood and sweat of calamity and trial" (1:16). Somewhere between supernatural and designed, this apparition seems simultaneously appealing and appalling to the governor. Combining stereotypical settler colonial descriptions in this scene, Neal highlights the physicality of spectrality inscribed in bodies marked as Indigenous. Not supernatural but hypernatural, these characters are described in association with the wilderness as enchanting—provoking not horror but fascination and terror.

Neal continues the literary tradition of writing spectrality into the national gothic canopy in relation to Shakespeare's famous scenes, a tradition initiated by Brown and Irving. The next chapter is introduced with the epitaph: "Great God!—what art thou? Speak!" (1:21). This intertextual reference to Shakespeare's *Hamlet* refers to the moment when the Prince sights the apparition of his dead father. Like the ghost of the dead King of Denmark in *Hamlet,* Logan's "phantom" enters and exits the scene the first time around without speaking. The governor simply faints, and the next day he can only remember having seen "an apparition" (1:42). In this early scene, the extinction narrative is already undergoing a critical turn through a spectralization of the living body that will keep reappearing throughout the novel in all its physicality. Neal consciously plays with the idea of a ghost, yet this Logan is not dead but dangerous and will certainly return, marking the scene as a promise of violence rather than a haunting.

At the outset, the intradiegetic narrator develops themes of extinction: "The sun of their glory set in darkness. I myself have seen the last of that valiant race, the very last, descending majestically to the chambers of death" (1:3). Offering a document of the Vanishing Indian project vividly set in the prerevolutionary period, the narrator claims with his testimonial to provide an outright piece of evidence. However, shortly after this decisive statement, the narrator admits: "I knew them. The last time that I was in my country I paid them a visit, and they all assembled to meet me, for—and why should I conceal it? I, myself, am of the same blood" (1:4). Further members of the Logan clan, including the narrator, keep reappearing despite the seemingly continuous sighting of the last representative. Furthermore, Logan, the last man, turns out to have offspring. Significantly, Logan's son Harold continues the paternal legacy of avenging the injustice suffered by but not restricted to the Logan clan. Even the future does not imply erasure: "The blood of this race was afterwards mingled with that of their white neighbours, and produced, in their remote descendants, a family neither Indian nor white, neither savage nor civilized" (1:9). The early emphasis on extinction is thus immediately revoked in images of miscegenation, continuity, and transformation, suggesting that US America's past, present, and future are not only multicultural but intrinsically intertwined.

Marking his hero at the very beginning of the novel as the last man who is at the same time not the last, Neal turns the screw one notch further, refusing to follow up with a simple eulogy for the wronged Other. In fact, this Logan turns out to be not only alive and healthy but also of Anglo-Saxon descent and therefore not much of an Other after all. Logan is the famous Mingo chief, but as we find out early in the novel, he is also a British nobleman called George of Salisbury, who emigrated to the US and married into the Logan clan. Questioning both British nobility and Indigenous savagery, Neal's fictional refiguration of the historical Logan demonstrates the prominence of violence that dominates what was supposed to be a transcultural meeting ground. Exposing the "contact zone" at the heart of American democracy (Pratt), Neal questions the ability of the new republic to neatly segregate settlers from those who have been there before. In fact, there are indications that the historical Logan's father was a Frenchman (Seeber 135). Neal's decision to rewrite the history of Logan as the history of a Mingo leader with an English heritage confirms this text's project of transculturation situated between the English and the Iroquoian-speaking group of North American Indigenous people renamed by French colonists as the Mingo people (primarily Seneca and Cayuga). "Mingo" is an Anglo-American colonial term for all the Iroquoian-speaking people, which *Logan* extends to include British nobility.

Other than Brown, who put spectral Indigenous voices into settlers' minds, Neal spectralized settler bodies in all their corporeality. From the white settler governor's perspective, Logan is "an Indian," an apparition, not fully human, because he lies outside of the scope of his narrative ideal. As argued by Sylvia Wynter among various other scholars, colonial settlers need this story to invent or, in this case, establish their "own matrix Christian identity as Man" (292). Through the spectralization of Indigenous bodies, a biopolitical subject is created so that the symbolic body could replace the empirically existing one. From the governor's perspective, Logan can only exist as a memory. This image of "the Indian" as a spectral, animalized creature is so deeply ingrained that even Logan's own son cannot see him any differently. Harold describes his father in a move from the present absence of a "spectre" to the insistent physicality of a predatory animal: "Logan—accursed be the recollection!—It rises like a spectre before me, and menaces me even now. Look! Look!—Spirit of the wilderness! ** Man of blood! ** whence art thou? ** why comest thou upon me? ** I feel thine unhallowed approach *** Oh, shield me, love—his cold hand is near me:—oh, how cold!" (1:231). Passages like this establish Logan as something that will not remain dead. The classic ghost-story reference to the touch of a cold, disembodied hand insists on an immaterial presence that is here to stay. Convinced that Logan, even in death, "walks the earth" (1:234), Harold, like the governor, can conceive of Logan's presence only as that of a wild predator at home in the wilderness: "He [Logan] met, and tore asunder, the jaws of the bear, and the catmount. He swam torrents, forded rivers, galloped the inaccessible mountain, played his archery above the clouds, bathed himself, over and over again, to drunkenness and delirium in the blood of the white men—ay, of the red men, too, in the unsparing bitterness of his wrath—a creature, born and baptized in hot gore" (1:235). Yet, these hyperbolic depictions of violence, animalization, and spectralization are not, as common at the time, reserved for the Indigenous characters. Turning Logan into a British nobleman, Neal extends the extinction narrative to the settler population. Amply, the material-immaterial characterization is presented as deeply disturbing even to Logan himself. As a violent creature trapped in his own body, either feared or idealized, he seems disturbed and repeatedly in danger of madness.

Introducing such a furious yet ephemeral, disturbing, and disturbed character, Neal exposes the original violence at the heart of the inauguration of his nation. Logan's irruption from the outside (the forest)—his entrance into the regulated space of the governor's office—marks an interruption that is quickly spectralized away but cannot be erased. Neal turns the outside space into the inside on various levels by marking his "phantom" as British and rewriting the colonial trope of the Vanishing Indian as a gothic travesty. His "phantom" is "an iron aspect of a man," an Englishman who murders the English dressed as a Native and, like Theodore Wieland, eventually loses his mind. And like Wieland, his vitality is most prominently exhibited in his violence. Within the biopolitical coding of Indigenous bodies at the time, the real body receives a representative presence only in relation to disappearance. In Neal's rewriting of this trope, the so-called phantom keeps returning not to haunt but to murder, not to die but to sow death. Neal's Logan marks the paradox of settler colonial representations of Indigenous people as *super natural* ghosts—brave but always the dead or dying warrior. Constructing a character that oscillates between erasure by spectralization and hyperphysicality by way of animalization, Indigeneity, and European nobility, Neal exposes both poles as reductive, ultimately damaging to the makeup of the new nation, and lethal for all.

Haunting and the Spectral Forest

Neal attends to various narrative registers to express his dissatisfaction with his government's treatment of the Indigenous population, the ongoing tolerance of slavery, and the, in his opinion, calamitous push for English supremacy. Upon insisting that this is an "American story," he confronts the reader with gothic scenes steeped in violence, gore, infanticide, and incest. As a patriot who believed in reform, Neal actively fought for female suffrage, prison reform, and the abolition of slavery throughout his life. The unconventional use of orality, a promotion of an intrinsic transculturality by way of linguistic code-switching, and even the inclusion of full passages in French, Spanish, and Italian in *Logan* are all narrative elements employed in service of this aim.

Part of Neal's reformation efforts was also a recoding of "the American forest," which, in this novel, is "steeped in the hot vapour of blood" and full of "specters" (1:185; 1:218; 2:84). Like Brown and Irving before him, rather than writing a ghost story, Neal chooses the aesthetics of ghostliness. This is established on two levels. On the one hand, central protagonists marked as "Indian" (but actually either British or transcultural) oscillate between life and death by disappearing and seemingly dying in the forest only to suddenly appear in other characters' lives. On the other hand, the novels' dominant setting, the forest, is presented in an eerily sentient manner, as if it were controlling the characters' actions. This setting, in what is described as "the green wilderness rising behind," is central to establishing a liminal space between life and death (1:147). Nature, rather than characters, is spectral. "Rising behind" settler characters, "wild" nature threatens to absorb anyone bold enough to enter this contact zone. Already in the opening pages, the narrator informs the readers that Logan has "journeyed to the wilderness, to hold communion with the GREAT SPIRIT. He abandoned his tribe" (1:8). "Wilderness" therefore is a restricted spatial category that can be entered and exited at will and is visited for higher purposes. Significantly, before allegedly disappearing Logan left his son in the custody of the forest. As a baby, Harold is left by his father at the foot of an oak tree. This scene is presented as a "tremendous rite" of offering the child's body to the forest, which will raise and educate him (1:8). Logan enters into a pact with the forest while putting down his son's body. He asks his natural environment for a last confirmation that his child will become a warrior: "His prayer was heard. There was a dark commotion in the turbid blue sky, as of a host hurrying away, appeased and conciliated, by some tremendous rite" (1:8). The forest's parental function is retained throughout the novel in repeated ecogothic scenes alternating between dread and nourishment.

Nature, thus, is represented as a sentient entity that in its parental function serves as a character. Both Logan and his adult son remain in continual conversation with natural elements, which they hope will direct their actions. Alas, they lead to more confusion. An exemplary scene can be found when Harold decides to follow his love interest, who is "journeying with a tribe towards the remote Spanish possessions," perhaps even to "Mexico," and leaves the landscape that has been his home up to this point:

He turns toward the home of his childhood. He invokes the Great Spirit of the place. He descends to the nearest running water. He kneels, scoops up a handful, and throws it over his head; an awful rite that, on a departure like this, was not to be omitted. He listens for the expected answer. He hears, or fancies that he hears, a shrill cry in the firmament. His blood runs cold. He gazes all over the heavens. [. . .] not the shadow of a shade is to be seen. He leaps backward! Something has passed him—he is chilled to the heart—and see! the top of yonder blasted pine bends for a moment, as with the weight of something that alights from heaven. And yet, nothing is to be seen—nothing!—was it in homage to some passing creature of the elements? or did it stoop with the weight of some descending shadow? Whatever might be the cause, Harold's heart felt cold and heavy, and he could not stir from the spot. How was he to interpret such omens? (1:194)

The ceremony described is reminiscent, among many others, of the Cherokee purification ritual called "Going to the Water," commonly performed by the edge of a creek by pouring water over oneself (Blackstock 5). Far from a romantic curiosity, descriptions of nature such as this suggest that there is more to characters' actions than their intention. Harold performs the rite and expects an answer. The novel does not provide clues as to the function of what to Logan and Harold are signs; they could indicate divine providence, or spectral guidance, or even the wreath of evil spirits animating this natural environment. Whether referencing the Invisible World in Puritan tradition or sentient nature in Cherokee teaching, the characters understand nature's performance as a sign language. Yet, rather than interpreting it, they are succumbed by it.

The silent but dynamic dialogues between members of the "Logan clan" and trees, wind, rivers, or clouds could be discarded as a popular romantic narrative tool were it not for the consistency in its application and the insistence on Indigeneity. Throughout the very long and confusing text, much more than harnessing nature into a romantic background for the Byronic hero to contemplate important steps in his life, these scenes attest to Neal's life-long effort to promote a diverse nation, training his readers to engage with Indigenous American perspectives. The forest plays a central role in his promotion of diversity in that it becomes a medium for transculturality. Neal was highly involved in promoting Cherokee cultures throughout his life. Kerin Holt writes about Neal's excitement about the publication of *The Cherokee Phoenix,* a new magazine that was to be published in both languages, English and Cherokee, "conducted by a native-red-man, printed in an Indian-town, and party in the Indian character" (Neal quoted in Holt 201). Rather than a guide or a punishing power as in the Puritan concept of the Invisible World, nature is depicted as a sentient entity in communication with the Logans, which makes the Cherokee culture a more likely source.

More than anything else, Logan and Harold are looking for signs. Nature, according to colonial Puritan teachings, is the visible part of the Invisible World and, in the phrasing of Cotton Mather, it "has an astonishing share in the Government of Ours [world]" (*Voice from Heaven,* 6). Yet, for the Puritan tradition, the study of the natural world was in large part a matter of interpreting signs sent by God to guide one's own life.

Numerous scenes in Neal's *Logan* present the forest in ways that replicate the understanding that such guiding principles are found in nature, but neither Logan nor Harold know how to interpret them, nor is a divine ruler ever mentioned as the source. Particularly Harold's hallucinations, which appear throughout the first and in much of the second volume, venture far beyond prophetic visions and dreams.

As an ecogothic element that finds its sources in traditions other than European, the spectral forest in *Logan* is presented as an unknown space that demands attention and engagement. The alliteration in the passage above stresses the ritual character of the scene: he kneels, he listens, he hears. Harold "invokes" the great Spirit of the place and receives an answer. In their introduction to *Romantic Gothic: An Edinburgh Companion,* Angela Wright and Dale Townshend argue that what had been viewed as separate modes, "the Romantic" and "the Gothic," in fact often overlap in texts that demonstrate mutual implications of both literary traditions (4–5). The intersection of these two traditions in settler colonial texts that borrow from Indigenous sources are yet to be accounted for. The almost frantic search for signs supposedly provided by natural environments, to which Harold repeatedly returns in utter confusion, creates an atmosphere of unsettling irritation, which unites a romantic quest for guidance with a gothic refusal of the same. Harold's resulting confusion points at missed opportunities and the absent commitment to communication on the side of the settler population. A refusal replicated in current scholarship.

Neal's romantic Gothicism departs from European narrative structures and borrows from Indigenous cultures, as it comes to the fore the strongest in images of seemingly sentient nature, particularly trees and rocks. In fact, it is these two characters that hold the most interpretive power, which is why I will now turn to arboreal matters and petrography. In a reversal of the sacrificial scene performed by Logan as he laid the body of his infant child at the foot of an oak tree, Harold, many years later, stumbles upon his dying father in the middle of the forest, under the very same tree: "All was deathlike, silent, motionless" (1:98). As if attached to earth by a magnetic power, Logan lies pressed into the green bed of leaves in this one particular spot and cannot move. As if reterritorializing his restless body, he is physically immersed in the landscape. This seemingly restful gesture bears no recuperating power. On the contrary,

> he had not the power to tear himself away; or even to change his position. The ghastly lineaments could not be shut out. They were forever before him. Turn

which way he would, with his shut eyes; quivering swollen lips, naked teeth, and clotted blood were pressing against his face, a hateful, detestable vapour rose, like a hot steam, about him. He felt pressed down and weighed upon by a contracting solidity, as of massy walls, like a prison, shutting him in on all sides, and compressing his huge frame as into a mold. Why should he abide there? (1:99)

This important scene, and in particular the narrator's question at the end of it, demonstrates an insistence upon the agency of a forest that seems to control the actions of its inhabitants. As a "Mingo chief," Logan is a member of the Haudenosaunee. Logan and Harold, with his Cayuga mother, would certainly be familiar with the spirit forces and the Great Spirit, and the Haudenosaunee concept of a life force is explicitly mentioned on various occasions. Robert W. Venables explains the Haudenosaunee's concept of "the woods": "the Haudenosaunee believe the trees and all the beings within the forest have spiritual components that are equal to human spiritual identities ('souls')" (40). Logan, whose preternatural strength can combat any human or animal, cannot fight the spirit forces. The tree's seemingly magnetic root seems to be pulling and fixing his body without Logan having a choice in the matter. A strong power radiating from the tree petrifies Logan's body in this position, preparing his deathbed for a final encounter with his son. Everything but accommodating and serving, nature's insistent agency marks the tree as an index to—or the tombstone of—an always already dead father.

It is difficult to determine if Neal was actually intending to quote specific rites, yet the Haudenosaunee were "the dominant Indigenous social formation of the Northeastern woodlands" (C. Prior 2). Given his interest in Indigenous cultures living in the Northeastern region, it is at least safe to say that Neal's engagement with those cultures must have influenced his writing. Scenes that explore the power of nature over the human abound in this novel. While Logan is fixed in this position under the tree, Harold, also as if remotely controlled by a secret power, stumbles upon his father's dying body. The next quotation describes the moment when Logan, in what seems to be his dying hour, discloses his identity as Harold's father:

Harold disengaged the naked arms of his father, and arose, and seated himself upon a rock under the tree. There was an insupportable stillness about him. [. . .] The stars were literally dropping in pale streams of light, and rippling upon the dark water at his feet. The whole dominions of heaven were bounded by piled up and broken ramparts of the blackest midnight; while, from horizon to horizon, sprang an arch of dazzling vapour, like a bridge, wavering and shining as if mid way between earth and immensity. Away beyond him flowed the river, in transparent blackness; and yet further, were measureless and undulating shores, darkly wooded: beneath him a sky, yet blacker and more brightly begemmed. (1:112)

The forest here yet again appears as a mediator. Magically attracting the father and his lost son to the same spot, the forest immerses both in a tightly knit structure of sky, river, and earth, elements which are together enveloped in "dazzling vapour." The color dominating this romantic ecogothic scene is black. Roland Barthes uses the concept of "emanation" to describe how a photograph does not "copy" but "emanate of a *past reality:* a magic, not an art" (Barthes 88). Various descriptions of nature in this novel, while trying to reach a romantic ideal, not only seem to describe a past reality but also *emanate* feelings of something dreadful and wrong about that past reality, creating a gothic atmosphere within which the natural environment seems to consume human bodies. As in Brown's *Wieland,* the father and the son return to the same sacred spot. A source of dread, beauty, and fascination, this sublime image of nature captures and possesses the characters within a flow of darkness. Logan's body is literally glued to the earth below him, while Harold drowns in a sky "yet blacker" just before his father appears to die in his arms.

Haudenosaunee or not, Neal's effort to depict conceptualizations of spirit forces is recognizable as a space that delivers scrutable signs interacting with human interests, albeit neither in a religious nor in a strictly supernatural sense but rather animated, literally as a life force. The "darkly wooded" realm is described as a sentient organism in control of characters' actions. As such, it remains unintelligible, suggesting a dominion of the natural environment over the human actors. In fact, this frustrating relationship with the sentient forest is at the center of Harold's characterization. He, who had spent most of his life in the wilderness, is described relative to his youthful attempts to interpret the voice of nature, which he explains himself:

O Nature! Is it sympathy between ye and me, ye winds! clouds! and thou, sky of the Almighty! dwelling of the unapproachable—thou! the self-upholden vault!—

O Nature! my passions awake and are rebellious with thee; and thou, O moon! who holdest thy continuity of march, forever and ever, whence is *thy* dominion over me! With thee, I wax and wane! With thee I conjure up the elements—holding communion with spiritualities, broad and boundless. With thine, *my* light is diminished and shut out, and I am doomed to accompany thee, in thine eternal pilgrimage of shadow and change. (2:119)

Neal is therefore invested in constructing a character who is not only immersed in nature but is of nature. In an esoteric entanglement of human and nonhuman bodies, the magic of the forest emerges in relation to the protagonists it controls, erasing the separation between not only European and Indigenous but between human and nonhuman.

The ending comes somewhat as a surprise, as the novel reverts to European gothic structures. What seems like the death of Logan in his son's arms marks the spot at the foot of a tree as haunted. Again, reverting to Indigenous rites, the narrator explains Harold's superstitious attitude as part of his upbringing among "the Indians": "the Logans particularly, to whom the preternatural visitations of their bold ancestry were common; so common indeed, that the stranger, nay the passing traveller, sometimes felt, in his proximity to the haunted places of the tribe, a shivering in his very bones, of which he knew not the cause until he was told by the experienced, and made to participate in the unwilling and awful communication of them that muttered and wrought there" (1:113). Accustomed to the presence of the spirits, Harold consequently runs away, leaving this Oedipal scene to looming panthers and birds of prey. The grounds are haunted and those walking the earth know where not to go. Knowing the secret power of the haunted spot to possess him were he to remain there at night, Harold evades the sighting of a ghost. Even the reader is warned not to trespass at night: "Stranger, beware. Intrude not upon the dominions of Logan, if thou lovest sleep. Touch not their confines if thou wouldst not be haunted forever and ever" (1:114). The haunted spot in the forest extends its control over any individual. The novel is thus less invested in spectralizing the Indigenous population than it is in spectralizing the forest:

> Wo [*sic*] to him that trespassed at midnight, upon their council, as they assembled in seasons of calamity—all the living and dead generations of the Logan! Wo [*sic*] to him! for go where he would, [. . .] he would see shapes and faces passing before him, and hear voices above and below, in the air and the earth and the water; upon the mountain top, in the deepest midnight, with shut eyes, he would see gigantic shadows, gesticulating fiercely against the sky, and walking all over the tents and water, and through the hunting grounds of Logan. [. . .] Go where he would, a shadow would precede him; stalking onward from height to height, looking at him from the tangled thicket, with

a dim and terrible face; or gazing upward from the depth of the water, over which his canoe was flying. (1:113–14)

Assembling all the dead Logans in this image, haunting marks an area as off-limits to all human inhabitants. Haunting restricts a particular part of the forest, reserving it for the dead and making it unavailable for trespassing and habitation. The potentially present spirits are guarding a dedicated territory. Even Logan's body disappears in this haunted environment. Anxious to recover the body of his dead father, Harold returns the next day only to discover an empty tomb. As if absorbed by the forest, "no track was in the dew—none upon the leaves. The dry moss and the withered herbage told no tale" (1:118). This spot was abandoned by Harold the night before, because, as he insists, it is haunted. In this scene, haunting effectively erases the history of this place rather than reactivating it, as a haunting would in a traditional ghost story. There is "no tale" to be passed on. While bodies are conceptually integrated in the environment, the forest functions as the space of erasure, where stories (and bodies) are immersed to the point of disappearance.

How did the forest become a space that tells "no tale"? The original meaning of the word *haunting* that indicates a habit or recurring practice is helpful in understanding this convoluted development. The noun *haunt* shares the same root with the English word *home*. Both stem from the English *hám*—"a village, a town, a collection of dwellings," which in turn marks the haunt as a place to return to ("Haunt"). The French etymology from the Old French *hanter*, with its meaning "to frequent, resort to, to be familiar with," confirms the context of intimacy ("Haunt"). This quality is also recognizable in the related word *familiar*, which can refer to both "a frequenter of a place" and "a spirit, often taking the form of an animal which obeys and assists a witch or other person" ("Familiar"). *Hám* and *haunten* merge at the end of the thirteenth century at a time when the verb *haunten* was also recorded, with the meaning of "to resort to frequently or habitually; to frequent or be much about (a place)" ("Haunt"). Consequently, haunting has always been strongly connected to a habitual return to a familiar place, demonstrating not only a strong spatial connotation but also an intimate connection. Haunting thus indicates a return, a revisitation; it relates to a spatial and temporal displacement that does not necessarily rely on the human mind.

Marking the spot as haunted without giving the reader an opportunity to engage with the ghosts, the agents of history, Neal, in fact, repeats Irving's method of preventing the past from being integrated in the future.

The spot is marked as haunted, yet the homecoming of the spirit never takes place. This crucial omission marks an erasure of the past in the present. What haunted ecologies such as forests can express better than other concepts is the more-than-human agency exerted by those places. The complex plot of *Logan* follows a particular pattern: in the forest, trees and rocks index important episodes. While no ghosts of the human dead appear, trees and rocks seem eerily animated. They haunt the Logans in their dreams and while awake. Entangling rocks and trees with human histories, haunting in this novel marks the forest as a character in need of appeasement. A character whose ghosts are not at peace. The forest is haunted by ghosts of the "lands that were our inheritance" (1:140).

Neal's admittedly excessive prose, also described as "a fermented syrup of romanticism" (Martin and Savoy 458), employs a common trope of the frontier gothic: the grounds are haunted. Yet by whom? In a complex entanglement of gothic extravaganza, *Logan* transfers spectral agency to nature itself. The ghosts that haunt the characters are those of trees, landscapes, seas, and rocks. Harold, significantly, keeps having visions of "all the boundless landscape so still," yet it is an ecohorror image: "the darkness was crowded with livid faces—shuddering with swollen lips—eyes bursting from their sockets, and dropping with coagulated blood" (1:294–95). Entangling the dead with the ground that the living characters inhabit exposes the violence involved in the inauguration of the new nation. Neal proposes an ecogothic understanding of the new country that is built on blood-soaked fundaments. In a typical gothic embodiment of violence, the forest is populated with fantastic images of death and destruction. In the following central scene, a whole forest that merges into the sea is presented to the reader in the classic gothic manner of an apparition: "Anon, forests of green and waving trees, in all their pomp and magnificence, slowly emerged from the far off horizon—parted—with brighter spots of agitated green; here, and there, between them—faded and vanished. Anon, the blue waters appeared, and spread themselves, hither, and thither, as though the bowels of the great deep were giving forth again, their cold treasures to the moon—and behold! These waters were covered with painted specters—great ships and sails. And then!—the air darkened—it thundered!" (1:140). Throughout the novel, characters are overcome with visions of natural environments, often at very inconvenient moments, suggesting that they have no control over them. The structure supports this argument: staccato language, ghostly aesthetics, dramatic speech, auto-diegetic narration and psycho-narrators create a feeling of utter restlessness. Following Logan–George of Salisbury and his descendants' paths, the novel suggests, is a doomed endeavor.

Consequently, the second volume ends in death and destruction. There, yet another Logan is discovered, this time in England. Harold's long-lost half-brother, Oscar, Logan's "English" son, joins the cause of *helping* the American Native population regain what has been stolen from them. Upon meeting Harold in England, Oscar decides to board the ship with him and leave for "America" (2:326). Yet, the night before the trip, he has a "strange, and terrifick [*sic*] dream" of a tree. Shaken by the images, he draws a sketch for Harold, who remembers: "That tree!—yes, I remember just such a tree as that somewhere; but, for my life, I cannot tell where I have seen it. It is associated, too, with something terribly indistinct in my fancy, something that turns my heart cold when I look upon it. But the rock, I know nothing of the rock" (2:329). The rock and the tree mark the spot in the forest where Logan put down his infant child and where the same child as an adult found his dying father. They return in Oscar's dream, haunting him. Foreshadowing doom, the rock and the tree will soon reappear in a very real—if gothic—setting. Oscar's interpretation already steers the novel in this direction: "I feel a strange oppression at my chest. This dream has affected my spirits. [. . .] Somewhat dark and threatening seems to be connected with it, and to me, appears continually flitting about me" (2:329).

Before appearing in Oscar's dream, the tree appears at the most significant moments in Harold's life, beginning with the tree at the foot of which his father leaves him as an infant. It is this very tree, next to the same rock, that Oscar somehow manages to sketch after they appear in his dreams. The tree and the rock magically connect all the Logans, no matter how scattered they are across the world. Oscar had not been to "America" before, but the tree and the rock are impregnated in his mind. What in Brown's *Wieland* was a transgenerational connection manifested in doom is in *Logan* inscribed in the natural environment.

Seen in this light, it is only consequent that the one proper ghost in this novel—in the sense of a body that is dead but appears to be alive—is a tree. While the characters are only ghostlike, an oak tree is depicted as undead. I quote the passage in its entirety, as it is crucial to understanding the role of spectral nature rather than human ghosts in creating the specifically US American gothic aesthetics so common to most now-canonical antebellum narratives:

And yet, there had he been, there! out under the midnight heaven—under that scathed tree, to whose history, and that of the bleak and barren solitude about, were allied ten thousand frightful stories of Indian superstition—a place that, for ages, the beast and the bird of prey had haunted for food—a tree that had been there—the same, unchanged, unshattered, unbowed—with never a branch, nor a leaf the less (so said the oldest red men, [*sic*]) from beyond time—centuries had rolled away—storm after storm had beaten upon it—rain after rain—and yet was it, forever, unworn and unwet—again and again, had it been in a blaze, from head to foot with the lightning of heaven—again and again, had the thunder and the earthquake shaken all the trees around, root and branch—nay, the very fountain that crept round it, so darkly and sluggishly, *that* had been dried up again and again, by the hot storming of the skies; and yet this tree, this old and awful, sapless and withered tree, had withstood it *all*—*all* the elements—*all* the principles of decay—had stood there, like an indestructible shadow, undiminished, unshaken, unsubdued! Not a blade of grass lay within its shade. The very soil was brown, and hot, and arid, like pulverised iron. (1:157)

In spite of continued extermination attempts, the tree survives, but only as the undead. As the narrator insistently specifies, it is "the very fountain that crept round it" that "dried out." The barren land that the tree stands on suggests that it is not alive, yet the green branches indicate the opposite. Like Logan himself, the tree, even if marked as dead in the beginning, sparks with glimpses of life within the project of death. Both alive and dead, civilized and uncivilized, sovereign and barbaric, not only Logan but also the tree are living relics. While the tree warns in its undead silent presence, Logan keeps appearing to his son, to the governor—the representative figure of the settler colonial society—or to anybody who might presume him to be dead, in a phantom-like manner, long after he is believed to have died. Just as the barren land does not imply that the tree is dead, the insistence on the ghostliness of "the Mingo chief" does not imply social erasure but rather an insistent presence in other characters' lives. In this image of the undead tree, Neal thus deconstructs the "darker forests" so firmly established by Freneau. His "Indian" is also an Englishman and is entangled in an ecogothic embrace with the destiny of the undead tree. He, just like the tree, can neither be safely deposited nor erased. Neal's narrator provocatively asks: "How then shall you read the Indian!" (1:87). (Note that there is no question mark at the end of this sentence.) The answer follows immediately: "You may not" (1:87).

◦◦

A specter always marks the visibility of a body that is not present in flesh and blood. In an interview with Bernard Stiegler, Derrida offers something that comes close to the definition of a specter as "the visible invisible" (Derrida and Stiegler 121). Neal's spectral visions of landscapes make it clear that claiming territory was at the center of the so-called "Indian problem."[9] The specters in this novel are "green and waving trees and blue waters," providing an imaginary complicity with the nonhuman world of trees and rivers missed by Harold. He interprets his vision himself: "God of the red men! Be thou, O! be thou with me! The lands that were our inheritance are returning to us. I saw them; I!—moving off upon the track of our retreating nations! Here! Here! oh thou spirit of our worship! thou who art hunted, even as thy children are hunted, from these, thine immeasurable solitudes—thine appointed places—here!" (1:140). Bergland reads the presence of spirits marked as Indigenous as a "discursive removal of Indians from American physical territory and the Americanization of the imaginative territory into which Indians are removed" (5). While this interpretation might come closest to Neal's text, *Logan* does not offer a version of the past that can be integrated into the present in order to construct a presentable future. By spectralizing the land itself, Neal suggests that all of its inhabitants are doomed and dying, including the colonial settler population and the nonhuman environment. The forest is a site of erasure, perhaps a site for new beginnings, albeit without the presence of the human population.

Literature published in the years following the War of Independence demonstrates an increased effort to simultaneously exclude Indigenous bodies and include their spirits in the national imaginary. The proliferation of various nameless spectral Indigenous characters, as well as those who are only singled out while perishing, must be understood as a biopolitical reconfiguration of the concept of race in the spectral tale. Feeling the pressure to unify the racial profile of the nation after the Revolutionary War, early American writers were invested in relegating the presence of the Indigenous population back into the forest, this time around as ghosts. Rather than an investment in *being* the "Native American" (Deloria), this is an investment in claiming Indigeneity through an intimacy with the land that only haunting can provide.

As the "last of his race," the historical figure Logan is, to quote Jonathan Elmer, a "*hyper*-territorialized creature: his mythic element is the land, or more specifically the new world territory as that must be overcoded by its European invader" ("Melancholy" 120). Yet, in Neal's version, this "European invader" meets his end in madness and isolation, and the landscape itself is spectral in very different ways. Rather than haunted, it is haunting, suggesting that territorial appropriation has lethal consequences for all. With his novel, Neal offers a near-apocalyptic reading of the extinction narrative in which only nature halfway survives, suggesting that postrevolutionary American national politics are, in fact, a failed necropolitics. In Achille Mbembe's definition, necropolitics defines "the capacity to dictate who may live and who must die [...], to kill or to allow to live" (11). Extending "the work of death" to both European and non-European inhabitants as well as human and nonhuman actors, Neal suggests that the necropolitics of the settler colonials constructs an uninhabitable space for all. Only, the forest might survive, as even this sentient entity is marked by necrosis: "There may be no places of pilgrimage in America, unless it be some lonely battle-ground, already forgotten by the neighbourhood, overgrown with a new forest, and overshadowed with a perpetual deep darkness, or covered far and wide with a sea of weltering herbage—the frightful vegetation of death" (Neal, "Critical Essays" 253).

In accordance with the rules of biopolitics as described in Michel Foucault's theory of racism, race operates not based on polarity but instead as something that is "ceaselessly infiltrating the social body" (Foucault 289). Instead of an understanding of two distinct races, Foucault writes about the splitting of a single race into a "superrace and a subrace" (83). Neal's writing is an attempt to break this cultural supremacist mechanism in place in the early republic. Extending its scope to spectral nature, Neal inscribes both settlers and Indigenous inhabitants into the landscape. As an Anglo-Saxon immigrant who presents himself as a murderous Cayuga leader, Logan, in this rendition, disturbs normative racial hierarchy, but he does not escape it. As a British nobleman driven by rage and practicing extreme violence geared towards anything or anybody alive, he ends up killing his son and is shot at by his other son. Throughout the novel, he remains a confused, lonely, and tired character, offering little in terms of national heroism. Like the protagonist in Brown's *Wieland*, Logan is, above all, self-destructive. Without offering an alternative version of the future, *Logan* can only function as a warning. Removing the borderline to the Beyond, only the "frightful vegetation of death" survives.

Between Indigenous Cosmology and European Alchemy

The sentience of the forest that comes to the fore not in actual acts of haunting but rather in the sense of animation transforms the forest from a potentially threatening sublime environment into a mysterious park where settler colonial characters come to reclaim their humanity. Brown, Irving, and Neal, the most successful writers of the early national period, set a standard with their settler male characters who seek to affirm their moral intactness. With their ecogothic forests infused with the remains of the Indigenous dead and settler ghosts, they have extended the project of colonization to nature itself. This trope comes to prominence most insistently in the writings of one of the most canonical writers of the succeeding period, Nathaniel Hawthorne.

I have written more extensively about Hawthorne's repeated return to nonhuman agents in the forest in a different publication ("Lithic Corporeality"). For the present context, suffice it to mention that Hawthorne continues the tradition of exploring his characters' mindset through narrative conceptualizations of trees and stones. In "Roger Malvin's Burial" (1831), for example, a specific granite rock central to the short story not only opens and closes the narrative but also appears nineteen times throughout the text, with every reference further underlining its significance.[10] Further narratives that feature rocks are "The Great Carbuncle" (1835), which revolves around a gemstone and the peculiar powers of attraction it exercises over a gallery of prototypical (human) characters. First published in the *New England Magazine* in 1835, "The Great Carbuncle" was included in the collection *Twice-Told Tales* in 1837. In the short story "The Great Stone Face" (1850), correspondences are drawn between features of a rock and those of various protagonists, establishing yet again a direct relation between humans and stones.[11] Spread across two decades, the publication of these narratives attests to Hawthorne's continuing and deep-seated interest in lithic materials and the ways in which they organize human communities. While this focus on landscape and nature is typical of the romantic period, the detailed attention that Hawthorne devotes to the corporal or material aspects of specific elements without engaging the perspective of his characters is rather unusual. Hawthorne's treatment of stones, in fact, corresponds to a certain degree with the teachings of both European alchemists and North American Indigenous cosmologies. As such, it departs from the more common romantic treatments of nature that imagine the human entanglement with the environment as a poetic mental capacity. Rather than a metaphysical correspondence between characters and nature, writings from Brown to Irving to Neal to Hawthorne repeatedly indicate a material, transcorporeal relation by employing a ghostly aesthetics of possession and animation that stands in the animist tradition as it was to be found in numerous Indigenous cultures at the time.[12]

A specter is that which acts without physically existing; in its material presence, a ghost relies on borrowed bodies. These can be the bodies of a tree or a stone. The spectral transcorporeality that extends to the natural environment comes to the fore in scenes of haunting, unintentional and seemingly forced returns of those who function as a medium to the unappeased dead. The mysterious, supernatural, spiritual aspect of Hawthorne's tale "Roger Malvin's Burial" is inscribed in the main character's body's attraction back to the rock where he let his father-in-law bleed to death. Decades later, in spite of his intention to follow a different path, Reuben steers his whole family, as if they were remotely controlled, right to the haunted spot, "a region of which savage beasts and savage men were as yet the sole possessors" (Hawthorne, "Roger Malvin" 28). Again, the Indigenous intimacy with nature is juxtaposed with settler colonial alienation. Reuben's return to the haunted spot has the same outcome as in the central novels by Brown and Neal analyzed in previous chapters: patricide, filicide, sibilicide; early American literature is full of familicide. Hawthorne advanced this topos to include nature as an actor even more directly than Neal. Like Irving's and Neal's characters, Hawthorne's protagonists are ghostly in their return to scenes that mark unfinished business. Reminiscent of mesmerist practices, which revolve around the idea that an invisible natural force flows through all living beings, his characters' compulsive returns are presented as something that they cannot comprehend. But in the final act, they do understand. Grounding his protagonist in the forest at the rock, Hawthorne connects animism with mesmerism to highlight more-than-human histories.[13] Those practicing mesmerism, also known as animal magnetism, were commonly referred to as "magnetizers" for their effort to demonstrate the power of attraction connecting all living matter, a power considered to be both material and beyond human comprehension. Their bodies were never randomly chosen. Indicating a higher order, their fate is entangled with the spot that marks an ethical call to remember, thus, extending agency to sources outside of the human.

Forests in all these texts appear as agents in their own right and as the final perpetrators. As a complex sentient entity, a tree is not a mere witness, nor does it only appear in the role as the executioner: "The dark and gloomy pines looked down upon them, and, as the wind swept through their tops, a pitying sound was heard in the forest; or did those old trees groan in fear that men were come to lay the axe to their roots at last?" (Hawthorne, "Roger Malvin" 28). The environmental concern voiced in this arboreal anthropomorphization hints at deforestation. Even without communication, the lives of trees are intricately intertwined with those of humans. The epiphora that closes Hawthorne's short story finalizes this human-nonhuman link in a simile that likens Reuben's eyes to rocks: "Then Reuben's heart was stricken, and the tears gushed out like water from a rock" (32). The deep temporal imprint on the rock that is evoked in the beginning of the story as "veins" is juxtaposed in the end with a biblical image of smiting a rock for water, wherein Reuben's eyes became the rocks. Finally immersed in the ecology of the landscape, Reuben feels relieved for the first time in his life. The slow movement of time visible in the inscriptions on the rock ceases to imply a nonhuman scale. Reuben is now inscribed in the temporal schema of the world.

Depictions of nature during the romantic period commonly bifurcate into either the dark and gloomy or the restorative and nourishing. But the wilderness in Brown's, Irving's, Neal's, and Hawthorne's narratives is neither. The exchange with nature is established as an inner voice, entangling characters' fates with rocks, oaks, and pines. This narrative element has sometimes been interpreted in an ethical context.[14] Suitably, in colloquial language it is the *voice of conscience* that initiates ethical action. Mladen Dolar discusses the long-standing association of voice with ethics: "We should pause at the extraordinary fact that ethics has often been associated with the voice, that the voice has been the guiding trope of reflections on moral questions, both in popular reasoning and in the grand philosophical tradition" (83). The focus on hearing a voice as if not one's own and on its peculiar relation to the body, which it appears to occupy but not exit, reorders assumptions not only about knowledge based on perception but also about responsiveness, relation, and most of all, responsibility. A voice implies that somebody is speaking to someone. Sound permeates the body that holds the voice of the other, and a resonance with the other serves to shift the focus to the place of production. Yet, in the examples above, the voice of the other appears to belong to the silent rock, the oak, the forest itself. The voice of consciousness becomes the *voice of nature* in early American settler writers' narratives, a voice that calls for death.

Early American settler writing tells ecogothic morality tales that explicitly refer to the transferential quality of the (inner) voice that connects nature not only with human conscience and consciousness but also with human corporality. In this way, the late eighteenth-century link between morality and spectrality is instrumentalized for a transcendental distinction between reason and understanding that decentralizes the role of the human, particularly the human mind. This shift out of the mind into the body relegates the voice to the realm of environmental ethics. It is the rock that is linked to the heart. This transcorporeality broadens the scope to a human-nonhuman interpsychic interaction and an ethics beyond the human.

So what does this mean for the conceptualization of the "American forest" in early nationalized US American literature? If one accepts the proposal made by Harrison in his study *Forests: The Shadow of Civilization,* that "a historical age reveals something essential about its ideology, its institutions and law, or its cultural temperament, in the manifold ways in which forests are regarded in that age" (115), the question as to the meaning of the spectral forest in early American narratives comes to the fore. Judging by representations in literary examples here analyzed so far, it is possible to conclude that there is a magical component to the forests portrayed, one which determines characters' actions. This mystical and mythical element is repeatedly associated with unspecified Indigenous histories and cultures. In Neal's and Hawthorne's texts, the forest is in control of the settler colonial protagonists, who end their lives as murderers in self-provoked violent deaths. Trees and rocks—just as introduced by Freneau—remain in the function of survivors. If a specter borrows the body of another to animate the dead, the forest in these settler colonial narratives becomes the spectralized body of the Indigenous population. Settler colonial characters who decide to enter that body and perhaps even mix their physical remains with those who have been there before fertilize the soil of the "American forest" for further settler generations to come. In this way, the space is recodified as settler colonial ancestral land.

Recently, "sentient landscape" has been at the forefront of anthropological research.[15] Scholars such as Julie Cruikshank and Elisabeth Povinelli are engaged in the effort to move away from theories of individuals autonomously shaping an outside world, to an understanding of agency as always co-constituent with human and nonhuman environments. Their studies reveal that looking at land as sentient is common to most Indigenous or Aboriginal peoples. Writing about the inhabitants of the Cox peninsula west of Darwin, Povinelli observes: "The everydayness of their labor-action is swept within the superhuman realm of a sentient landscape populated with ancestors and totemic beings" (133). Similarly, in *Wisdom Sits in Places: Landscape and Language among the Western Apache,* Keith Basso writes about the Apache concept of a sentient landscape that demonstrates itself even in place-naming. The human, in this theory, is understood to be merely a vessel for the place to name itself. This type of shared agency, as Michael Marker points out, as well as similar expressions of sentience relating to places and landscapes, is understood to be a ritual that interlocks human and nonhuman destiny and, thus, an environmentally conscious approach, across various Indigenous cultures. In most, if not all, representations of a sentient landscape, this concept is presented in a thoroughly welcoming and appreciative manner. Yet, as human/nonhuman binaries gain attention in academia, it is necessary to complicate the history of animated nature. The above examined examples of early American literature demonstrate how the subversive politics of the sentient landscape are aligned with settler colonial purposes.

Placing more recent theories of Indigenous philosophies in conversation with non-Indigenous representations of sentient nature in US American literature of the 1820s demonstrates that ancient metaphysical understandings of land have been replaced in early American literature with colonial modernist regimes of division. Indeed, to extract the settler character from nature, as has been described by Arendt and Wynter, forests fuse with Indigenous bodies in a spectral embrace that offers a national imaginary solidifying into effective replacement narratives. Written at the point of friction between a hopeful nationalism and devastating genocides of Indigenous populations, early romantic writing in this context instrumentalized images of the forest as sentient nature to mediate between the two. Infused by those dead bodies, the forest signified Indigeneity in these texts as a social construct that never exceeds what Mark Rifkin calls "settler time." As a concept that describes the temporal dimension of elimination practices that are at the center of settler governance, settler time circumscribes not only genocide but also symbolic erasure, displacement, and assimilation. The source for the trope of sentient land as it is employed in the above literature, therefore, is precisely not to be found in any Indigenous conceptualizations but rather in colonial efforts of land appropriation.

Avoiding to mention their Indigenous sources in search of cosmologies that permit mystical conceptions of the universe, US American writers from the romantic period were often drawn to European mysticism, particularly the writings of Emmanuel Swedenborg, Jakob Böhme, and Paracelsus. Hawthorne was indirectly influenced by mysticism through at least four German writers that he admired, namely E. T. A. Hoffmann, Ludwig Tieck, Novalis, and Friedrich von Schlegel. Robyn Schiffman even speculates in her article on Hawthorne how he "might have written the German romantic novella" (41). She particularly foregrounds Novalis' *Heinrich von Ofterdingen* as a source for Hawthorne's "Rappaccini's Daughter." What she does not mention, however, is that Novalis had plunged himself deep into the world of Paracelsus while doing research for and writing this novella. In fact, Hoffmann, Tieck, and Novalis too had found kindred spirits in Böhme and Paracelsus. Both Hawthorne himself and Edgar Allan Poe have pointed out the resemblance between Hoffmann's and Tieck's writing on the one hand and some of Hawthorne's more famous publications on the other.[16] Robyn Schiffman more recently added Novalis and Schlegel to the discussion as further influences on Hawthorne by way of German Idealism. She, too, failed to mention that all four of these German romantic writers shared a profound interest in the writings of Paracelsus. We can thus assume that not only German Idealism but also German mysticism had a direct or indirect influence on all the abovementioned writers' choice of topics and particularly on their understanding of nature.

Hawthorne's oeuvre most prominently exemplifies the entanglement of Indigenous sources and German mysticism.[17] In two of his most-quoted works, "The Birth-Mark" and *The Scarlet Letter,* one will find explicit mentions of Paracelsus, but only via "customs of the Indian" ("Roger Malvin" 22). In *The Scarlet Letter,* Roger Chillingworth claims that he has learned as much from Paracelsus as he did from Native American shamans (71). Borrowing from Indigenous cultures and medieval mystics is a successful endeavor. After impressively relieving Pearl of her pain with a poison he had brought to the prison cell, he explains: "I have learned many new secrets in the wilderness, and here is one of them—a recipe that an Indian taught me, in requital of some lessons of my own, that were as old as Paracelsus" (72). The replacement narrative enacted in "Indian" costume is here presented as a scientific replacement narrative that does not shy away from magic.

In "Roger Malvin's Burial," the narrator reverts to Indigenous philosophy to correct what should not have happened. From the outset, the missing burial of Roger Malvin is described in opposition to the customs of the Native population: "An almost superstitious regard, arising perhaps from the customs of the Indians, whose war was with the dead, as well as the living, was paid by the frontier inhabitants to the rites of sepulture; and there are many instances of the sacrifice of life, in the attempt to bury those who had fallen by the 'sword of the wilderness'" (Hawthorne, "Roger Malvin's Burial" 22). Not accustomed to "Indian" traditions, Reuben failed to consider the agency of the dead in his plans for the future. The energy and influence that a dead body that binds with other elements in the earth might exert on the living is yet another telling intersection of various Indigenous and alchemist cosmologies. Indeed, Charles Swann describes how the relation between "Indian knowledge" and practices of alchemy is persistently evoked in Hawthorne's *The Elixir of Life Manuscripts* (372).[18] Hawthorne's characters repeatedly suspect the power of nonhuman agents, seeking out or assuming they will be able to find a missing explanation in Indigenous customs. Much more than a simple example of a racial stereotype, these passages point at an awareness of deep history that was experienced as absent in the settler colonial society. At the same time, settler colonial characters in Neal's and, more insistently, Hawthorne's texts pose as the guardians of all knowledge, Western and Indigenous. While "Indian customs," like Indian costume, could serve as a supplement for a settler society in need of spiritual consolation, actual Indigenous concepts remain buried in obscurity. In their fiction, Neal was writing against "Indian Haters,"[19] while Hawthorne followed the agenda of ironic detachment, ambivalence, and quietism when it came to politics,[20] yet a search for spiritual balance inscribed in the promise of "going native" is recognizable in the works of both authors.[21]

Avoiding the stench of spiritualism, Hawthorne simply skips spirits but continues to explore the Paracelsian inscription of humans into nature. Paracelsus was particularly devoted to understanding the relation between microcosm and macrocosm—a grand unifying theory of nature that includes the human. In *Astronomia Magna* (1590) Paracelsus explains his dedicated intention to combine medicine with theology in astronomy. In this universe, all matter is animate, and all elements exert energies that create and sustain life. For Paracelsus, the familiar distinction between the animate and inanimate is a false one; minerals, plants, animals, and stars are all vital systems. The human body is connected to a cosmic network through a certain type of energy that Carl G. Jung named "cosmic matter" (8). The human—just like anything else in the world—is an aggregate of animate matter: "The human body is elemental and sidereal," whereas the material body is constructed from elements of the earth, and the "sidereal" body from the stars (Paracelsus 96). The human system (microcosm) can therefore only be understood in relation to its environment (macrocosm). Very similar cosmology is described by numerous Indigenous scholars; for example, Leanne Betasamosake Simpson writes in relation to Mich Saagig Nishnaabeg knowledge: "My Ancestors are not in the past. The spiritual world does not exist in some mystical realm. These forces and beings are right here beside me" (192–93). And like Paracelsus, she includes the "plant nations, animal nations, insects, bodies of water, air, soil, and spiritual beings" into this equation (38).

Neal's romanticism, too, oscillates between Cherokee animism and European enchantment. Paul Gilmore recently demonstrated that Neal's writing manifests significantly more parallels with Schlegel's Jena school of poetry and philosophy than with the national cause within which it had been situated thus far. Schlegel—who, as has been mentioned, was strongly influenced by Paracelsus' writings—encouraged a re-enchantment of nature through poetry, which he believed provided access to a transcendental knowledge necessary for freedom. In this theory, reality is knowable as creative nature that eludes full comprehension. Schlegel's *Frühromantik* (Early Romanticism) considered the efforts of Enlightenment to create an—in his opinion—dangerous disenchantment (*Entzauberung*) of nature, which consequently is in need of a re-enchantment (*Verzauberung*).[22] The function of the poet is accordingly similar to that of a sorcerer or a witch, whose work acknowledges the mysterious and unintelligible aspects of nature. In Schlegel's view, the mystification of one's environment is valuable in that it eventually leads to a harmonious unity with nature through the acceptance of its illegibility. Ludwig Tieck asserts, in this vein: "Well then, a good disorder is worth more than a bad order."[23] Neal's *Logan,* with images of animated nature and an excess of confusion and disarrangement in relation to it, certainly attests to a feeling of disorder and corresponds with the ideals of German *Frühromantik.*

The spiral of references from German early romantics to North American Indigenous customs uncoils throughout most canonical texts of early American literature. Though often only mentioned in passing, parallels to Indigenous traditions of land-based knowledge forms were much closer historically to Hawthorne's and Neal's times than was German mysticism. In *Teaching Spirits,* Joseph Epes Brown and Emily Cousins warn against romanticization but at the same time suggest that "Native American cultures share some fundamental principles in their relation to the land. [. . .] Because the land has spiritual power, many tribes look to the land for assistance and guidance" (13–14). Understanding the land as alive and as a moral force thus connects numerous North American Indigenous cultures. It is in the creation of a mixture of what settler colonial writers deem to be alternative cosmologies that their resulting assertions of freedoms are located. Hawthorne and Neal wrote their novels during a period pronouncedly dedicated to a schism between anything relating to magic and the realm of science. Both were aware of the difficulties involved in enacting this separation. The narrator in Hawthorne's "The Birth-Mark" refers to this period as "those days when the comparatively recent discovery of electricity and other kindred mysteries of nature seemed to open paths into the region of miracle" (36). Rather than the supernatural, this realm covers the domain of the natural or the sentiency of nature. The narrator in "The Birth-Mark" explains his theory of interaction in nature: "The crimson hand expressed the ineludible gripe in which mortality clutches the highest and purest of earthly mould, degrading them into kindred with the lowest, and even with the very brutes, like whom their visible frames return to dust" (39). Here, again, dust is the all-connecting concept. The "crimson hand" is a reminder that we are animals, we are earth, we are dust. Understood as a narrative structure of multispecies kinship that involves rocks (water and dust), the magic perceptible in Hawthorne's and Neal's writings becomes a holistic perception of the world referred to in relation to the teachings of European mystics and Indigenous philosophy alike.

None of the writers spell out the rich conceptualization of nature in the corresponding Indigenous cultures. The holistic approach that was appropriated in their work, finally, even if against the authors' intentions, promoted yet another colonial version of a specific *human* sovereignty in antebellum romantic literature reserved for European settlers. Nature is not simply animated; its sentience is exclusively Indigenous. What is repeatedly referred to as "stories of Indian superstition" (Neal, *Logan* 1:157) is a framework for colonial replacement narratives. The magnetic attraction that stones and trees seem to exert on settler colonial characters in Hawthorne's and Neal's writing functions as a colonial cleansing of the natural space.

In the subjectivation of what was believed to be inanimate matter and the objectivation of thinking subjects, Neal and Hawthorne postulate a world within which the category of the nonhuman equals Indigenous. In this way, nature, and particularly spectral nature, was instrumentalized for the establishment of a very specific category of *human,* one reserved exclusively for settler colonials of European descent. In spite of the effort to instrumentalize a romantic view of nature as enchanted and to endorse freedom, criticism, and egalitarianism by doing so, the aforementioned tales are some of the earliest US American examples of a biopolitical racial divide that relies on images of spectral forests. Borrowing from alchemist holistic theories and Indigenous cosmologies alike, writers of the 1820s tried to produce counternarratives to the colonial settler racial divide, only to affirm it.

～6

Feminist Colonialism
Emancipation and Cultural Appropriation

The settler colonial desire to adopt what was marked as an "Indian" lifestyle went through various stages throughout early American literature. Stories of intermarriage held a particular fascination for readers at the turn of the nineteenth century. As early as 1790, Sarah Wentworth Morton published her little-discussed epic poem "Ouâbi; or, The Virtues of Nature: An Indian Tale, in Four Cantos" based on the true story of a French officer who, in 1667, left his post and went to live among the Abenaki on Penobscot Bay. According to Gordon Sayre, such cases were not uncommon in the southeastern colonies in the eighteenth century ("'Azakia'" 319). Morton assures her readers in an introduction to the poem:

> I am aware it may be considered improbable, that an amiable and polished European should attach himself to the persons and manners of an uncivilized people; but there is now a living instance of a like propensity. A gentleman of fortune, born in America, and educated in all the refinements and luxuries of Great Britain, has lately attached himself to a female savage, in whom he finds every charm I have given my Azâkia, and in consequence of his inclination, has relinquished his own country and connections, incorporated himself into the society, and adopted the manners of the virtuous, tough uncultivated Indian.

Along with the obvious "noble savage" agenda that forces a celebratory yet diminishing perspective on all local Indigenous cultures, this passage demonstrates an acknowledgment of an existing society functioning at the intersection of settlement and wilderness. In Morton's poem, this space is experienced and represented as an alternative to the strict lifestyle practiced by European immigrants and their descendants. Almost half a century and numerous ethnic conversion stories later, in the wake of the Indian Removal Act signed by Andrew Jackson in 1830, this idea of an alternative way of life became a contested ground (Cave). Even the wilderness becomes wilder as the fundamental violence of settler-native relations escalates. To an antebellum observer living in the 1820s, "wilderness" and "Indians" were interchangeable, or, as Spence puts it: "forests were wild because Indians and beasts lived there, and Indians were wild because they lived in the forests" (10). As demonstrated in the analysis of *Logan* and "Roger Malvin's Burial," forests, having fused with the Indigenous dead in literary representations, increasingly came to circumscribe a liminal and dangerous space that could not be entered and exited at will, at least not alive. Forests became a place associated with death even if only within the settler colonial logic of a moral corrective. Either way, turning to an Indigenous lifestyle in search of meaning in the 1820s cannot be compared to the same desire in the 1790s. When Charles Brockden Brown decided to explore the idea of "spectral evidence" in his novel *Wieland,* the wilderness surrounding "the hut" served as a protective space where the Wieland children were able to pursue their intellectual lifestyle. The same is true for *St. Herbert—A Tale,* written before *Wieland,* where the titular character prefers a life in the forest to the hypocrisy of the settlement. Like the Wieland family, St. Herbert's search for meaning is fulfilled by a life in isolation, which is what wilderness represented at the time. In the 1820s, entering the forest was more likely to result in death than in a calm and fulfilled life. And while the forest could hold the promise of adventure and adversity for male settler characters, for female settler characters, it almost certainly meant captivity and possibly death.

It was within this literary landscape that Lydia Maria Child joined the growing number of writers engaged in recoding the demonized Puritan wilderness and challenging the dominant Vanishing Indian mythos, by prominently placing a narrative centered on miscegenation between a Puritan woman and her Pequot lover. Within this story, wilderness is tamed by means of magic and transformed into the heroine's safe space. This chapter challenges the interpretation common in current scholarship of Child's narratives as simply progressive, by offering a careful analysis of the often-employed trope of the transfiguration of characters marked as Indigenous into trees and flowers. In addition, I analyze Harriet Beecher Stowe's seldom-discussed tales of the supernatural to demonstrate ways in which the colonial framing of Irving's and Child's stories was taken up by the succeeding generation of writers who claimed to write in the name of equality and emancipation.

Necropolitics in Lydia Maria Child's Writing

In the preface to her most famous novel, *Hobomok, a Tale of Early Times, by an American,* published in 1824, Lydia Maria Child spells out her aim to write a "new England novel" in the style of "Sir Walter Scott, or Mr. Cooper," with noticeable differences (*Hobomok* 3). Writing against Cooper and his model, Walter Scott, Child inscribed herself in the tradition of what at various stages has been termed "frontier romance," "national romance," or "domestic frontier romance." The designations imply that corresponding authors set out to write fiction with US American characters and with the aim of producing a national narrative. Child also promises "an American story," yet she offers an alternative to the violent, xenophobic, and often misogynistic narratives of the frontier romance popular at the time. She also departs from the familicide that was so firmly established by her male colleagues.

Instead, as Child explained on various occasions, her writing was dedicated to a fight against the violence and, most of all, the dominant extinction narrative, preferably through stories of intermarriage. She explains this intention most clearly at the end of *The First Settlers of New-England; or, Conquest of the Pequods, Narragansets, and Pokanokets* (1829): "It is, in my opinion, decidedly wrong, to speak of the removal, or extinction of the Indians as inevitable; it surely implies that the people of these states have not sufficient virtue or magnanimity to redeem their past offences, by affording the sad remnant, which still exist, succor and protection" (*First Settlers* 281). In this publication, which was written for parents and children for educational purposes, Child explains her goal: to expose "the general misapprehension in reference to the conduct of the Indians" and the unjust treatment that they have suffered "from the usurpers of their soil" (*First Settlers* iii). Like Neal, Child understood her profession as a writer to be a form of her social activism and a tool for an alternative form of nationalism that includes rather than excludes the original inhabitants in its makeup. It is in this vein that she sets out "to explore the viability of cultural syncretism and intermarriage with Indians," which, according to Carolyn L. Karcher, was "promoted by the French" and was supposed to present an "alternative to the genocide practiced by the English" (Karcher quoted in Child, *Hobomok* 233). This interest, more than anything else, shifted Child's fictional settings into "the woods" (Child, *Hobomok* 13). In what follows, I will demonstrate how the forest served this aim to redefine settler-colonial relations, and what role spectrality and the supernatural played within these revisions.

It is in "the thicket" of the forest that the reader encounters Mary Conant (Child, *Hobomok* 13), the heroine of *Hobomok,* with the help of whom Child rewrites the spectral Puritan forest as a space of emancipation rather than dread and horror. The Invisible World remains the dominant reference, yet the magic of the forest, so thoroughly dark and threatening in Puritan narratives of the seventeenth century, is transformed in this text into a recuperative and protective space.[1] The first chapter sets the tone in spectral matters. Here, a first-person narrator, a pious Puritan man, walks into the night to pray undisturbed, hoping to free himself from his erotic desires and "the childish witchery of Mary Conant" (12). Opening with the theme of repressed Puritan male sexuality, the reader is immediately transferred to a place "everywhere surrounded by dark forests" (12). The nocturnal setting in the forest creates an alternative space veiled in secrecy and possibility. It is there, while kneeling down to pray, that his "heart might be kept from the snares of the world," that the narrator spots a shadow that he first mistakes for a ghost but soon discovers to be no less than the very Mary Conant whose presence he feared so much (12–13). The narrator nevertheless decides to follow her secretly into "the thicket" of "the woods." There, he observes her performing a pagan magic ritual in the light of the "full moon" (13). Upon cutting the skin on her hand, Mary Conant drips her own blood onto a feather, uses it to write on a carefully prepared piece of cloth, and then draws a magic circle on the ground, into which she steps while continually chanting. The narrator reports to have understood one passage only:

> Whoever's to claim a husband's power,
> Come to me in the moonlight hour.
> And again,—
> Whoe'er my bridegroom is to be,
> Step in the circle after me (13)

As if responding to her magic, "a young Indian spring[s] forward into the centre" (13). It turns out to be Hobomok, "the savage, who seemed scarcely less surprised than herself" (14). The titular character is thus not a spectralized Indigenous person but rather a Cayuga man who happens to be caught in a magic ritual performed by a heterenormative Puritan woman for purposes of finding a romantic partner.

This seemingly innocent episode recording a young woman's sexual awakening and her playful, proactive magic in what she believes to be the isolation of the forest sets the tone for the novel. Magic can provide access to power, and Mary Conant is aware of her conjuring potential. Literarily encircled within this narrative, Hobomok, indeed, ends up in a conjugal relation with Conant. Yet, Hobomok's incidental stumbling upon the larger story of a young woman's desire is programmatic. Their relationship is present as nothing more than an accident. The marriage is initiated by Conant in a rather convenient and fleeting moment. She eventually resigns herself to her fate at a moment of weakness and depression caused by what she believes to be the death of the man that Conant actually loved, Charles Brown. Believing Brown to be dead, she succumbs to her desperation and decides during another nocturnal chance encounter with Hobomok, while crying at her mother's grave, to marry him. A "blind belief in fatality" makes her decide: "I will be your wife, Hobomok, if you love me" (121). The concept of preordination is a premise of the Puritan religion, and Conant decides to comply with rather than fight her fate. Hobomok, therefore, functions as a convenient placeholder rather than the object of her desire. When Brown, to everyone's surprise, returns from captivity alive, Conant simply divorces Hobomok, leaves her wigwam, and continues her life in the settlement with Brown.

Set in Salem in 1629, the scene in the forest inevitably evokes a history of witchcraft. Child thus effectively recalls the painful history of unjust persecution, only to neutralize its effect in the present. At the same time, her "ritual" exposes the continued fascination with the unknown, the unrepresentable, and, on the side of the settlers, the related anxiety involved in "the supposed occult properties of the natural world" ("Magic"). Both Mary Conant and her friend Sally are insecure as to whether they should take the ritual seriously, preferring to err on the side of caution. "There's no telling what may come of asking the devil's assistance," explains Sally (20). Mary's "wicked" magic does much more than simply mark witchcraft as impish (20). Apart from confirming her belief in her own powers, the ritual connects Conant to what in the scene before has been described as the "dark forest" around her, which she had carefully chosen as the setting for her ceremony. Practicing magic is a "ritual activity" intended to "manipulate the natural world" ("Magic"). By engaging with this procedure, Conant extends her dominion over the forest while creating a space that enables her to step out of her restrictive Puritan environment. The fact that Hobomok happens to "spring" into her "circle" marks her as the liminal figure and him as the character that is manipulated into this space, thus effectively inverting the roles of the European woman and the Indigenous man common in captivity narratives at the time. Furthermore,

Hobomok's arrest in Mary Conant's magic circle does not end that night, as he eventually falls in love with her.

Indigenous religious rituals were often interpreted by Christian missionaries as magic. This reductionist view quickly morphed into a stereotype. A much-discussed prime example is Henry Wadsworth Longfellow's epic poem *The Song of Hiawatha* (1855), which, according to Nickerson, is one of the most popular literary works of the nineteenth-century United States. The image inaugurated in this poem of Hiawatha as an Iroquois leader from the Lake Superior region who has magic powers was imitated by various writers and soon after became the dominant narrative concerning this historical person (Nickerson). The short scene at the beginning of Child's novel effectively challenges this, at the time already established, myth of the "magic Indian" while simultaneously neutralizing the image of female witchcraft in the forest. Child's Puritan heroine not only feels at ease in the wilderness but also, most significantly, practices pagan rituals without being persecuted, thereby rewriting the US American stereotype of the threatening and potentially deadly witch. Moreover, when Hobomok, who himself is presented as a "high souled child of the forest," becomes her short-term husband, Mary joins him and his family in the wilderness and raises a son with them without being accused of transgressing Puritan moral and social standards (Child, *Hobomok* 141–42). Mary Conant is "turning the Puritan errand into a female quest," as Christopher Castiglia put it in a different context ("In Praise" 10).[2] What's more, Mary's life in the forest productively denounces the separation between the "city upon a hill" and "the howling wilderness," exposing its artificial makeup.[3]

But where does this leave Hobomok? Child's is a feminist take on the spectral forest, which, even more than Neal's transcultural focus, continues to build on the topic of noble savagery and supremacist psychology.[4] Reading Sedgwick's *Hope Leslie,* a novel published in 1827 and therefore only three years after *Hobomok,* Stacy Alaimo exposes how "the very valorization of Indians" was central to the text's feminism (*Undomesticated Ground* 37).[5] Alaimo suggests that Sedgwick, in envisioning "nature as the ground of female individual liberation, stands as somewhat of an anomaly in the nineteenth century" (*Undomesticated Ground* 38). Yet, the same is true for *Hobomok.* The configuration of Mary Conant as a strong female character depends on the scenes in the forest in opposition to those in the settlement. Life in the village is oppressive: "Even Hobomok, whose language was brief, figurative, and poetic, and whose nature was unwrapped by the artifices of civilized life, was far preferable to them" (Child, *Hobomok*

121). During a vulnerable period in her life, Conant inhabits "the woods" together with her husband Hobomok and his family. Yet, the plot presents Mary's Pequot family only as a nourishing environment that helps her regain her health and her strength. Upon her successful regeneration, the Indigenous characters fuse with the wilderness that she leaves behind. To construct a return to the now reformed society, Mary Conant needs to dispose of Hobomok, who, as in so many previous extinction narratives, conveniently decides to leave and then simply disappears in the forest. What Hobomok significantly leaves behind, yet again, is a tree: "the tender slip which he protected, has since become a mighty tree, and the nations of the earth seek refuge beneath its branches" (150).

Despite Child's effort to present Hobomok as a full character worthy of identification and sympathy, he serves Child's feminist purposes and is eventually abandoned, dying silently and secretly. Reminiscent of so many dying "Indians" in Freneau's poetry, before leaving "forever," Hobomok laments his faith (141), declaring: "And now, I will be buried among strangers, and none shall black their faces for the unknown chief" (149). In the next moment, he dutifully and conveniently disappears into the yet again darkened woods. Even in his hopes for an afterlife, prompted by the painful separation from his family, Hobomok hopes to meet "the Englishman's God" so that he can reunite with his wife and child (149). Postponing a happy life to a period after death while praying to a foreign God, Hobomok turns out to be simply yet another element in the growing colonial project that helps to build the trope of the regretful yet inevitable extinction of the Indigenous population.

Child had intended to avoid the dreaded trope of the Vanishing Indian, yet her reconfiguration of the spectral forest led the narrative exactly there. The novel certainly provided what Ann Douglas has described as an "*ex post facto* protest against the masculine solidities of the past" (185). As these have included the erasure of the Indigenous population, Mary Conant's romantic involvement with Hobomok presents an alternate history. The fact that this relationship ends in divorce only adds to the narrative's reconfiguration of power, as Puritan law at the time did not recognize any type of marriage annulment outside of its own courts. Yet, Mary instrumentalizes the "wilderness," taken to include her Indigenous husband, to demonstrate control over her own life. This relation only exposes that without an intersectional perspective that includes the environment, even the feminist liberation only enables further exploitation. The ease with which the protagonist moves between the settlement and the wilderness directly relates to her relationships with the Indigenous and the Puritan lover respectively. Hobomok, in this taxonomy, is the wilderness, a metaphor for her untamed nature, therefore for freedom. Brown stands for culture that she cannot enjoy without her freedom. In spite of all societal restrictions that contextualize both public spheres, settlement and wilderness, in her manipulation of visible and invisible forces, Mary, in the end, is in control of both.

The majestic reference to a global community that is protected by the branches that Hobomok became upon his death is supposedly signifying reverence. The tree, essentially, encapsulates the presence of the departed Hobomok, transforming the forest into a mortuary. This ecogothic signum, the undead tree, is an elemental part of Mary's freedom, as it circumscribes a space where she was able to live out her individuality. Mary and Hobomok are interconnected in a colonial embrace that both characters deny. Having cleansed herself of the hypocrisy of a life in the Puritan settlement through her time in the forest, Mary can go back and enjoy her newly discovered freedom enveloped in lightness and sunshine: "Her father clasped her in a long, affectionate embrace, and never to the day of his death, referred to a subject which was almost equally unpleasant to both" (149). Hobomok, however, never comes back. The forest, meanwhile, turns into an even darker space than it was before.

In his study *Forests: The Shadow of Civilization*, Harrison links the continuity of heathen traditions with the survival of the forest: "If certain elements of pagan culture survived the Christian revolution in covert forms, leaving their legacy in popular legends, fairy tales, and traditional folklore, it was thanks in part to the fact that Christian imperialism did not take it upon itself to burn down the forests in a frenzy of religious fervor, despite the enjoinder of certain ambiguous passages from the Old Testament" (62). In this theory, the persistence of the forest grants the persistence of non-Christian traditions. Writing against established patterns of frontier romance that designate the wilderness as a space for white men to establish their masculinity or Indigenous men to die,[6] Child's novel confirms Harrison's proposal, yet only under the erasure of those very "pagans" whose rites are being negotiated. Not only was Mary practicing a pagan ritual on the night depicted in the opening scene, but Hobomok and even the male narrator in the first chapter were themselves busy with their own rituals. Asked about the reason for his walk in the middle of the night, Hobomok explains his intention of performing an act of devotion by throwing a stick on "Manitto Asseinah," which the author explains in a footnote to be the term for "Spirit Rocks" (14). To this end, he, too, performs a short incantation and a specific ritual. And here it is again, the rock animated in relation to the Indigenous character, and the settler colonial character attracted by the same. Yet, Mary Conant practices her own magic, a pagan, proactive fertility rite, and survives.[7] Hobomok, on the other hand, dead at the end of the novel, fuses with the natural environment that once was his home. The forest is a space for moral cleansing for settler characters and remains a place to die for the Indigenous population.

Even the Christian narrator performs a type of magic with his secret act of cleansing through prayer. All three seek the forest to perform their rites, thus suggesting that this is both a sanctuary and a space that marks the limits of the knowable. Yet, only the settler characters survive. In the United States at the time, the forest already functions as a restricted pagan space itself. As trees and stones in settler colonial literary representations are one by one infused with souls of the Indigenous dead, the forest itself becomes "pagan," providing a space for European settlers to mark their independence from prescribed norms and restrictions, rather than enabling pagan cultures to survive.

As Hobomok and his family are effectively absorbed into the forest, their cultures are not preserved but erased. What is often referred to as "the woods" or "wilderness" in the novel is a spectral space that Mary Conant, as Hobomok's former wife, easily navigates, effectively replacing him and his family. She does not end up in captivity, nor does she die in childbirth as was common for female characters in sentimental novels of the time. This certainly affirms the (white) feminism of this text. By not complying with the doctrine of separate spheres and extending this space to "the wilderness," Mary Conant produces an alternate conception of living as a woman in a Puritan settlement.[8] This is a radical recoding, as the heroine is not only free to enter a self-determined bond with an Indigenous man but also to terminate it when her affection turns to another, at which point she effortlessly returns to the settlement. In this way, parts of the novel that are set in the forest challenge some of the most fundamental contradictions of American society at the time. Yet, the Indigenous protagonist, as centrally as he might be placed in this novel, providing even the title, receives a resolution only by disappearing in the woods. Rather than vanishing, he is transformed into a tree, giving his ghostly character a material presence. The act of transfiguration prevents his ghost from returning to haunt the living.

Bergland interpreted the opening scene with the magic ceremony in terms of its spectrality in *The National Uncanny*. As she points out, Mary Conant at first mistakes Hobomok for a ghost, and before that she herself is mistaken for a ghost by the Puritan narrator, who happened to see her run off (Bergland 64). This leads Bergland to conclude that "Child's description of a Native American man as a ghostly figure connects her to a tradition of Indian spectralization" (70). True, both Mary and Hobomok are at first mistaken for ghosts and thus "united by the fact that they are both perceived as ghostly beings" (Bergland 64). Mary Conant appears ghostly as a woman to a Puritan man, and Hobomok appears ghostly to Mary as a Puritan woman. Both characters do their part in spectralizing the other. Yet, there is more at stake in this scene than a simple spectralization, which, significantly, is not effective. Hobomok is not spectralized away in this scene. Instead, he becomes Mary Conant's husband. And Mary Conant has a very material presence herself; she is nursed to strength by Hobomok's family; she then effortlessly receives the divorce she wants and marries the man she loves, thus properly starting a new life. Even Hobomok does his share of spectralizing in this novel. While walking in the forest, he is the first to encounter Charles Brown, who is trying to find his way back from captivity to the settlement. Hobomok runs away, "his knees trembling against each other in excessive terror" while "casting back a fearful glance on what he supposed to be the ghost of his rival" (Child, *Hobomok* 138). After understanding that Brown, in fact, just returned from imprisonment "on the coast of Africa" (145), Hobomok "plunged into the thicket and disappeared" (140). Spectralizing does not emerge in the context suggested by Bergland in this novel, as it does not erase the characters' presence. Instead, the mutual act of mistaking each other for ghosts exposes the ways in which the characters are trained not to see each other. What's more, replacing visible bodies with the immaterial signs of those bodies is a mechanism that keeps their desires for the other in check.

What is productively spectralized in this novel is the forest. It is within this space that Hobomok's presence is erased and reconstituted in the form of a tree. The focus on the setting of the forest exposes the ways in which Child was reinterpreting the Puritan concept of the Invisible World. Puritans carefully cataloged various natural phenomena, such as fire, famine, and meteors, that they experienced as terrifying and interpreted as messages from God. To this list they added the Indigenous population, which in Puritan depictions appears demonized and often in the shape of the devil. Puritans were thus, as explained in the first chapter of this study, trained to see ghosts. Mary's fear of Hobomok and her eventual rescue that night by Brown demonstrate that she is subject to the same social upbringing. Cotton Mather was explicit in his assessment of the wilderness as the devil's natural habitat. In *Wonders of the Invisible World,* he writes: "Where was it that the Devil fell upon our Lord? It was when he was Alone in the Wilderness" (21). The devil was often accompanied by witches, who sought to covenant with the devil and were consequently potentially forming alliances with the "Indians." Mary Conant, as the figure of a witch, performing magic alone in the wilderness, demonstrates that navigating this space for a Puritan woman is always both a supernatural and a natural journey. Her seeing a ghost in Hobomok is a reaction that she knows how to unlearn. Through the performance of the magic ritual in the forest (witchcraft), Mary Conant claims the wilderness as a private space of freedom into which she invites the Indigenous man.⁹ Marrying him afterwards and forming a family with him is part of her unlearning. As this is not a bond made in love, it breaks. Seen from Mary Conant's perspective, this is a progressive move towards emancipation. She has successfully instrumentalized the magic of the forest for a feminist recodification of the doctrine of separate spheres that confined women to a domestic and passive role. For Hobomok, this reconfiguration of the settler power structures changes nothing, producing yet another lethal situation. Mary invites and discards him at will, reproducing the xenophobic structures that the author sought to challenge with this text.

Racialized Transfigurations and Environmental Degradation

Child's pronounced interest in European mysticism is well recorded. At the age of twenty, the author left Calvinistic Congregationalism and converted to Swedenborgianism.¹⁰ She was particularly interested in the denomination's teaching about a special correspondence between the natural and the spiritual world, which translates into some of the most notable passages in her writing. In *Hobomok,* she compares "spiritual light" to the "natural sun": "Spiritual light, like that of the natural sun, shines from one source and shines alike upon all; but it is reflected and absorbed in almost infinite variety; and in the moral, as well as the natural world, the diversity of the rays is occasioned by the nature of the recipient" (69). This and similar passages, in which the natural world serves the function of bringing one closer to a better understanding of the human intellect and reason as embedded in its environment, corresponds with central aspects of mystic teachings. In *The First Woman in the Republic,* Carolyn L. Karcher writes about Child's religious conversion and how it is reflected in *Hobomok:* "the attraction Mary feels for her Episcopalian and Indian lovers is at bottom the same. Both represent a fusion of nature and culture. Both foster the aesthetic impulses Puritan society condemns" (29). It is this lack that, in Karcher's opinion, has driven Child towards mysticism. Yet, it is important to filter the colonialism out of this progressive theory.

Already the excerpt above demonstrates that in Child's writing, not all recipients of the spiritual light have the same ability to absorb it. In fact, confirming Swedenborg's theories, some absorb it, and some are the light. Hobomok is more nature than human. The actual colonial process of spectralization in the moment when Hobomok is transformed into a tree is therefore effortless. Rather than being demonized, the Native character is now transfigured. Given the popularity of Child's *Hobomok* and similar narratives such as Sedgwick's *Hope Leslie,* these transfigurations that fuse the Indigenous population with the natural environment eventually produce images of national significance. While Child's mysticism might be grounded in the desire to fuse nature with culture in her feminist protagonists, it also creates antagonism between Indigenous nature and settler culture in a similar way as was done in Swedenborg's dualism between spiritual beings and those corrupted by reason. To demonstrate that this is systemic in Child's writing, I will add yet more examples that prove my point.

Child's insistent fear of environmental degradation, which she addressed in relation to the dispossession of the Indigenous population, produced numerous narratives that must finally be read as extinction narratives, in spite of the author's intention to produce counternarratives. In fact, nature, and particularly nature animated by the remains of dead Indigenous characters, is central to the extinction agenda in Child's writing. In the short story "The Lone Indian," for example, Powontonamo, the son of a Mohawk chief, "sighed to hear the strokes of the axe levelling the old trees of his forests. Sometimes he looked sorrowfully on his baby boy, and thought he had done him much wrong, when he smoked a pipe in the wigwam of the stranger" (Child, *Hobomok* 156). Powontonamo continues to mourn both the disappearance of his people and of "his forests": "the young oak and the vine are like the Eagle and the Sunny-eye. They are cut down, torn, and trampled on. The leaves are falling, and the clouds are scattering, like my people" (160). Even in well-intended laments like this, one can recognize (both male and female) settler colonial writers' inability to disentangle the Indigenous population from their conceptions of the forest. Before Powontonamo "depart[s] forever," he sighs: "I wish I could once more see the trees standing thick, as they did when my mother held me to her bosom, and sung the warlike deeds of the Mohawks" (160). Child's short story opposes dominant extinction narratives in relation to the Native population but leaves the extinction narrative in relation to nature uncontested. Associating the Indigenous population with deforestation confirms their supposed disappearance.

Child's texts that focus on Indigenous characters successfully reject the common separation between settlement and wilderness and even expose the hostile relationship that settlers exhibited towards nature;[11] and yet, it is through spectralizing forests with the bodies of the dead Indigenous characters that this effect is produced. This necropolitical conjunction becomes even more exposed in the short story "Chocoroua's Curse," first published in *The Token* in 1830. Child uses the framework of the explained supernatural to refer to settlers' conscience: "A curse upon ye, white men! May the Great Spirit curse ye when he speaks in the clouds, and his words are fire! [. . .] The Evil Spirit breathe death upon your cattle! Your graves lie in the war path of the Indian! Panthers howl, and wolves fatten over your bones! Chocorua goes to the Great Spirit—his curse stays with the white men!" (Child, *Hobomok* 166). These are the last words of Chocorua, a man formerly acknowledged as a prophet, who is shot and whose bones are left "to whiten in the sun" (166). His curse is effective: "the winds tore up trees and hurled them at their dwellings, their crops were blasted, their cattle died, and sickness came upon their strongest men" (166). Yet again opening a space situated somewhere between the natural and the supernatural, the narrator concludes: "To this day the town of Burton, in New-Hampshire, is remarkable for a pestilence which infects its cattle; and the superstitious think that Chocorua's spirit still sits enthroned upon his precipice, breathing a curse upon them" (167). The ghost of Chocorua is not an apparition. It materializes in the form of a local pandemic. The supernatural, once again established in relation to land, productively enables a national imaginary that not only seals the disappearance of the original inhabitants but even manages to demonize them again. The exposure of the settlers' dependence on their nonhuman environments takes place in relation to the fusion of Indigenous spiritualities with this habitat.

Child further develops the motif of nature animated by Indigenous spirits in relation to settler colonial characters in her subsequent publications. Rejecting Irving's European recoding of grounds haunted by European spirits, she proposes visions of forests infused with the spirits of dead Indigenous characters, whose stories are recalled in her writing. In a peculiar ghost story, "She Waits in the Spirit Land," for example, the narrator follows the awakening physical love between Wah-bu-nung-o (Morning Star) and O-ge-bu-no-qua (Wild Rose). First published in 1846 as part of *Fact and Fiction: A Collection of Stories*, this text records the happiness of the two lovers: "Fortunately for the free and beautiful growth of their love, they lived out of the pale civilization. There was no Mrs. Smith to remark how they looked at each other, and no Mrs. Brown to question the propriety of their rambles in the woods" (Child, *Hobomok* 193–94). It is again in "the limitless forest" where "the tall trees were of noble proportions, because they had room enough to grow upward and outwards, with a strong free grace" that the two "handsome" lovers live out their sexuality freely (195). The feminist effort at redefining society is prominent in this text as well. Legal marriage is exposed as superficial in the context of love and sexuality: "There was no person to object, whenever he chose to lead her into his wigwam, and by that simple circumstance she became his wife" (196). Exposing Christian romantic bonds as procuring sin where there is none, civilization is deemed "artificial" and "filthy" (194). Different than Neal's confused warriors, these lovers speak the language of nature, completing the visions of freedom for Euro-American Puritan women. The visions of non-Euroamerican women and men, even in this celebratory context, are tuned to tragedy: "Indian music, like the voice of inanimate nature, the wind, the forest, and the sea, is almost invariably in the minor mode; and breathed as it now was the silent moon, and with the shadow of the dream interpretation still resting on their souls, it was oppressive mournfulness" (196). Child romanticizes the wilderness as a utopia where nature and "Indians" are not only in sync, they literally fuse. The two lovers, pronouncedly celebrated as uncivilized, merge with a rosebush when they, one after the other, lay down to die in "the Isle of Willows," where one's "loved one had lain upon his breast" (198). The "rose-bush" that became a symbol of their love is still there, even after "the human Rose had passed away, to return no more" (198). The character with the programmatic name Rose thus literally transforms upon death into the plant. Transformed into a decorative ornament, she will "return no more," not even as a ghost. Tired of the "filthy" civilization, her lover lays down under the very same rosebush in the Isle of Willows and dies. Finally, they reunite in "the spirit-land" (201). Even while celebrating the purity of love, including its physicality, Child's "Indian" bodies can exist only as figurations of nature. The hyperphysicality of Cooper's Indigenous and settler characters and Neal's tragic mixed-blood warriors is replaced in Child's oeuvre with images of *natural* sexuality transformed into yet another version of "the vegetation of death" (Neal, "Critical Essays" 253), thus affirming rather than revising exclusionary visions of colonial settler-native relations.

The publication of *Hobomok* hit a nerve at the time, turning Child into a new star of American literature. Writing in the 1820s, a period marked by the promise generated among the European population by the Monroe

Doctrine and an air of reform, Child's recoding of the forest is primarily concerned with white feminism. In 1821, only two years before *Hobomok* was published, Emma Hart Willard founded the first endowed school for girls, the Troy Female Seminary in New York. The education of women was proposed most prominently by Catherine Maria Sedgwick, a writer that Child is often paired with in current scholarship. It is within this cultural sentiment that Child reclaims both the natural and the supernatural as a space of settler women's empowerment in her novel. Its central topics of miscegenation and community-building in the wilderness set the tone as a feminist agenda for future writers, which is confirmed in the success of Sedgwick's *Hope Leslie; or, Early Times in the Massachusetts,* published only three years after Child's novel, in 1827. Sedgwick takes the issue of female individualism as "rooted in nature as an alternative ground of values" even further (Alaimo, *Undomesticated Ground* 16). In outright scenes of supernatural possession, healing rituals that include rattlesnakes and chanting, various demonstrations of Invisible World agency, all taking place within the protective space of the forest, *Hope Leslie* provides its heroines with supernatural agency away from patriarchal oversight, but only to unwillingly affirm "Indian Removal" in images of the fusion of dead Indigenous bodies with the wilderness.[12] Spectralizing the forest is thus a trope of the early feminist frontier romance that occupies a central place in efforts at redefining gender relations in settler colonial constellations, but only at the cost of affirming the trope of the Vanishing Indian.

To conclude, analyzing Child's use of the supernatural in the context of the forest raises important questions about ecofeminism, the defining claim of which is that the destruction of nature is linked to the oppression of women.[13] The ecofeminist effort in Child's narrative cannot serve as a corrective with a potential of breaking down the binaries of human/nature and nature/culture, because Hobomok marked as natural is excluded from her category of the human. Tracing how the spectralization of the forest with disappearing Indigenous bodies in this and similar narratives is grounded in these very dualisms foregrounds the crucial role of an intersectional approach that renegotiates whose freedom and thus humanity was constructed against the centrality of the nonhuman.

Drawing magic circles around "Indians" in the "American forest" establishes a very different image of the haunted forest to those proposed by Washington Irving and John Neal. In Irving's oeuvre, settler characters collect "Indian" and "African" bones that they find in the haunted ground of New England to perform their own private rituals, inscribing themselves in the land as stewards and thus replacing the Indigenous population. In Neal's writing, warriors of mixed Anglo-Saxon and Indigenous heritage, and a British nobleman passing as "Indian," are associated with the wilderness they inhabit and in which their lives end. These grounds are haunted by their ghosts, the act of which does not necessarily replace the Indigenous cultures but, in its transcultural haunting, proposes a shared doom. Analyzing the element of spectral forests using an ecogothic lens in Child's texts, rather than focusing on her feminism, makes clear that as much as she insists to the contrary, her works do not correct the "general misapprehension" about "the conduct of Indians." In contrast to Irving and Neal, Child installs a spectral forest in order to reclaim this space for white female emancipation. She repurposes and thus extends the genre of the national romance popular at the time, exclusively in the service of Euro-American feminism under the exclusion of the colonial framework within which she writes. Spectrality here serves the function of emancipating Puritan women at the cost of codifying nature as "Indian," with the effect of further solidifying the colonial nature/culture antagonism. Far from an acknowledgment of an Indigenous relationship with land, this codification of nature is part of the colonial effort to excuse the dispossession and genocide of Indigenous populations as *natural*.

Harriet Beecher Stowe's Tales of the Supernatural

While Harriet Beecher Stowe's novels are certainly not lacking in scholarly interest, her ghost stories are seldom the subject of literary analysis. Taking a closer look at her tales that include the supernatural reveals telling congruities with Irving's ghost stories. Juxtaposing Irving's with Stowe's ghost stories discloses specific settler colonial patterns that complicate the few scholarly interpretations of Stowe's tales, most of which claim an emancipatory framing. Barbara Patrick deems Stowe's "The Ghost in Cap'n Brown House" to be one of the three "best tales using the conventions of the ghost story to veil feminist concerns" (75). In "Stowe and Regionalism," Pryse argues that Stowe skillfully employs the comic "do-nothing" Sam Lawson "to write sketches that shift the center of perception to marginal and socio-economically disenfranchised characters" (148). Likewise, Jeffrey Weinstock ascribes feminist intentions to Stowe's ambiguous construction of a "ghost," who may be a real woman held captive in the house as a way to "foreground the unsettling realities of women's lives—the entrapment and subjugation of women to patriarchal, legal, and class structures that systematically confine and disempower them" (*Scare Tactics* 41). Again, all of these readings lack an intersectional approach, with the result that none of these critics considers the racially marked characters in Stowe's ghost stories. In this section, I analyze those characters and compare Stowe's narrative style to Irving's tales and Child's trope of racialized transfiguration in order to demonstrate the extent of their influential topicalization of the blackened spectral informant and its settler colonial purposes.

Mostly narrated by the character of Sam Lawson, who first appears in *Oldtown Folks* (1869), Stowe's ghost stories in many ways resemble the tales by Irving already analyzed in chapter four. The collection of stories *Oldtown Folks* introduces the reader to Oldtown, "originally an Indian town," where "the great apostle of the Indians had established the first missionary enterprise among them, under the patronage of a society in England for the propagation of the Gospel in foreign parts" (Stowe, *Oldtown Folks* 887). Native American towns are introduced in markedly colonial terms as the past rather than as the present or even as a heritage. Narrated in the manner of Irving's Knickerbocker tales, the collection is a manuscript presented as a historical study of Oldtown by the amateur historian Horace Holyhoke. And just like Knickerbocker, Holyhoke assures the reader of being an objective observer and knowing the neighborhood intimately: "I have tried to maintain the part simply of a sympathetic spectator" (884). After introducing the origin of the town in an Indigenous past, Holyhoke very quickly moves on to propose that "the children of the forest, [are] a race destined to extinction with the progress of civilization" (890). It is pronouncedly "civilization" that advances the Native population toward extinction. As in the previous texts, civilization here stands for the settler population, qualifying *Oldtown Folks* as a proper replacement narrative.

Stowe is even more pronounced than Irving and Child in her narrative fusion of the Indigenous dead with US forests. Her narrator claims that the people who originally lived in the region simply could not "avert the doom which seems to foreordain that those races shall dry up and pass away with their native forests, as the brook dries up when the pine and hemlocks which shaded its source are town away" (887). As in Child's short stories, Stowe's narrators promote a vision of forest degradation or loss as the reduction or extinction of the Native population. Both are seen as needed to clear the way for civilization to spread. The, at that time already firmly established, myth of the Vanishing Indian is presented in its common style as part of a natural cycle that is inevitable and unstoppable. Along with this established myth, narratives such as this one regularly promote the inevitability of forest loss. Even worse, the forests need to go in order for the settlers to be able to account for the lack of Indigenous presence.

Like Irving's narrators, Stowe's ghost storyteller is the "village do-nothing," a character who is fully integrated in the small-town community and at the same time an outsider to its rules and regulations—he is the anomaly that proves the existence of order. It is from this informed and objective position that her narrator claims the interlocked disappearance of nature and those inhabitants perceived as part of nature. Their humanity is therefore of a different kind; the type that is receding in the face of civilization, which is represented by the settler population.

The concentric narrative structure is retained as well: Sam's ghost stories about "Indians" are collected by Holyoke and preserved for posterity. Keeping most elements in place, Stowe moved from Irving's fantastic spiritual encounters that insinuate extinction, to plain extinction in the name of progress. Repeating and affirming the topos of the Vanishing Indian only marginally in the introduction, the narrator, Holyhoke, quickly moves on to tell his personal story. The collection opens with the death of Holyhoke's father, which the narrator uses as an opportunity to introduce the inhabitants of Oldtown, a small part of which are "four or five respectable Indian families" and "a few negroes" (927–29): "let me not forget dear, jolly old Caesar, my grandfather's own negro, the most joyous creature on two feet. What could not Caesar do? He could gobble like a turkey so perfectly as to deceive the most experienced old gobbler on the farm; he could crow so like a cock that all the cocks in the neighborhood would reply to him; he could mew like a cat, and bark like a dog; he could sing and fiddle, and dance the double-shuffle, and was *au fait* in all manner of jigs and horn-pipes" (Stowe, "Oldtown Folks" 930). As in Irving's tales, in order to establish a background against which a Euro-American "well-regulated New England family" could be presented in a joyful domestic setting, animalized African American characters are framed by stories about Native Americans vanishing "with their native forests" (903). Stowe's narrator makes no effort to conceal his social hierarchy based on racial markers: "And now, having taken my readers through the lower classes in our meeting-house, I must, in order of climax, represent to them our higher orders" (931). The introduction continues with a presentation of European settler colonial families.

The title of the chapter "In My Grandmother's Kitchen" already marks the importance of the domestic setting, as grandmother's house on a Sunday afternoon becomes the meeting ground for neighbors involved in politics as well as gossip, wandering and hungry "Indian women," the

ghost-storyteller Sam Lawson, and the servant "black Caesar." These detailed and didactic domestic introductions are, similarly to Irving's tales,
the settings for ghost stories to be told. And again, it is the "village-do-
nothing" of Oldtown, Sam Lawson, known to spend much time with "Indian families," who has access to Indigenous knowledge. Like Irving, Stowe
is using detailed descriptions to establish the absence of Indigenous characters by insisting on the presence of their "friends" who can relate their
stories. Aside from Lawson, the grandmother fills this role. A repeated jux-
taposition between a settler colonial community and "them" (Indigenous
inhabitants) is the common narrative structure in these tales. The reader
learns that the grandmother "not only gave *them* food but, more than once
would provide *them* with blankets, and allow *them* to lie down and sleep
by *her* great kitchen fire" ("Oldtown Folks" 902; emphasis added). The
narrative structure insistently separates the population of Oldtown into
benevolent settlers and native recipients.

A ghost story once again proves to be the perfect framework for this
binary strategy. While grandmother decides to feed "two hungry Indian
women" with "snaky eyes gleaming with appetite" (958–59), Sam Lawson
happens to be present and asks the women about the "haunted house" (961).
Even after marking them as spectral informants, the animalized women
never receive the opportunity to respond. Their bodies are only there to be
fed by the grandmother. Instead, Sam tells the story of the haunted house
in which a man lived with his servant in a romantic relationship because of
which he was expelled from society. Only "people that wanted to be splen-
didly entertained, and that were not particular as to morals, used to go out
to visit them" (963). The first haunted house is thus a house placed outside
of the common moral restrictions of a New England small town. Again,
the ghost that materializes is of European descent. The apparition turns out
to be "a figger of a man [...] in a long red cloak," a feature which helped to
identify him as Sir Harry Frankland, the amoral ambassador. No headless
apparitions or chain-clanking ghosts appear to entertain the assembled
group of villagers; the haunting is solely a prerequisite or rather a framework that holds ethnic and racial constellations of a typical New England
town in place. Holyhoke concludes: "So passed an evening in my grandmother's kitchen, where religion, theology, politics, the gossip of the day,
and the legend of the supernatural all conspired to weave a fabric of thought
quaint and various" (965). In this way, Stowe's tales continue the tradition
established by Irving in his ghost stories, of grounding the binarism between rational settler characters who listen and tell ghost stories and racialized characters as spectral informants and the supernatural themselves. Just

like Irving's tales, they serve the didactic purpose of establishing exclusive living conditions based on racial distinctions.

Various characters from *Sam Lawson's Oldtown Fireside Stories* (1881)— the collection by Stowe that contains numerous ghost stories—are first introduced in *Oldtown Folks*. Keturah, "a regular old heathen Injun" and a "witch," is one of these reappearing characters (1067). In *Oldtown Folks,* she is introduced on the side of her husband, "the praying Indian," as "a creature" who "had retained in most respects the wild instincts and untamed passions of the savage" (927). No church or baptism could encourage her to abandon "the practice of her old heathen superstitions" ("Oldtown Folks" 928). It is with "terror and delight" that the narrator remembers "Old Keturah," who he introduces as "one of the wonders of my childhood" (928). Not her actions but Keturah herself *is* the wonder. Congratulating himself for his charitable inclusion of nonsettler characters in a communal space experienced as exclusive, the narrator creates a formal structure within which the population is separated in binary opposites and arranged within a mutual space fixed in oppositional social roles: "But such as we were, high and low, good and bad, refined and illiterate, barbarian and civilized, negro and white, the old meeting-house united us all on one day of the week, and its solemn services formed an insensible but strong bond of neighborhood charity" (940). Again, working under the premise of inclusive exclusion, the narrative structure of *Oldtown Folks* is based on first-person accounts and dialogues. This allows for a seemingly objective experience placing the reader in the position of an onlooker who learns about the communal life in a New England town. Keturah is the wonder within this structure.

Stowe returns to the character of Keturah in *Sam Lawson's Oldtown Fireside Stories.* The first story of the collection, entitled "The Ghost in the Mill," features Ketury, an Indigenous woman solely defined in association with the supernatural and the "Devil" (*Oldtown Fireside Stories* 16). In spite of the slightly different spelling of the name, it is clear that Stowe intended to recreate the same character in her descriptions of Ketury's resistance to common values and to those of her Christian husband. The narrator explains that despite her marriage to "one o' the prayin' Indians you couldn't no more convert *her* than you could convert a wild-cat or a panther" (*Oldtown Fireside Stories* 16), leaving no doubt as to the correspondence between the two characters.

It is in this, so far little interpreted, tale that we can find the most important features of Stowe's ghost stories. Ketury's story is introduced as part of America's uncontrolled and uncontrollable history that nevertheless is

tamed within the colonial domain of the supernatural. Ketury's disobedience to the system in place is transformed into a supernatural voice of
morality that corrects the settler colonial population, reducing her presence
to a defining characteristic of settler colonial lives. Extending her characterization as the Noble Savage to the domain of the supernatural restricts
her scope of influence to that domain.[14] Her ontology as the irrational
is absorbed within the settler colonial self-image as "civilization" that leaves
no one behind:

> I've seen her sit and look at Lady Lothrop out o' the corner o' her eyes; and her
> old brown baggy neck would kind o' twist and work; and her eyes they looked
> so, that 'twas enough to scare a body. For all the world, she looked jest as if she
> was a-workin' up to spring at her. Lady Lothrop was jest as kind to Ketury as
> she always was to every poor crittur. She'd bow and smile as gracious to her
> when meetin' was over, and she come down the aisle, passin' oot o, meetin';
> but Ketury never took no notice. (16)

Far from social inclusion, Ketury's presence in the church is a welcome opportunity for reinforcement of racial and colonial attitudes and ensuring
their lasting effects into the future. At first presented as a source of amusement and information, this "chimney-corner story-telling" is framed as a
way of preserving narratives about the past for posterity: "Then, the aged
told their stories to the young,—tales of war and adventure, of forest-days,
of Indian captivities and escapes, or bears and wild-cats and panthers, or
rattlesnakes, of witches and wizards, and strange and wonderful dreams and
appearances and providences" (2–3). The Puritan link between "Indian captivities" and "appearances and providences" is here reactivated for purposes
of postcolonial romantic primitivism and settler colonial cultural authority.
"Indians" appear next to panthers, witches, and ghosts, embedded within
tales that the "aged" are passing onto the next generation. One of these
stories told by Sam Lawson contains an introduction of Ketury, an outsider within: "Her father was one o'them great powwows down to Martha's
Vineyard; and people used to say she was set apart, when she was a child, to
the service o'the Devil: any way, she never could be made nothing' of in a
Christian way" (16). Here too the Puritan association between the Indigenous population and the Devil is reconfirmed, just as it was in Irving's and
Hawthorne's writing. The village inhabitants obviously not of Indigenous
origin do not know how to associate with such a satanic being as Ketury
except through witchcraft: "Everybody thought that Ketury was a witch: at
least, she knew consid'able more'n she ought to know, and so they was kind

o' 'fraid on her" (16). Imposing a recognizable order across social experiences, Ketury is marked in the Puritan tradition as a satanic spiritual being able to impose harm on others. By describing a small settler community that integrates the Indigenous character Ketury as an outsider to one's own habits and regulations, Stowe's narrative renders the Indigenous character unintelligible. This, in turn, is helpful when affirming one's own postcolonial distinctiveness. Transcultural relations between Christian settlers and satanic Indigenous characters are presented as simply impossible. A comparison between the characters of Mary Conant and Ketury can forward the understanding of this trope. Both Mary Conant and Ketury are at first presented as witches. Conant's engagement with the supernatural is playful and therefore in control, whereas Ketury exists exclusively in relation to the supernatural. Rather than as a source of power, the reader perceives her access to magic rituals as a distinction.

One night, Ketury appears to two drunk villagers. Presented in the manner of a ghost, she arrives "on the wind" and leaves no traces in the snow (Stowe, *Oldtown Fireside Stories* 19). Literally nature itself, she is disembodied but visible. Cack and Cap'n Eb had just made a fire in a remote old mill in which they planned to spend the night to wait out the bad weather and high snow, when they heard her knocking at the door. Shortly after being let in, she placed herself in front of the chimney and began calling out loud: "'Come down, come down! Let's see who ye be'" (19). With the help of this incantation, Ketury slowly pieces together one fragment after another of a complete human body. Commencing with the feet and closing with the head, she assembles the body of a peddler, a stranger who used to frequent the village twice a year. As a consequence of Ketury's frightful appearance and her supernatural performance, Cack admits to having helped his father bury the dead body of the peddler Lommedieu. His father murdered the man for his money. The assembled body is the ghost of Lommedieu. Even though Cack was only an assistant to his father when he helped to hide the corpse in this very chimney out of which the body was taken out by Ketury, he commits suicide a couple of days later.

What is the role of Ketury in this narrative, who appears on the wind and disappears after exposing the murder of the father? I want to propose that Ketury presents the disembodied morality theorized by Swedenborg as non-European. In the settler colonial US American context, this type of ghost appears in the figuration of an Indigenous woman. As a married woman who is integrated in the local community as an anomaly, she is presented as an immaterial body that leaves no trace and has no trouble surmounting severe weather. Fusing with the image of nature, she is neither the ghost nor the host. Her assembling of the spectral body marks her presence as a corrective to the erroneous behavior of the two settler characters guilty of murder. After the exposure of the ghost to the ghost-seer, order is reinstalled in the picturesque settlement. Like the animated forest that appears to have a will of its own, Ketury is a medium through which settler characters reinstall their moral integrity. Sam Lawson explains to the reader: "So there you see, boys, there can't be no iniquity so hid but what it'll come out. The wild Indians of the forest, and the stormy winds and tempests, j'ined together to bring out this 'ere" (22). The nameless spirits of Indigenous provenance in Irving's forests receive a full-bodied characterization in Stowe's Ketury, who materializes only to merge with atmospheric disturbance into a magical tool for the reinstallation of settler colonial earthly justice.

Ketury's function within a carefully constructed New England community exceeds that of the African spectral informants introduced by Irving. Ketury marks a settler colonial fantasy not only of an Indigenous presence stripped of humanness but also of nature stripped of sovereignty. Both serve settler colonial purposes: as a supernatural being in convergence with nature, Ketury literally unveils the corpses hidden in New England's closets (or chimneys). This seemingly marginal character encodes important tropes of antebellum literature: the irrepresentability of Indigenous femininity and a geographical, ontological, and historical lack inscribed in Indigenous characters "too 'alien' to comprehend."[15] The socio-spatial denial that Ketury experiences in her spectral travels are a building block in settler colonial fantasies of contractualness. Other than in everyday life, as a nonhuman creature belonging to a parallel reality, Ketury not only complies with but even promotes the earthly laws prescribed by the settler community. She is thus yet another settler colonial fantasy of internal exclusion, of Indigenous life accepted only in relation to death.

Stowe was a spiritualist. This, in no small part, was due to the constant presence of death in her life. Harriet Beecher was five years old when, in 1816, her mother died after having given birth to nine children in fifteen years. When she reached the age of nineteen, her best friend, Eliza Ellis Stowe, passed away. Only one year later, Eliza's widowed husband proposed to Harriet, and she accepted. After marrying into a family marked by death, the young woman gave birth to a child that she named Eliza in honor of her deceased friend and her husband's former wife. On July 6, 1843, a few weeks before the birth of her third daughter, Georgiana May, Stowe received notice that her brother, the Rev. George Beecher, walked out into his garden to shoot birds and soon after was found dead of a gunshot wound. Six years later, in the early summer of 1849, cholera broke out in Cincinnati.

Among the hundreds of victims that the epidemic claimed daily was Stowe's infant child Charley. In 1857, her oldest son, Henry Ellis, drowned while bathing in the Connecticut River close to his dorm at Dartmouth College. Stowe was to lose another daughter to morphine addiction, and another son, who vanished at sea in California. Out of seven of the children that Harriet Beecher Stowe cared for and raised, only three survived her legacy: Hattie Beecher, Eliza Tyler, and Charles Edward.

To cope with the immediate and constant presence of death in her life, Stowe became a devoted spiritualist who fervently engaged in theories about communicating with the dead.[16] Even before calling herself explicitly a spiritualist, Stowe had formulated ideas that resembled spiritual thought. In 1849, the year when her first child died and one year after the Fox sisters initiated the institutionalization of spiritualism in the United States, Stowe published an article in the *New York Evangelist* entitled "The Ministration of Departed Spirits": "as we advance in our journey, and voice after voice is hushed, and form after form vanishes from our side, and our shadow falls almost solitary on the hill-side of life, the soul, by a necessity of being, tends to the unseen and spiritual, and pursues in another life those it seeks in vain in this" ("Ministration" 98). In this article, later republished by the American Society for Psychical Research, Stowe develops her theory of spiritualism, which centers upon the question of how emotional strength can be gained through a voluntary belief in the postmortal existence of deceased family members and friends. She proposes that with the help of imagination, one could find peace, understand the necessity of death, and cope with the shortcomings of one's own life by hoping for a life after death. Although the question of proof was of central concern for intellectuals at her time, Stowe is not concerned with the validity of her emotional support system. For her, the belief in the existence of spirits is a "necessity of being." Without pretending to follow scientific method, she presents her conclusion as a "beautiful belief," thus a matter of personal choice. People who have not "familiarized themselves with that unknown" she simply pitied as "poor." Her theory proposes that the work of imagination allows for integrating the unknown into the sphere of the familiar. Seeking to combine her Christian beliefs with these spiritualist affections, Stowe explains in the same article that even the Bible indicates "that there is a class of invisible spirits who minister to the children of men." This theory of spirits ministering to the living remained at the center of Stowe's literature for the rest of her writing career. Stowe's biographer Nancy Koester even shifts spirituality into the center, claiming that it was a defining influence on Stowe's work and her life alike.

Given the centrality of spirituality and the importance of at least meta-physically providing a space in life for the presence of the dead, it is striking that Stowe chooses a living Indigenous woman to "minister to the children of man" in the character of Ketury. As an act of alienation rather than ac-commodation, Ketury's supernatural practices depart strongly from spiri-tualist genealogies. Also, in spite of numerous correspondences between Indigenous and spiritualist practices, these two belief systems never merged in Stowe's work nor life. In his study of late nineteenth-century spiritualism, John Kucich proposes a broader definition of spiritualism, one that includes non-European sources: "The genealogy of American spiritualism includes, I will argue, not merely European occultism, but the myriad African and Na-tive American religions that mingled on this continent; its manifestations include not just the Rochester rapping, but a broad array of creole spiritual-isms, from hoodoo to Santería, from the Virgin of Guadalupe to the Ghost Dance, and from faith healing to angelmania" (4). Apart from perhaps "angelmania," none of these features are acknowledged in Stowe's version of spiritualism. Instead, there is a clear separation in her writing between those ghosts that, for example, Holyhoke *can see* versus the ghostly charac-ter of Ketury, who *is* material but leaves no trace. Holyhoke is presented as a typical spiritualist ghost-seer, whereas Ketury is ghostly herself. As a ho-modiegetic narrator, Holyhoke receives the opportunity to share his feel-ings about seeing ghosts: "The peculiarity of my own mental history had this effect on me from a child, that it wholly took away from me all dread of the supernatural" (*Oldtown Fireside Stories* 1066). Ketury, on the other hand, not only never receives a voice of her own; she *is* the dreaded supernatural. Not a ghost proper nor fully human, she bursts all common registers. Her appearance does not acquaint the reader with the Indigenous spirituality or with European spiritualist manners. On the contrary, her knowledge of the spirit world is setting her apart while putting the reader at a distance. Even as devoted a spiritualist as Stowe drew a stark colonial line between settler ghosts and the ghostly Indigenous characters. The double structure introduced by Irving that separates illegible Indigenous ghostly characters from familiar European ghosts, therefore, only further highlighted this imaginary line of separation. In spite of her spiritualism, Stowe's writing is not only repeating but pronouncedly enforcing the narrative structures laid out by Irving and Child, reminding us that even immaterial bodies are not safe from cultural erasure.

The Politics of Presence

Ghosts in Slave Narratives

> In this world which we enter, appearing from a nowhere, and from
> which we disappear into a nowhere, *Being and Appearing coincide.*
> [...] Nothing and nobody exists in the world whose very being
> does not presuppose a spectator.
> —Hannah Arendt, *The Life of the Mind*

Henry Louis Gates Jr. discovered Hannah Crafts' *The Bondwoman's Narrative* at an auction; when he published the text in 2002, the prominent scholar of African and African American literature introduced it as "the first novel written by a woman who had been a slave" (Crafts xxv). What qualifies this text as the "first" work of literary fiction, rather than autobiography, by a female enslaved person is, among others, the intentional gothic framework that asserts its fictionality. Until the discovery of this manuscript, Harriet E. Wilson's *Our Nig,* published in 1859, was considered the first novel written by an African American woman and formerly enslaved person. The discovery thus created quite a stir in the literary community.

Critics and scholars disagree about the generic typology of this text. The Nigerian scholar and novelist Adebayo Williams calls the text, which was likely completed in 1853 and never previously published, "an engrossing literary paradox," for its genre oscillates between fact and fiction (139). There is still no consensus on how to read the text appropriately. The African American literary scholar Hollis Robbins, who together with Henry Louis Gates Jr. edited the collection of critical essays on *The Bondwoman's Narrative,* opted for "something completely new" (Robbins 82). Gates saw in Crafts' narrative "a source of fascination as a testament to the will of a black woman determined to utilize fiction both to indict her oppressor and testify to her own irresistible desire to be free" (Gates quoted in Crafts xi). In his reading, fiction yields to autobiography and becomes an instrument of personal expression. Others, such as Robert S. Levine, have defended the craftsmanship and poetology of the text, even going so far as to propose that the discovery of Crafts' text calls for a redefinition of slave narratives in general, since it testifies to an unacknowledged, yet lively and functioning, literary culture among enslaved people. As succinctly summarized in a review of the publication: "The market reader is contradictorily seduced by a text which is offering very different things: a black woman's true story or a novel; a raw, unmediated narrative; or a work guaranteed by a reputed editor and authority" (Bernier and Newman 150).

Harriet Jacobs' *Incidents in the Life of a Slave Girl* is another important slave narrative written by a woman that has introduced voices and perspectives in the text other than that of the narrator (Yellin). Her specific style had already sparked long-lasting debates about the fictionality—or rather, the untrustworthiness—of the text. This led William L. Andrews to introduce the phrase "novelized slave narratives" to describe narratives that allow multiple perspectives and as such venture away from autobiography towards fiction (275). Crafts' publication sparked the debate yet again, in particular for its application of gothic elements. Even if adjusted to fit a slave narrative, gothic paraphernalia feature prominently in the novel: haunting, ghosts, animated portraits, a family curse, villains, and a maiden in distress. In addition, structural elements, such as narrative cliff-hangers and an intradiegetic narrator who determines the rhythm of the narration, recall classic structures of gothic novels. Various passages either resemble or directly quote from famous gothic texts: Horace Walpole's *The Castle of Otranto,* Charlotte Brontë's *Jane Eyre,* Walter Scott's *Rob Roy,* and most prominently, Charles Dickens's *Bleak House.*[1]

This chapter responds to the much-debated question, is *The Bondwoman's Narrative* by Hannah Crafts a gothic novel? As a slave narrative written probably sometime in 1852 or 1853 and discovered at an auction only in 2002, the text raises an important question: how does a gothic novel written by a racialized and enslaved person fit into a genre which, as the previous chapters have established, rests upon a racialization of the Other, either "Indian" or "Black"? Answering this question is particularly important because it not only illuminates even more clearly the fundamental function of race as a motif and structural element in the American gothic but also the role of nature in establishing the same. Perhaps precisely because this narrative mode is founded upon a racialization, numerous scholars have assumed that the gothic is an exclusively white genre. Others, most prominently Maisha L. Wester, read the American gothic even as race theory ("Gothic"). Focusing on ghosts and ghostliness, this chapter demonstrates that Crafts' text offers a unique opportunity to both revise the narrative authority of slave authors and recognize the central role

African American antebellum authors have played in what has come to be called US American gothic literature, by acknowledging the constitutive role African animism has played in slave narratives and the cultures of enslaved people.

The Gothic Slave Narrative

Dale Townshend offers the most thorough reading of the gothic mode at work in *The Bondwoman's Narrative*. Tellingly, his analysis includes not only the manuscript but also paratextual elements, most importantly the spirited introduction written by Gates. In his poignant examination, Townshend recognizes a gothic device in the framing of the text. This device was also employed in Horace Walpole's *The Castle of Otranto;* indeed, it has been present since the very inception of the gothic novel. Like Walpole, who claimed his role as a "textual editor, curator and translator and insisted to be making available to his enlightened, late eighteenth-century readership a documentary trace of the 'darkest ages of Christianity'" with the help of a found manuscript (Walpole quoted in Townshend 142), Gates claimed that his random discovery from "'the depths of the black past' of nineteenth-century American culture and political history" would enlighten the current readership in regard to US American history (Townshend 142). The gothic, thus, to a certain degree relies on the framing rather than on the content, which is why it is often discussed as a mode rather than a genre.

Intertwining fact and fiction on various levels, Townshend's reading proposes the gothic not only as a narrative element, or even a genre, but also as a network within which the slave narrative is conveniently nestled. Teresa A. Goddu was one of the early voices among literary scholars who attested to an intrinsic connection between the gothic mode and not only this narrative but slave narratives in general (Goddu *Gothic America*).[2] Yet Goddu remains careful regarding the instrumentalization of the gothic in addressing slavery: "by recasting history in the terms of a familiar fiction, the Gothic had the potential to dematerialize those horrors by turning an historical reality into an imaginative effect" ("African American Slave Narrative" 73). Her conclusion leads to the assumption that writing fiction is not helpful in escaping prescribed roles: "In the end, the slave remains stuck playing the terrified victim in the antislavery movement's Gothic story line" (79).

The English literature scholar Priscilla Wald went so far as to deny the text its gothic quality altogether, insisting in the opening sentence of her essay on Crafts' slave narrative: "it is not a haunted text" (213). In doing so, Wald follows scholars such as Laura Doyle, who argues that any choice within writing a slave narrative "was constrained because the story line of slavery was already possessed by whites" (255). The slave's story was "already-framed on arrival" and "overwritten" as a gothic text (Doyle 255–56). In the interpretations of Goddu, Doyle, and Wald, the character of the slave is reduced to a categorical placeholder prescribed by the gothic "white" framework. Moreover, the author is restricted by the implicit racially marked structure and consequently loses control over the text.

Although restricted to her role as a slave, Crafts' narrator, Hannah, and the author herself were far from "playing the terrified victim[s]" within a "white" world, as Goddu suggested.[3] Instead, the protagonist reached a state of sovereignty through imaginative agency working within a transcultural framework that is both African and European. In doing so, she reclaimed the right as an African American writer to define literary values and social arrangements. The mode of narration and the protagonist's behavior attest to a strong capacity for self-governance and emotional control, made possible through what the philosopher Judith Butler called "the force of fantasy": "The so-called deconstruction of the real, however, is not a simple negation or thorough dismissal of any ontological claim, but constitutes an interrogation of the construction and circulation of what counts as an ontological claim" ("Force of Fantasy" 105). In what follows, I will demonstrate that Crafts' use of fantasy is her deconstruction of the real, as it released her from the bondage of her social position and allowed her to interrogate and reconstruct her role with her own ontological claim. Interpretations like Gates' insistence on the authentic writing of a "female slave" neglect the poeticity of the text, produced within a complex intertextual structure that includes a wide-ranging set of intercultural references that are at the center of my interpretation. Craft's text bursts the confines of a slave narrative and, in certain ways, even the dualism of the "Black" and "white" context. A careful analysis of the elements relating to "fantasy" (in Judith Butler's sense of the word) can redress the neglect of Gates Jr. and others.[4] Relying on an epistemology that refuses the racial restrictions imposed on her, Crafts constructs a transcultural web of fantastic gothic devices that include West African concepts of animated nature as well as European gothic elements popular at the time. In this way, Crafts does not necessarily rely on the "master's tools" and thus escapes even Gates' well-meaning but nevertheless reductionist reading of the text as an authentic antebellum document of slavery.[5]

In light of the lively discussion that Crafts' use of the gothic provenance has generated among scholars of the slave narrative, the question arises: why are critics so reluctant to classify this work as a gothic novel? Even scholars who support the novel's gothic origins do so only cautiously and express their discomfort when granting *The Bondwoman's Narrative* proper gothic characteristics. In an illuminating and long overdue study on the African American gothic, Maisha L. Wester sees potential in Crafts' gothic framing of her slave narrative: "Haunted by the dead and built upon torment, slavery proves the fitting setting for any gothic novel. The lives, struggles and complexities of the beings suffering within the institution reinforce the gothic as a mode of reality" (*African American Gothic* 66). Yet, Wester, too, warns of the incorporation of dominant oppressive views by enslaved and formerly enslaved narrators (*African American Gothic* 52). Why would the positioning of the author within an oppressive system render the text less gothic? As John Carlos Rowe has pointed out in his reconsideration of the task of literary criticism, even canonical writers such as William Faulkner, for example, "must confront the dilemma that his own style is inevitably trapped within a Western cultural tradition that is very much part of the social and human problems he wishes to remedy in his fiction" (*Literary Culture* 225). The problem for the enslaved author is her position within a literary analysis that is suspended between a "white" gothic tradition and the "darkening," or the "Africanist presence," of the same (Hack). As she is neither white nor African, Crafts is barely authorized to develop a particular aesthetic in these interpretations.[6] Consequently, this chapter argues that more attention should be paid, first, to Crafts' individual choices—including the likely Yoruba influences that are key in her text—and secondly, to West African–influenced elements of magic in US American literature more generally. As will be seen, the influence of African American traditions in the creation of the US American gothic mode is more significant than scholars have so far acknowledged.

Reading the gothic in *The Bondwoman's Narrative* as a subscription to a "white" genre (Castronovo, "Art of Ghost-Writing"), or as a "white" genre that has been "Africanized" by Crafts (Hack), does not do justice to this complex, hybrid, and multivalent text, which explores the heteroglossia of literature and highlights relationality. In particular, the concept of "black magic" is, to date, missing from the discussion.[7] Scholars like Doyle and Goddu, and to a certain extent even Wester, propose that the gothic simply provided a framework that made slave narratives intelligible to a suggestively *white* readership in antebellum United States. Russ Castronovo proposes that "Crafts' ghost-writing is not that gothic after all but is rather a critical aesthetic response to the everyday horrors of slavery" ("Art of Ghost-Writing" 195). Yet, gothic writing is often exactly this—a critical aesthetic response to the horrors of everyday life; consequently, the slave narrative should not be an exception. If a central trope of the US American gothic has always been slavery, as Teresa Goddu and many others have argued, it should be possible to consider intentionally gothic structures of slave narratives. Marquis de Sade explained of the gothic novel in Europe in the eighteenth century already "that this kind of fiction, whatever one may think of it, is assuredly not without merit: 'twas the inevitable result of the revolutionary shocks which all of Europe has suffered" (109). There is no reason to assume that a former slave would not have reacted in the same way to the shocks of experiencing slavery in the United States.[8] Rather than a simple framework that secures cultural legibility, the gothic is a mode of expression. The racial conflict might have haunted settler colonial writers, but as Robert Levine remarks: "there is no reason to believe that African American writers couldn't be haunted by race as well" (278). The gothic mode is suitable for capturing this form of being haunted on both sides of the spectrum, but it only defines one of the many possible modes of expression that might be met in any given novel, and it certainly does not discard the craftsmanship of the authors.

If we accept that the early British gothic "normalizes and naturalizes a modern subject defined by its autonomy and interiority and so works hand-in-glove with the sentimental tradition to modernize kinship relations at the level of the individuated subject and the contractual household," as the gothic scholar Siân Silyn Roberts proposes (4), it can be argued that the same holds true with the African American gothic and with slave narratives. Narratives that pertain to the domestic setting of so-called houseslaves are particularly important resources for any study of subjectivity and kinship relations. As a testament to systematic torture and traumata, slave narratives are necessarily works of psychological fiction. Depending on their focus, they lend themselves to the framework of the gothic within an emergent modernity that recognizes the autonomy and interiority of the individual. As such, gothic slave narratives are yet to be acknowledged in their capacity for reading, constituting, and performing the modern subject with all its contradictions and complexities. The gothic as a mode that corresponds with the demands of Crafts' slave narrative does not hark back to an exclusively racialized tradition; rather, it allows for an epistemological inquiry situated at the intersection of conflicted cultural elements. It can even be understood as a testing ground for competing positions, all of which might not prove adequate to describe individual experience under slavery. As a mode, the gothic is by definition an open structure, which is not reducible to existent literary parameters and develops an aesthetic of its own, which may or may not remain within prescribed genre boundaries.

In conclusion, Crafs was working within an Africanist cultural tradition and influenced by the late eighteenth-century British gothic aesthetics. Even if published only recently, her writing must be understood as a contribution towards a literary mode that eventually merged into the US American gothic. As will be shown in the following, Crafs as an author had authority over her transcultural gothic project, which is characterized by complex interpolation and interaction between West African and European cultural influences.

Horrorism

Readers of *The Bondwoman's Narrative* gain a sense of the novel's gothic ambience as observers of the protagonist's ongoing and insistent stream of conscience, which offers flashbacks as foreshadowing. This classic gothic pastiche, which accentuates the firsthand experience of a character and invites the reader to judge the reliability of the narrator, reaches its peak fifteen pages into the novel. Hannah is sent to the house's portrait gallery. "Threading the long galleries which led to the southern turret," she begins to contemplate:

> There is something inexpressibly dreary and solemn in passing through the silent rooms of a large house, especially one whence many generations have passed to the grave. Involuntarily you find yourself thinking of them [. . .]. Then all we have heard of or fancied of spiritual existences occur to us. There is the echo of a stealthy tread behind us. There is a shadow flitting past through the gloom. There is a sound, but it does not seem of mortality. A supernatural thrill pervades your frame, and you feel the presence of mysterious beings. It may be foolish and childish, but it is one of the unaccountable things instinctive to the human nature. (15)

Echoing eighteenth-century musings of German and British philosophers on the nature of apparitional sightings, Hannah's potential spectral visitors are presented as "instinctive to the human nature," an involuntary reflex common to all human beings. Far from frightening impositions, the ghosts are very accommodating "mysterious beings" in this gothic setting.

Through Wheeler's library, Craft would have had access to the works of the Scottish writer Sir Walter Scott, which she was most likely well familiar with, since he was highly regarded in the antebellum United States.[9] One of the first scholars of the supernatural in literature, Scott stated: "It is, I think, conclusive, that mankind, from a very early period, have their minds prepared for such events by the consciousness of the existence of a spiritual work, inferring in the general proposition the undeniable truth, that each man, from the monarch to the beggar, who has once acted his part on the stage, continue to exist, and may again even in a disembodied state, if such is the pleasure of Heaven, for aught that we know to the contrary, be permitted or ordained to mingle amongst those who yet remain in the body" (Scott, *Letters* 45). Scott suggests that the idea of ghosts, or what he terms "the abstract idea of apparitions," allows humanity to engage in the fantasy that death is not the end (45). These are not the "terrible spirits, ghosts in the air of America," English writer and poet D. H. Lawrence claims to have sensed everywhere (Lawrence 85). Rather than being an American or even otherworldly presence, ghosts are imaginary mediums enabling participation in a community comprised of all human beings: visualizing a ghost is a common cognitive ability. The haunting quality of the long passageway offers the narrator an opportunity to reflect on what is "behind us"; in doing so, she is placed in relation to a larger community "of all thinking beings," creating a mutual historical memory (Kant, *Dreams* 64). The embrace of the plural "we" created a community strong enough to trespass the identity border between enslaved and enslavers, as it split both categories and permitted Crafts to take the musings of her heroine a step further. Hannah considers her reaction to be exemplary for humankind and concludes: "for there surrounded by mysterious associations I seemed suddenly to have grown old, to have entered a new world of thoughts, and feelings and sentiments. I was not a slave with these pictured memorials of the past" (Crafts 17). The gothic framework allows the protagonist to take a step outside of her reality as a slave.

It is the "mysterious associations" and "supernatural thrill" that allow the narrator to move beyond her present restrictions into a "world of thoughts, and feelings and sentiments" (Crafts 17). This key passage signifies a determining moment in Hannah's life as an enslaved person: she asserts her humanity through an affirmation of a cognitive activity in an environment that insistently denies her ability to do so. This empowering work of fantasy gives her a new sense of presence—one not determined by her current situation. The presence of the images recalls "memories of the dead" that gave "any time a haunting air to a silent room" (Crafts 16). The dead, whose images Hannah is attentively studying, are those of former enslavers and their wives. Aware that she ought to feel differently, Hannah admits that "though filled with superstitious awe," she "was in no haste to leave the room" (17). The haunting presence of the past is experienced as a leveler—a feeling that both the enslaved and the enslaver succumbed to: "As their companion I could think and speculate. In their presence my mind seemed to run riotous and exult in its freedom as a rational being" (17–18).

This philosophical conclusion is reminiscent of Immanuel Kant's concept of freedom as "the key to explaining the autonomy of the will" (Kant, *Groundwork* 41). In *Groundwork of the Metaphysics of Morals,* Kant wrote: "*Will* is a kind of causality that living beings exert if they are rational, and when the will can be effective independent of outside causes acting on it, that would involve this causality's property of *freedom*" (40). Kant proposed that all human beings are free by virtue of being rational. The narrator in *The Bondwoman's Narrative* establishes herself as a rational person and concludes that she, as a rational human being, is free. This freedom could be restricted by outside causes, as Kant and Crafts both concluded; yet, it exists prior to and independent of those influences. John Hill Wheeler's library most likely held no translations of Kant's writing (Crafts, "Appendix C"); however, both Kant and Crafts conceptualized the presence of the spirits of the dead as a cognitive activity that asserts one's inscription into a larger community of thinking beings and, axiomatically, freedom.

Imagining ghosts is an acknowledgment of one's own involvement in the presence of the other. This relationality shifts ghost-seeing to the realm of ethics. Allowing the past to penetrate the present, the homodiegetic narrator in *The Bondwoman's Narrative* conceives of historiography as a space into which she can inscribe herself after being erased from it. She can now put herself in relation to those who have deemed her unrelatable. The haunted room brings the past back into the present and allows for a reconfiguration, transforming the supernatural into a warrant for a different future, this time on Hannah's terms.

Andrew Smith concluded his study of Charles Dickens' ghost stories with the notion that ghosts are abstractions and, as such, "not so otherworldly after all but [they] constitute new attempts at encoding an understanding of the changing relationships between the subject and the economy of the time" (Smith, *Ghost Story* 47). Hannah Crafts, an avid reader of Charles Dickens, approaches ghosts similarly in *The Bondwoman's Narrative.*[10] In her text, ghosts do not visit mystically from the Beyond but act in accord with the ghost-seer. Thus, ghosts initiate an ontological perspectivism that allows the Self to be situated, even under conditions that deny ontological certainty. Ghosts do not even need to materialize; perceiving their possibility suffices to define ghosts and ghostliness in a highly specific manner. A ghost is not perceived as an interruption that generates a context; rather, the context determines the presence of the ghost. Surrounded by family portraits, the narrator is surprised by the energy the mere idea of the presence of the dead evokes: "my mind seems to run riotous and exult in its freedom as a rational being, and one destined for something higher and better than this world can afford" (Crafts 18). Rather than marking the domain of the unnatural, ghosts initiate an epistemological inquiry.

The euphoria induced by the environment of a seemingly haunted room has led scholars to conclude: "the story does not go where literary conventions suggest that it should" (Wald 218). But Crafts is establishing those very literary conventions. The empowering quality of a haunted room has been explored repeatedly since Crafts' publication. Recalling a classic gothic tale, such as Shirley Jackson's *The Haunting of Hill House,* exposes parallels that suggest a literary gothic slave narrative is no more a contradiction than a literary gothic feminist narrative. In spite of generic and periodical differences, both narratives demonstrate telling congruities that allow for Crafts' novel to be placed at the beginning of a feminist tradition of haunted tales. The narrator in Jackson's 1959 novel *The Haunting of Hill House*—intended as a ghost story by the author, yet often marked as gothic horror by scholars and critics—feels equally comforted by the haunted walls of an old mansion. Eleanor, a depressed middle-aged woman and a social misfit, learns to enjoy living in a haunted house. Outside of her former social environment, her state of mind improves considerably: "I would never have suspected it of myself, [Eleanor] thought, laughing still; everything is different, I am a new person, very far from home" (Jackson 27). Like Hannah, who experienced herself as a "different person" in the haunted room, Eleanor found solace as "a new person" within the confines of a haunted mansion. Eleanor, like Hannah, derived joy from having stepped outside of the social structure and class mechanisms that caused her exclusion in the first place. The haunted room marked a space apart from her previous life, because there her existence mattered. In the end, Eleanor concludes: "I can't picture any world but Hill House" (Jackson 27).[11]

Jackson's narrative belongs to a different tradition but points at the potential of protection within the confines of haunting, harking back to the original meaning of the word as a return to a home of something rendered nonexistent. Hannah creates a space where she can reminisce and be free: in the haunted room, if only for a fleeting moment. This understanding of haunting as an empowering mechanism that creates a sense of personhood is retained throughout *The Bondwoman's Narrative*. To provide one example: when the family portrait of Sir Clifford falls off the wall while the haunted tree is creaking in the middle of a wedding ceremony, the narrator begins to daydream about death, "the great leveler who treats the master and slave with the same unceremonious rudeness, and who touches the lowly hut or the lordly palace with the like decay" (30). Hannah's imagination is a source of solace that, with the help of the supernatural framework, connects her to (a community of) all thinking beings, which, at least imaginatively, relieves her of the restrictions of the enslaver's household.

Hannah's pondering upon the nature of haunting exposes the horror of the situation outside of the supernatural framework. The horror that marks this novel is corporeal, material, and quotidian. A representative, if disturbing, example is the scene that depicts the slave-holder's wife after the discovery of her husband's infidelity. Determined to search the mansion for proof, she discovers children that her husband must have fathered with a number of "beautiful female slaves" (Crafts 177). Hannah explains: "no Turk in his haram [*sic*] ever luxuriated in deeper sexual enjoyments than did the master of Lindendale" (177). Reacting to her husband's nocturnal activities, his wife, "the English woman of aristocratic family and connections," organizes a house auction to sell both the enslaved mothers and the offspring her husband had fathered (177). When the slave traders arrive, one of the young mothers reaches for a knife and stabs her infant son. She then thrusts the body into his father's arms before committing suicide, "bathing them in her blood" (183). The scene is very short and nestled marginally at the end of a long description concerning the irate mistress. It is misleading to assume that this scene is not exploring the specific potentiality of literature merely because of its conditions of production. The novel was written before Margaret Garner's infamous case of infanticide as a protection from a life in slavery, suggesting that scenes like this might not have been an exception in the antebellum United States. Toni Morrison, after all, constructed one of the most important ghost stories in US American fiction based on a similar atrocity.

As a typical gothic scene of horror, this scene produces the effect of repulsion. Horror designates a scene that provokes such total repulsion that it paralyzes the body. Whereas terror can provoke a psychological reaction, horror induces a physical immobilization similar to torpor.[12] The Medea situation of an infanticidal mother allows for no contemplation, escape, or rescue. It is an act of unilateral violence on the helpless. Furthermore, it replicates the helplessness of the enslaved position the mother has been subjected to. Turning herself into a perpetrator and murderer of the only possible victim, the mother marks her struggle with agency and resistance.[13] The mother's horrific act calls the act of enslaving her into question, yet it also imprisons her in the role of the perpetrator. Neither the language of terror nor of horror can adequately grasp the situation.

The problem when interpreting this scene is not located in Crafts' text but rather in the way contemporary scholarship has been reading the gothic. So far, gothic scholarship has made no distinction between violence inflicted upon the helpless and violence carried out among equal partners. Beyond the context of literary studies, the political philosopher Adriana Cavarero proposes the designation *horrorism* to differentiate between regular horror and the violence against the helpless. This distinction is necessary in literature as well, particularly in reading the gothic. Finding a language for the violence inflicted upon those who are not in a position to respond moves the violence beyond questions of death. It is not primarily the homicide that evokes the reaction of repugnance, but rather the many-layered offenses against defenseless and vulnerable victims. Adding horrorism to the vocabulary of the gothic enables a reading of literary slave narratives such as *The Bondwoman's Narrative* in their literary and historical complexity.

The abrupt and shocking bloodbath is immediately followed by a vocative, accusatory address by the reader to those in power. The author used a metalepsis to expose those responsible for deaths of the mother and the child by calling out the president, politicians, and ministers: "A slight spasm, a convulsive shudder and she was dead. Dead, your Excellency, the President of this Republic. Dead, grave senators who grow eloquent over pensions and army wrongs. Dead, ministers of religion, who prate because poor men without a moment[']s leisure on other days presume to read the newspapers on Sunday, yet who wink at, or approve of laws that occasion such scenes as this" (Crafts 183). This is one of the passages with strong resemblance to Charles Dickens' *Bleak House*. In a joint article, the literary scholars Gill Ballinger, Tim Lustig, and Dale Townshend claim that this passage is ineffectual, because Hannah is not speaking "in her own person." Instead, these scholars perceive a "forcing of Dickens' third-person voice into the interpolated first-person narrative of Lizzie," which, in their opinion, allowed Crafts to let "Dickensian charity begin abroad" (228–29). Yet, their argument does not go far enough. Borrowing from Dickens, Crafts not only subscribes to an acknowledged literary environment that she imports to the United States; her intertextuality also exposes the entanglement of literature with the injustice of US slavery. This narrative staccato at the end of the chapter effectively leaves the reader with the image of the young bodies of enslaved people, dead and covered in blood, while ministers stand aside reading newspapers. Making space for an activist and didactic stance within her literary narrative, Crafts exposes the horrorism at the center of the British and the American gothic, and the silence of writers who fail to address it. In this way, Crafts is working with and against the gothic as well as with and against Dickens. This dynamic enables her to simultaneously develop gothic suspense and social polemic. Rather than pointing out the importance for "black writers" to write with and against "a Western canon," as proposed by Gates Jr. in his introduction to *The Signifying Monkey* (xxiiii), this element in Crafts' text, as has been suggested by Ann DuCille in a different context (discussing William Wells Brown and his literary influences), functions as a "complex nexus of literary cross dressing and back-talking" (24). *J'accuse,* exclaims the narration and not the narrator, effectively instrumentalizing the literary complexity that enables an intertwining of political motivation, literary experimentation, and classic intertextuality.

The Bondwoman's Narrative, in conjunction with other similar texts, foremost among them Harriet Jacobs' *Incidents in the Life of a Slave Girl* (1861) with its domestic horror or rather horrorism of the protagonist's entrapment in the garret, demonstrate how the political visions of the formerly enslaved, expressed through the dynamic of the gothic, articulate the worldliness of literature. Rather than recounting the history of slavery, they explore the specific potentiality of literature in its capacity to participate in larger intercultural polylogues. Pheng Cheah's *What Is a World?* is an important contribution to a growing field of literary scholarship that works to rehabilitate the ethical and political work of literature. Crafts' text should be part of this discussion as the transculturality and intertextuality of the text alone already expose the inscription in ethical and political frameworks. Crafts' narrative structure, which instrumentalizes the European gothic for the purpose of constructing a slave narrative, demonstrates that the gothic sensibility is a global network of literary exchange, influences, and sensibilities based on a wide range of literary and nonliterary factors, the intersection of which can only be taken into account if we do not restrict the text to the author's personal history.

The experience of being enslaved is dominated by a sense of personal erasure from social life and thus history. One's persona, culture, and identity are negated. Into the annals of history, an enslaved person enters only as a number, if at all. Orlando Patterson famously used the concept of "social death" in order to analyze and expose this form of existence (Patterson). Most of Crafts' critics similarly propose a form of authorial death. Juxtaposing "social death" with Roland Barthes' famous theory of the "the death of the author" in the context of *The Bondwoman's Narrative* is revealing. Whereas Barthes' famous theory confirms the body of work independent of its author, these attempts at theorizing the production process of *The Bondwoman's Narrative* erase the poetics of the work.[14] However, through the instrument of the fantastic, the slave narrative is able to connect the past with the present and reclaim the slave's historical agency. A. Timothy Spaulding, one of the early scholars of the now growing field of the African American fantastic, has proposed ways in which "postmodern slave narratives" participate in a "re-formation of the historiography of slavery" through their "representation of time" (25).[15] Hannah Crafts proves this theory long before postmodernism's breakup with threadlike chronology. In Crafts' *The Bondwoman's Narrative,* the Self connects to a network of historical relations by rejecting linear time. Her ghosts mark a future that is the past. The reader follows the unfolding of the narrative in which the protagonist Hannah asserts her subjectivity, which prevents the denial of her identity, her presence, and her relevance. Hence, neither the protagonist nor the author, Hannah Crafts, can be considered socially dead. Relying on the parameter of the gothic that proposes a view of history that influences the present allows the narrator to authorize herself retroactively as a member of the community she has been previously excluded from—humanity. Hannah describes this act as a sensation of growth. Breaking up chronological time with the help of spectrality, Crafts' work challenges the universality of the interpretation that an enslaved person's body by default disappears within the gothic environment. Indeed, Hannah *grows.*

Nature and Spectral Transcorporeality

The confines of the ethical in interpretations of slave narratives have commonly been restricted to the confines of the human. In most slave narratives, however, just like in *The Bondwoman's Narrative,* the contours of the ethical have been stretched to include nature. Through ecogothic scenes of what I describe as spectral transcorporeality, Crafts' narrative exposes that in the face of slavery, there is nothing natural or self-evident about humanity. This study thus reads *The Bondwoman's Narrative* as a text that develops a human ethics beyond the human through the aesthetics of the ecogothic, which is the topic of this section.

The most striking gothic element in Crafts' novel is the bequeathed story of the house servant Rose, whose death affirms rather than erases her presence. The slave, who had nursed her current master, Sir Clifford, as a child, refuses to strangle a little dog that is her only reminder of the daughter who'd been taken away from her. As a punishment, Sir Clifford orders her gibbeted alive. In an appalling scene of torture, Rose is left hanging on a linden tree for three days without access to food and water, until "her rigid features assumed a collapsed and corpse-like hue and appearance, her eyes seemed starting from their sockets, and her protruding tongue refused to articulate a sound" (Crafts 23). The narrator describes Rose's situation as "suspended between heaven and earth," thus foreshadowing her ghostly presence even before the morbid and horrific moment her death occurs (23). Throughout this section, the dying woman and her dog are described in close relation to the weather: "After they had hung in this manner five days, and till their sinews were shrunk, their nerves paralysed, their vital energies exhausted, their flesh wasted and decayed, and their senses gone, a dreadful storm arose at night. The rain poured down in torrents, the lightning flashed and the thunder rolled" (24). The raging storm is followed by an even more horrifying scene, in which the narrator describes the revivification of the (almost) dead bodies through the fresh raindrops. The natural elements, wind and water, join together with the tortured bodies that now, with their renewed strength, have had their voices restored: "Through the din and uproar of the tempest could be heard all night the wail of a woman, the howling of a dog, and the creaking of the linden branches to which the gibbet hung. It was horrible: oh how horrible: and slumber entirely fled the household of Sir Clifford" (24). Nature appears synchronized with the tortured bodies of the woman and the dog, who join together in producing a shared sound. In an interpolation with the storm, Rose regains her last strength to place a curse on Sir Clifford's household. She exclaims "with a deep sepulchral tone": "I will come there after I am dead [. . .]. In sunshine and shadow, by day and by night I will brood over this tree, and weigh down its branches, and when death, or sickness, or misfortune befall the family ye may listen for ye will assuredly hear the creaking of its limb" (25). Upon her death, just like Rose herself before, the tree continues to wail and creak, marking the place forever with her absence. At the time of narration, Rose is dead and belongs to a previous generation of inhabitants in Sir Clifford's household. It was not only the creaking of the tree that reminded later generations of her ordeal, but also the sighs of the plantation inhabitants, who continued to whisper to each other: "Whether it laughed or shrieked the wind had something expressively ominous in its tone" (20). The wind and

the tree have become agents that warn visitors and residents alike of previous and future injustices.

A ghost makes absence present. The arboreal curse emerges at a moment of transmigration during which the tree continues the aural lament
Rose had initiated; the curse thus turned the tree into a supernatural agent.
Scholars who claim that there is no proper ghost in Crafts' narrative dismiss the wailing of the linden.[16] Yet, the creaking of the tree is a language
that all inhabitants of the plantation understand: "Then the linden lost its
huge branches and swayed and creaked distractedly, and we all knew that
was said to forbode calamity to the family" (20). The group of those who
see the ghost in the linden tree include the owner and all those enslaved at
the plantation.

Furthermore, the previous history of the tree is also known to the same
community of ghost-seers: "a wild and weird influence was supposed
to belong to it" (Crafts 20). The cruel enslaver Sir Clifford had planted
the linden, which grew strong and big and consequently "was chosen
as the scene where the tortures and punishments were inflicted" (20).
Rose was thus not the first to experience physical abuse and possibly even
death on the now haunted site. Sir Clifford cultivated and nurtured the
tree strictly as a tool to destroy the free will of those he enslaved. In this
way, the tree, too, was abused and misused.

The corporeal fluids nurture the roots of the tree, and the body and the
tree seem to begin to act in accord with each other. This transcorporeality
established between the tree and the dying body of the old woman and
her dog has lasting consequences, as it initiates the act of haunting. In *The
Bondwoman's Narrative,* the moment of transcorporeality created through
the exchange of the slaves' bodily fluids with the tree is affirmed in the enslaver's fear of the growing tree and his feeling of being haunted. Nature
becomes an agent in its own right. The commutation transforms the linden
into a Frankensteinian creature that returns to haunt its creator. "Many a
time had its roots been manured with human blood," explains the narrator (Crafts 20). The tree, nourished with the blood of the enslaved, slowly
morphs into an extension of the tortured bodies as the aural transformation
between the tree and Rose progresses.

The way the shrieks smoothly transition from those of the enslaved to
those of the tree shifts transcorporation to the center of the narrative. The
nonhuman force now has power over the enslaver. The tree, now an ally of
the enslaved, is reclaimed in this novel and transformed from a master's
tool into an agent that opposes him. The subsequent arboreal haunting
of the master, who eventually commits suicide, can be understood as an act

of resistance against the abuse of nonhuman nature within a settler colonial culture. Stacy Alaimo argues in her important intervention in environmental studies: "Imagining human corporeality as trans-corporeality, in which the humans are always inter-meshed with the more-than-human world, underlines the extent to which the substance of the human is ultimately inseparable from 'the environment'" (*Bodily Natures* 13). The act of haunting confirms the agency of this environment in the fear of the perpetrator. Acting together, the human remains and the nonhuman presence create a coalition recognized in the whispers of the future inhabitants and the death of the perpetrator.

Most sightings of ghosts take the form of spectral transcorporeality. A ghost acts through the body of another, be it in a human or a nonhuman form. Choosing a tree to make the presence of the past sensible, Crafts joins many antebellum writers in their attempt to recodify the Invisible World in the forest. It is therefore only logical that the narrative shifts from the slave plantation to the forest. In this text, the forest is neither a Puritan nor gothic environment; it is not a space of evil and gloom, nor a romantic space of nourishing escape from the thrills of urbanism and domesticity. In the succeeding chapters, the reader encounters long descriptions of unpredictable nature acting of its own accord. Hannah escapes with her mistress and hides in the forest: "We then retired still farther into the woods, making our breakfast on some wild fruits, and quenching our thirst at a small rillet, that meandered among the shades. Gloomy, indeed, was our walk, but gloomier were our thoughts. Serpents, wild beasts, and owls were our companions, yet our horror was of man" (Crafts 66–67). The forest, an alternative place of refuge and regeneration, is also a dangerous test of surviving in wilderness. Yet, in their desire to gain freedom, the two women initiate a change in relation to their environment. In her study of the African American gothic, Wester asks critically: "In a country where the slave body, the 'not-free,' provides the racially marked contrast of the 'not-me,' how can freed, yet still racially marked writers create such a unified, essentialized self?" (*African American Gothic* 46). Wester concludes that the fleeting structure of freedom becomes "a recognition of the instability of being and identity" (46). I would like to add that this instability is foremost expressed in exchange with nature. In the US American tradition, the creation of a (seemingly) unified self was imagined in relation to or in exchange with the wilderness and the forests—transitional spaces that accentuate self-awareness.

Crafts' narrative structure goes even further by exploring the interpolation of bodies with nature. The result is an acknowledgment of the fragility and porousness of the human body and mind. Upon their elopement, Hannah and her mistress discover a desolate cabin in the middle of the forest, overgrown with weeds. Yet, the cabin's only room, now windowless, features a bloodstain and a skeleton in its center. Simply discarding these insignia of the European gothic horror, the two women use the cabin as a safe haven: "There was mirth and music around us; there was youth, and love, and joy for all things, but our troubled hearts" (Crafts 67). Crafts uses the gothic forest to domesticate the instabilities involved in modern identities and reconstructs a representable and seemingly unified image of a Self positioned in relation to one's environment. Rewriting the gothic setting as nourishing yet again, the narrator presents the reader with a fractured individual, who, once broken by the atrocities of slavery, recomposes herself as a bewildered outcast in a cabin in the forest. The narrative is forming personhood in a transcorporeal exchange with nature, as the two women even begin to blend with nature in their feral looks. When their physical appearance begins to resemble the surrounding wilderness, Hannah wonders: "Had we indeed lost all resemblance to human beings?" (70). The scene insinuates that humanity in the face of enslavement is not a desirable subscription.

Henry David Thoreau's famous transcendentalized version of domestic economy, exemplified by a cabin in the woods in *Walden* (1854), receives a worthy antagonist in Crafts' gothic version of the same: "chocked with weeds," "forlorn and desolate," and "formed much as Indians formed their wigwams" (67). In both autobiographical texts, the protagonists desperately sought "Shelter" (Thoreau 11): Crafts for reasons of physical survival, Thoreau for reasons of psychological health. The two women fleeing bondage quickly recover their physical health: "We could gather our sustenance from the forest, we could quench our thirst at a neighboring spring, and at least we should be free" (Crafts 67). Yet, their mental capacities suffered from their isolation: "After a time my mistress became decidedly insane, and her insanity took the most painful character. She fancied herself pursued by an invisible being, who sought to devour her flesh and crush her bones" (69). While Hannah, who had been enslaved as a servant in the house, can restore her life and joy in the forest, her mistress, who had been living under the signet of whiteness, experiences gloom and desolation, suffers under delusion and schizophrenic attacks.

The tension in human relations with their environments demonstrates Crafts' original rejection of the romantic ideals popular at the time.[17] Crafts' depiction of cabin life gives the project of human self-transcendence an outspokenly material turn. In this way, Thoreau's reductionist and prescriptive depiction of a "life in the woods" receives a corrective in Crafts' insistence on the relationality. In many ways, racially marked writers make use of the same register of references available to nonmarked writers when exploring the resources at their disposal for the construction of a "unified, essentialized self" (Wester, *African American Gothic* 47).[18] Transcorporeality is a topic not exclusively reserved for white male property owners in New England, such as Henry David Thoreau and Ralph Waldo Emerson. In Crafts' narrative, we find as much of a transcendental positioning of the subject within an "original relation to the universe" as we do in some of the transcendentalist classics (Emerson, *Essential Writings* 3).[19] In contrast to those works, however, Craft's vision is material, as it involves the human and the nonhuman body and puts them in relation to each other. At the same time, it is spectral, as the bodies receive agency through the act of haunting. Depicting in her narrative both nature and women as active subjects rather than passive objects, Crafts transforms the power of literature to be of Nature first and Woman second, rather than a "reconciliatory of Man and Nature," as Emerson envisioned it (Emerson, *Collected Works* 203). Moreover, Craft's narrative directly counteracts transcendentalism. In Crafts' depiction of nature as a force in its own right that refuses to serve the human, both Thoreau's and Emerson's pantheistic fantasies of merging with a divine nature are exposed as yet another instance of colonization: the colonization of nature.[20]

As scholars such as Judith Butler propose, fantasy has been central to the feminist task of rethinking futurity. Crafts' contribution to the feminist tradition of instrumentalizing fantasy lies in the power of her ghosts who, dehumanized and decomposed, resist expropriation and come with an insistence that the living acknowledge the role they play in present injustices. In doing so, Crafts' ghosts gesture towards the materiality of colonized bodies. In Butler's words: "the deconstruction of the real [...] counts as an ontological claim" ("Force of Fantasy" 105). Crafts' depiction of a spirit that will not accept the world as it is, in the character of Rose, introduces a spectral panopticon within which the enslaver is exposed to something he cannot see. In his reading of Shakespeare's *Hamlet,* Jacques Derrida writes about the "vizor effect" as something that arises in the moment when one sights a ghost, and this is "to feel ourselves seen by a look which it will always be impossible to cross" (*Specters* 7). Suffering under this very "vizor effect," the enslaver is left without the ability to respond.

Animism allows Crafts to produce an authorizing discursive form, which is related to, but not defined by, European gothic guidelines set by writers such as Charles Dickens and Charlotte Brontë. Her writing also demonstrates a predisposition to a continual re-enchantment of the world that could not be reduced to religion. Nigerian writer and scholar Wole Soyinka describes this form of re-enchantment as "the African world view," which he describes as "an attitude of philosophical accommodation" and thus a dynamic always at work in African cultures (53). It is, in Soyinka's words, "a cosmic entanglement in the community" (54). It is this type of entanglement in visible and invisible communities that structures Crafts' narrative. The writer herself lived in a community that would not accept her as a living, thinking being; entanglement asserts her humanity. The novel's uncompromising style might account for its missing publisher, yet this did not prevent Crafts from contributing to the creation of the US American gothic.[21]

US American Haunts

Hannah Crafts inscribes her narrative in more than just a feminist tradition and Euro-American philosophical discourses. As an enslaved person, she is able to draw from more influences than just her enslaver's library. Most West African cultures include a belief in the spirit world and the power of magic as a healing form (Fortes). One shared belief among these different traditions is that spirits interfere in the daily life of the living, frequently in a positive way (Mbiti). Under conditions of slavery, the promise of healing through a recourse to the spirit world can turn into the only possible stronghold. The influential sociologist W. E. B. Du Bois demonstrated in his sociological study entitled *The Negro Church* how the roots of African American religion are to be found within "Obe Worship, or Voodoism" and not in Christianity. In Voodoo—one of the most widely spread religious concepts among African American slaves—the future is derived from the past. Life and death merge into one. And if death is life, the threat of extinction by the enslaver can be reevaluated with a set of references that exclude termination. While this assumption certainly makes neither death nor violent acts committed by enslavers acceptable, the belief in the ghost world becomes vital for a community facing the possibility of death daily.

According to Du Bois, the belief in ghosts and sorcery is part of the African American worship of nature (1). Coexisting among the living, the spirits of the dead materialize in the form of plants such as trees. Crafts' haunted linden tree could be a direct reference to this tradition. Furthermore, the presence of the spirits of the dead in nature is even more prominent in the context of slavery. It is due to the slave trade that "animal worship, fetishism and belief in sorcery and witchcraft strengthened their way and gained wider currency than ever. [. . .] The Negro priest, therefore, early became an important figure on the plantation and found his function as the interpreter of the supernatural, the comforter of the sorrowing, and as the one who expressed, rudely, but picturesquely, the longing, the disappointment and resentment of a stolen people" (Du Bois 3–5). Since ghosts often appear as soothing presences in the context of West African religions, offering comfort and advice or at least marking the absence of the dead in the present, it is very likely that enslaved Africans, upon their arrival in North America, held onto this source of strength. As spirits were believed to be noticeable only through the enslaved's own recognition, they were safe from detection by enslavers—the belief in the spirit world became a secret code (Du Bois 6). Furthermore, no records prove that pressure was applied in converting slaves to Christianity. On the contrary, while the archives consulted for this study held documents curiously and redundantly celebrating Christianity among slaves, records of actual conversion stories are rare.[22] It is telling that the English law, as Du Bois pointed out, never had a *Code noir*—a law that made baptism and the religious instructions of slaves obligatory. Accordingly, we can assume that both Christianity and African traditions of conjuration and magic were strong influences in Hannah Crafts' life and shaped the author's choice of haunting as spectral transcorporeality.

Considerations of the supernatural as a determining element of African American cultural and religious traditions have often been tainted by the rather depreciative tone in which it has been presented within settler colonial narratives. In his study *Matter, Magic, and Spirit,* the anthropologist David Murray analyzes the increasing systematization of race and belief in the eighteenth and nineteenth centuries. Following the US genealogy of the terms *conjure* and *hoodoo,* he demonstrates that this vocabulary originates in African American folk practices and was dismissed as superstition by preachers and missionaries in the eighteenth century (10).[23] In this way, colonizers marked superstition and ghostliness as an African American trait and devalued their function. At one point in *The Bondwoman's Narrative,* the narrator admits to being superstitious and refers to the African American tradition that she claims as part of her culture: "I am superstitious, I confess it; people of my race and color usually are" (Crafts 27). Crafts' decision to excavate superstition from the colonial context reevaluates and valorizes its presence within Africanist cultures.

The connection between African Americans and superstition is a topos of nineteenth-century American literature by Euro-American writers. In his introductory essay "How to Tell a Story," Mark Twain wrote that the humorous story is American, the comic story belongs to the English, and the witty story to the French. In the same vein, Twain used the ghost story as an instructive example of an African American text: "On the platform I used to tell a negro ghost story that had a pause in front of the snapper on the end, and that pause was the most important thing in the whole story" (342). The confidence with which Twain used a traditional ghost story, *The Golden Arm,* and claimed its African American origin to instruct his readers on how to properly install a break when aiming for suspense indicates that telling ghost stories in the antebellum United States was understood to be an African American practice. Juxtaposing "American" with "English," "French," and "negro" indicates that this rhetorical device was not perceived as a domestic tradition. None of the encyclopedias consulted registered *The Golden Arm,* a folktale that in fact appears in various cultures, as an exclusively African or African American tale. In the nineteenth-century United States, however, ghost stories were often presented in an Africanist context by default, which could explain Twain's taxonomy. Hannah Crafts must therefore have consciously operated within a stereotype; her narrative, in turn, carves out a legitimate space for the supernatural.

Looking into the genealogy of the word *haunting* in its US American usage reveals a telling history of racialization. This overlooked genealogy of the term *haunting* is significant for two reasons: (1) the racially marked and oppressed body mistaken for, or marked as, a ghost; and (2) the natural setting of a cave in a forest now marked as haunted. The original meaning of the word *haunt* simply refers to a frequently visited place, which may or may not demonstrate any connection to the supernatural. The first entry where the *Oxford English Dictionary* registered a connection between a frequently visited place and ghosts in the noun "haunt" specifies a "*local U.S.*" usage in the mid-nineteenth century: "The noun meaning 'spirit that haunts a place, ghost' is first recorded 1843, originally in stereotypical US black speech" ("Haunt"). Not revealing much, the entry reads as follows: "**1843** WINNEMORE & REPS *Cud's Wild Hunt* (song) 3 It am de hunt ob Cudjo dat nigger so bold." The entry is referring to a minstrel song about Cudjo—a common name for an enslaved man—who went on to gain more fame as the protagonist of the antislavery novel *Cudjo's Cave,* published by J. T. Trowbridge in 1864.[24] The haunt in this example is a cave—the home of a fugitive from slavery named Cudjo. In both the song and the play, the cave in the forest, Cudjo's haunt, becomes a place of refuge.

It is first in Shakespeare's plays that spirits become the agents of haunting. The *Oxford English Dictionary* records the application of the word in *A Midsummer Night's Dream* (1600), where the place to return to is the forest populated by spirits ("Haunt"). Like its English predecessor in Shakespeare's example, the first recorded US American example of a haunt is also located in the forest, yet this forest is haunted by living fugitives from slavery, marking Cudjo as ghostly even before his death. The haunt is thus neither a graveyard nor a castle in its US usage; it is a natural cavity in the forest that is used as a refuge by an enslaved person. Just like in Crafts' narrative, the forest is a space of revivification. The haunt, the place to return to, the familiar resort in its North American context, is, paradoxically, a place of survival—a natural cavity protecting abducted Africans and their sympathizers from violent European settlers. The last example in the 2018 edition of the *Oxford English Dictionary* that demonstrates how the noun *haunt* can carry the meaning of "a spirit supposed to haunt a place, a ghost" is also taken from a markedly African American context. It is an entry in the *Autobiography of Malcolm X* (1965): "It was spooky, with ghosts and spirituals and 'ha'nts' seeming to be in the very atmosphere when finally we all came out of the church" ("Haunt"). The "ha'nts" in this example circumscribe a protective space visible exclusively to African American visitors of the church and as such signify yet another refuge from oppressive environments.

At the very least, these examples demonstrate that, throughout the last two centuries, *haunting* in its US American usage has repeatedly been used in close proximity to living African American bodies. Commonly, haunting is defined in opposition to an intentional visit to the underworld (*katabasis*) as an interruption and intrusion from a person believed to be dead into the present of a living person. In the examples above, we encounter either living bodies perceived and represented as a spiritual interruption to the quotidian life or spirits that provide a protective space with recuperative qualities. In both cases, the meaning of *haunting* is close to its original usage as a protective space (home) to return to with one notable difference: those in need of protection are racially marked and alive. While from a settler colonial perspective, haunts might be rendering African Americans dead while alive, from an Africanist perspective, a haunt might be a place of recuperation.

Animation and the Unappeased Dead

The numerous biblical references in Crafts' text have been extensively studied, yet the elements of animism in the text, the source of which is most

likely the Yoruba tradition, has not yet received enough attention.[25] Both
religious traditions merge in the life of an antebellum enslaved person such
as Hannah Crafts, and both find expression in her narrative. Highlighting
the narrative influence of animism reveals an important set of references
beyond the everyday atrocities that came with enslavement. The African
incorporation of ghosts into everyday life shifted European settlers' perspectives on this omnipresent topos in literature and culture. Thus, the omnipresence of animism among the enslaved can, at least to a certain extent,
explain the common use of animated nature in the works of writers who
only partially subscribed to transcendentalism, as is the case with Nathaniel
Hawthorne, for instance.

One of the key characteristics of Voodoo is the emphasis on the actual-
ity and perceptibility of ghosts. A ghost is regarded as part of life, and it
manifests itself within the realm of the visible and the invisible. Theories
of natural energy transference between animate and inanimate entities became widely discussed topics among New England intellectuals in the 1780s
with the spread of theories and demonstrations of mesmerism.[26] Introduced by the German physician Franz Anton Mesmer and widely debated
in the United States most prominently by Benjamin Rush and Benjamin
Franklin, this theory of invisible natural forces connecting humans, plants,
and animals with the movements of the moon and the sun quickly became
a popular topic of science and gossip alike, shifting ghosts and spirits back
into the center of public attention. Separate, and most likely not unrelated,
to these discussions among influential politicians and philosophers, the African diaspora in the United States proposed a similar materialization of the
spirit in nature and objects animate and inanimate.

Animism offered African slaves in the antebellum United States a great
source of spiritual empowerment. Conjuration and haunting were often
used as a deterrent against an enslaver's oppression and violence. In her now
classic study *Black Magic: Religion and the African American Conjuring Tradition,* the theologian Yvonne P. Chireau has poignantly demonstrated a
lively coexistence between Christianity and magic that led enslaved people
in the antebellum United States to establish a particular system of communication with the spirits of the dead (12). Based on personal anecdotes and
interviews, Chireau's research convincingly shows that magic, particularly
communication with the dead, was an elemental part of the religion of the
enslaved, and that even in cases of conversion, there was no fixed dichotomy
between Christianity and magic (2). The connection between conjuration
and enslaved people, and the persistence of magic on slave plantations, can
be observed throughout the nineteenth century.

As late as 1899, the *Journal of American Folklore* printed a ghost story "by a negro man [. . .] who had come from Louisiana where he had been a slave" (Bergen 146). The nameless formerly enslaved person told the story of a haunted house inhabited by the ghost of an elderly woman that "cannot be laid." Neither Methodist nor Catholic priests were successful in their attempt to rid the house of evil spirits. The storyteller was amused by the rejection of closure or resolution offered in acts of exorcism. As if mocking his audience in alliance with the ghost, the narrator concluded: "the ain't no one ever tried to lay that ghost sence" (Bergen 147). By escaping closure and linear development, the ghost escaped historicity. Reports by formerly enslaved people who *see* ghosts, like this man, often attest to a coexistence of the living and the dead without providing further subtext.[27] The appearance of a revenant is experienced as pleasant and, in some cases, even triumphant. The following account by a formerly enslaved person is exemplary:

> Ghosts? I'se met plenty of um! [. . .] You jes' got to talk to 'em same as to anybody. It don't pay to be 'fraid of 'em. So he wheel 'round. (Spirits can wheel, you know.) [. . .] Dey sure is a t'ing, all right! Dey look jes' like anybody else, 'cept'n it's jes' cloudy and misty like it goin' to pour down rain. But it don't do to be 'fraid of 'em. I ain't 'fraid of nuttin', myself. I never see 'em no more. Guess I jes' sorta out-growed 'em. But dere sure is sech a t'ing, all right! (Federal Writers' Project)

The narrator is Isaiah Butler. In this interview, Butler affirms a familiarity with ghosts, a subsequent "outgrowing" of "them" and the resulting ability to vouch for their existence. Breaking the established convention of surprise through alienation, Butler's story and similar ghost stories by the formerly enslaved normalized the presence of ghosts and set the African American subjectivity in close proximity to spectrality. Unable to gain insight into ghostly habits, Butler's audience relied on the African American informant. In doing so, the African American narrator was marked as the unknown himself. Butler explained further: "De white folks'd see 'em, too," but they don't understand them (Federal Writers' Project). People who believe themselves to be in power have to rely on Isaiah Butler and his revelations when it comes to ghosts. While this is certainly a moment of exoticization on the part of the unmarked interlocutor, it is also an empowering moment for the formerly enslaved man, as spectrality is a field acknowledged by the oppressor though not understood. In this folkloristic tale, the formerly enslaved person explains the ghost as a symbol for an intellectual space that cannot be entered by the enslavers. Like the fictional character Hannah, he rejoices in the idea that there is a sphere more powerful than the oppressive society that surrounds him.

A collection of ghost stories by former slaves from North Carolina, South Carolina, and Georgia compiled by Nancy Rhyne confirms that numerous personal testimonies, interviews, and folkloristic tales repeated similar narrative structures. Conjuration was a psychological defense mechanism against oppressive and violent enslavers, and the supernatural realm served as a source of empowerment.[28] The realm of the supernatural not only provided a retroactive source of recuperation but also a means of active resistance against oppression.[29]

Given the importance of ghost stories in communities of enslaved and formerly enslaved people, and the influence of these stories on the cultural makeup of the antebellum United States, it is not surprising that there are numerous examples of enslaved people deploying ghosts against enslavers, not only in ethnographic studies and popular journals but also in fiction. Crafts' *The Bondwoman's Narrative* also contains a passage that describes enslaved people who take advantage of superstition to create a hiding place: "We had that day heard that Charlotte's husband, ~~having~~ after being severely, and as he thought unjustly punished by his master had run away, ~~and that he had been~~ that he had been gone several days, and that all effort to discover his place of concealment had signally failed. It occurred to me at once that some connection existed between his elopement and the appearance of this ghost, or was the man and the ghost identical? The conjecture was wild, though not beyond the bounds of probability" (Crafts 138; text passages crossed out in original). The slaves spread the rumor about the appearance of a ghost in order to keep the return of a fugitive secret from enslaver, Mr. Henry. As ghosts are a transcultural topos, taking advantage of masters' superstitious tendencies is a promising practice taken up in antebellum literature.

A well-known example can be found in Harriet Beecher Stowe's *Uncle Tom's Cabin* (1852). In the chapter titled "An Authentic Ghost Story," Cassy and Emmeline, both enslaved and both sexual victims of their enslaver Simon Legree, organize their escape by exploiting the Legree's and his assistants' fear of ghosts. They hide in a supposedly haunted attic until Legree gives up and terminates the search, knowing that no one would dare look for them there. Stowe's example vividly demonstrates why the enslaved could so easily rely on the performed sighting. The haunted attic merely provides the architecture that hosts the ghost who has already been haunting the enslaver Legree's mind—it was the ghost of "a negro woman who

had incurred Legree's displeasure" and was confined in the attic for several
weeks (346). "What passed there, we do not say; the negroes used to whisper darkly to each other" (346). Too horrible for words, even when offered
under the protective cloak of rumor, the story of the woman remains untold. Only her dead body is seen by a few inhabitants while being taken out
of the attic and buried. Yet, her story remains within the perpetrator's and
his henchmen's consciousnesses. "No one is so thoroughly superstitious as
the godless man," explains the narrator (347). Cassy, the antagonist of the
"godless man" Legree, links morality and superstition in his act of hanging
an empty bottle on the door to the attic. In high winds, the bottle produced
wailing sounds as if the woman's crying voice announced the return of her
abused body: "A superstitious horror seemed to fill the house; and though
no one dared to breathe it to Legree, he found himself encompassed by it, as
by an atmosphere" (347). Cassy did not stop here. To make sure to explore
every corner of this haunted mind, she wraps herself in a white sheet and
steps in front of Legree in the middle of the night. The enslaver's conscience
prevents him from seeing Cassy in plain sight—all he can see is a ghost: "After all, let a man take what pains he may to hush it down, a human soul is an
awful ghostly, unquiet possession for a bad man to have" (366). Stowe's and
Crafts' examples demonstrate that ghosts are always already on standby. The
architecture of the haunted house is the architecture of the haunted mind.

Both literary examples build on a long tradition of simulated haunting
based on mutual familiarity with spectrality. The European gothic version
of ghosts becomes only one of many. In 1925, the sociologist Newbell Niles
Puckett collected in his PhD thesis *Folk Beliefs of the Southern Negro* some
"thirty-five hundred" examples of "beliefs" and "lore" from formerly enslaved people in the southern states and juxtaposed them with traditions
that were either similar or the same as found among the European-American
population (Puckett viii). Though outdated, the study nevertheless contains
important documentation about the continuous intertwining of European
and African beliefs in ghosts and spirits. For instance, an enslaved person
in Puckett's study interpreted the custom of covering mirrors following a
death in a house: "the ghost will run you unless the glasses are covered"
(Puckett 82). Puckett explained that the English version of this practice was
rooted in the belief that seeing the reflection of a corpse in the mirror, or
even one's own body after someone's death, incurred bad luck (Puckett 81).
Further belief and habits are compared: "a belief European in origin, as is
also the common Negro belief that if you put your hand on the corpse the
ghost will not harm you" (Puckett 88). Puckett offered various examples

that affirmed the intercultural, or rather increasingly transcultural, quality of supernatural beliefs that connect the enslaved to the enslavers. In this way, customs and beliefs about ghosts have also always been a testament against the foundational fiction of pure whiteness. Seen from this perspective, it becomes obvious that Hannah Crafts could not have been writing in relation to an exclusively European gothic framework. Ghosts and superstition might be the pillars of the European gothic, but they had been firmly at home in other cultures long before *The Castle of Otranto* fell on ground ploughed enough to initiate a blossoming career of the gothic mode.

It is only with this tradition in mind that a reader can understand why the brave protagonist in *The Bondwoman's Narrative,* who had previously been confronted with the possibility of her own death on numerous occasions without even taking note of it, has such a strong reaction of fear when she is left alone with a corpse in yet another cabin in the woods. One night, Hannah is waiting for the return of a fellow fugitive in the cabin in the forest where they are hiding. She is left alone with his deceased sister: "I shuddered in every limb, great drops of sweat started to my forehead, and I cowered down in the corner like a guilty thing. [. . .] Mutterings, chatterings, and sounds of fearful import echoed through the gloom" (Crafts 228). Eventually, she begins imagining that the corpse is moving. The corpse demands that she come closer. Finally, towards the morning, exhausted, Hannah falls asleep. Her dream continues the vision: "The corpse seemed to rise and stand over me, and press with its cold leaden hand against my heart. In vain I struggled to free myself, by that perversity common to dreams I was unable to move. I could not shriek, but remined spell-bound under the hedious benumbing influence of a present embodied death" (229). In spite of the many atrocities Hannah describes in her life as an enslaved person, this is the only scene that the narrator experiences as a threat that causes a strong physical reaction in her. The episode ends with Hannah's companion returning to the hut and both of them filling up the entrance with brush and stones in order to create a tomb for the deceased woman.

The exchange between the living and the dead is one of the strongest African influences within the Christian spheres of North America. The mutual exchange of belief patterns, which renegotiate the interference of ghosts within intercultural spaces, can be retraced to funeral rites—highly performative and ceremonial matters that are key to all cultures. One of the most significant distinctions of African American funeral rites at the turn of the nineteenth century was the custom of a second ceremony or funeral, during which the soul took leave of the body. Enslaved people in America retained this African ritual even under the harsh conditions of slavery. A prototypical article published anonymously in New York in 1825 under the title "A Jumbus, or Negro Wake" recalls the happiness exposed at the funeral of a formerly enslaved person that was due to the attendees' belief that the soul would return to the home country in Africa. The article ends with the rhetorical statement: "Twelve months after death, they visit the grave with provisions and drink, and ask the dead how they do." Yet another much reprinted piece, a poem with the title "Ode on Seeing a Negro Funeral," asks:

> Why triumph o'er the Dead?
> No tear bedews their fixed eye:
> 'Tis now the hero lives they cry;—
> Releas'd from slav'ry's chain:
> Beyond the billowy surge he flies,
> And joyful views his native skies,
> And long-lost bower again.

These and numerous similar texts published in popular journals at the time demonstrate the engagement and interest of settlers in African American funeral rites that include a form of spectral dialogue between the living and the dead.

The omnipresence of African American death also led to significant adjustments in the ceremonies held by European settlers during the late eighteenth and early nineteenth centuries. In Virginia in the 1790s, the historian Mechal Sobel recorded numerous funeral services that were performed three weeks after a person had been buried. Detailing how seashells, inverted jars, and wine bottles were placed on graves, she documented the influence of African funeral rites and the rising significance of providing space for life after death on earth (Sobel 219). The rituals described by Sobel all served the purpose of enabling the living to remain in conversation with the ghosts of the dead.

Similar to most beliefs across the world, African rituals demonstrate a belief in the possibility of being haunted by the dead if the living fail to provide proper rites for appeasement. John Chitakure writes about the numerous types of "Ngozi" existing in African traditions. These are spirits of the dead who were treated badly in life or killed. These spirits return to seek revenge and demand justice (100). Again, far from being restricted to the domain of the spiritual, this belief receives material dimensions. Lieutenant John Matthews's widely distributed and often-quoted account of his voyage to the Gold Coast in 1788 records a funeral ceremony within which the living ask the dead how they should be properly mourned. In this way, during the second funeral, the deceased are given an occasion to communicate once more with the living. In particular cases, corpses are said to impart messages to the living in order to shape the future of the living. It is a part of leave-taking that distributes responsibility among both the living and the dead. Matthews reported: "When the deceased is designed for interment, the corpse is laid upon an open pier, decently wrapped in a white cloth, and born upon the heads of six young people, either male or female; for that is a matter left entirely to the choice of the corpse, who signifies his approbation or disapprobation of the bearers, by his inclination or disinclination to move (which they firmly believe it is capable of exerting) to the place of burial" (Matthews 122). When this procession arrived at the graveyard, one person addressed the dead body, informed it of its death, and inquired as to the cause: witchcraft or poison. Matthews explained that if one died without prior knowledge of their looming departure, these were the only possible causes. Natural death did not exist as a concept. Assuring themselves of the eternity of life in the face of death, the assembled bearers lined up and started asking the corpse questions. The corpse answered in the affirmative by "forcibly impelling the bearers several paces forward, by a power which they say they are unable to resist," and they denied forcing a "rolling motion" (Matthews 123). This was followed by an elaborate procession during which the corpse "judges" present and absent friends and relatives until the dead body "moves" with its most valued clothes and possessions into the earth. In this way, the death of a relative or a friend could be taken as an occasion to structure future relations among the living.

This detailed and much-reprinted description of conversations with the dead, presented by Matthews as an "African" funeral custom based on his voyage to Sierra Leone, is certainly a colonial view of a local tradition; it nevertheless exemplifies the familiarity of readers in the early republic with the physicality of the solid bond between the living and the dead in Yoruba traditions that is confirmed by current scholarship as well (Adéèkó). People belonging to Yoruba were some of the most heavily affected by the transatlantic slave trade. They imported their ceremonies within which the dead *move* the living and the living are *moved* by the dead; or, put another way, the dead and the living move together. Matthews' report was widely discussed in revolutionary America. Such strong images changed the understanding of death among the European settler colonial population, as European settlers willingly adopted from African newcomers the belief in death as a comforting state. Sobel describes the Black Creek Baptist Church, an interracial church founded in Southampton County, Virginia, in 1774:

"For half a century this garden was a black and white one, and blacks came to accept a personal Christ," while "whites" came to accept that "death was not a fearsome prospect but a step toward one's genuine fulfillment" (Sobel 226). African belief in the cohabitation of the living and the dead was embraced since the inception of the country, by at least parts of the settler population, for its ability to provide relief in the face of death. Death is presented as a homecoming and described in joyful terms that are meant to invite a peaceful coexistence with ghosts, who return to share the present with the living. The missing funeral rites in the scene described by Hannah Crafts and her subsequent fear of the consequences thus address both the potential African American and Euro-American settler readership.

While many scholars have confirmed that American gothic narratives cannot be separated from the history of slavery,[30] the importance of African spirituality, transcorporeality, and the strong presence of conjuration on slave plantations have not been sufficiently explored as determining factors in the genealogy of the gothic mode or of the antebellum slave narrative. West African traditions that rely on the coexistence of the living and the dead were widespread, recognized, and influential in antebellum United States. Consequently, spectral matters in their US American literary figurations can only be understood when these important influences are taken into consideration. Crafts was living and writing at a time when American spiritualism began to take hold of the country. She had access to works on popular ideas about animal magnetism and mesmerism, vitalist theories of an invisible natural force that relates to spiritualism.[31] At the same time, she most certainly had direct access to cultural practices of animism. Scholars such as Harry Garuba have suggested that animism, at home in Yoruba cultures, offers a different regime of knowledge—one that does not comply with the dualism of the modern. The writer Crafts is, indeed, creating alternative conceptions of modernity. Instead of the supernatural, Garuba asserts a "basically 'magical' worldview" in Yoruba cultures, which could not be interpreted by the Western colonizers (265). Crafts' use of magical elements, such as spectral transcorporeality, subscribes to this worldview. *The Bondwoman's Narrative* fuses these disparate influences with elements of the European gothic in shaping a specific spectral narrative that was not published for another 170 years, perhaps because it rejects a monocultural reading. The novel, nevertheless, demonstrates a style not untypical in antebellum literature.

Crafts' narrative was not the only one to redeem and explore the space of the supernatural as an important element in processes of subject formation. To name another famous example, in *Narrative of the Life of Frederick*

Douglass (1845), Sandy Jenkins presents Douglass with a "certain *root*" that protects slaves from being whipped (Douglass 73). Douglass brushed it off as superstition but kept the root to please Sandy: "On this morning, the virtue of the *root* was fully tested" (73). Magical or not, Douglass reports having felt a strange energy that provided enough courage for him to fight back for the first time. He succeeds in putting his enslaver at a distance, not only during this occasion but also in the future. Douglass began to wonder about the power of the root and always kept it close. The power of fantasy, yet again, receives a very material expression, marking a relational mode of being-in-the-world and a survival strategy.

This ontological instability as a source of strength that signifies an openness towards understanding the entanglement of the human body with its animate and inanimate, human and nonhuman environment is in fact a neomaterialist concept of animism. The human body is relational, affective, and incorporated in a larger nonhuman environment. Narratives such as those of Frederick Douglass and Hannah Crafts, with their minutely crafted transcorporeal elements, were interweaving the supernatural as an active agent within figurations of power structures and thereby forming a particular US American literary aesthetic within gothic confines. Animism, as a step outside of the matrix of modern dichotomies, occupies a central role within this aesthetic that allows for a positioning simultaneously inside and outside of the epistemic structures and languages of modernity. Ghosts, as a spiritual power of the dead, characterize ways of knowing and doing in relation to another; they might mark a metaphysical approach, though only in conjunction with a material component. In her interpolation of British gothic conventions and African traditions of animism, Crafts' text attests not only to the atrocities of slavery but also to a flourishing transcultural literary history among writers who achieved literacy and published under the severest of conditions.

Rather than just a generic reference or a tool for expressing the horrors of slavery, Crafts' use of the ecogothic can be understood as a search for a narrative form that avoids metanarratives. The writer succeeded in expressing the mixture of magic and Christianity that enslaved people in the US were exposed to daily. A ghost has the ability to interrupt historical chronology and binary thinking; "black" and "white" collapse into mortal humans; history and future collapse into a haunted presence. If historical chronology and binary thinking are understood to be essential to the early republic's quest to build a new nation, the ecogothic form becomes an alternative space within which to imagine future configurations of an inclusive society. Crafts' narrative exposes the narrativity of history. Having come to this conclusion while wandering through the long hallways of the enslaver's haunted mansion, Hannah recognizes her opportunity to revise the past and inscribe herself into it, thereby transforming the domain of the supernatural into a tool for political interrogation. The sociologist Avery Gordon has most impressively expressed the ghost as "a social figure" (8), but she didn't go far enough. The prosopopoetic creaking, the ghost that materializes aurally in the linden tree, is not merely one of those spectral social figures but one that performs the important work of decentering the huMan.

Beyond the Humanist Imagination

> Each of we have a special one who is we father or mother, and no
> matter what we call it, whether Shango or Santeria or Voudun or
> what, we all doing the same thing. Serving the spirits.
> —Nalo Hopkinson, *Brown Girl in the Ring*

Recent scholarship in the critical humanities has demonstrated an increasing interest in theories of what has been termed the human overrepresentation of itself as Man.[1] As theorized by the philosopher and novelist Sylvia Wynter, a focus on Man as the matrix of culture emerged in the fifteenth and sixteenth centuries with the dawn of the Enlightenment. During this period, a certain "ethnoclass Man" was self-designated, establishing whiteness, masculinity, cis-ness, and ability as the *civilized* "human" in a long process of disentanglement from the nonhuman environment (Wynter 291). Consequently, anyone not belonging to this category was relegated to "a secular slot of Otherness," wherein simple biological organisms merged with nature to form a "subhuman" background for Man.[2] Nature was essential to such processes of othering, as it provided the necessary structure against which fantasies of domination could be established.

This study demonstrates how spectrality in general and ghost stories in particular aided this violent colonial project of constructing both the "ethnoclass Man" and the "subhuman." Haunting in its current sense was established around the same time Sylvia Wynter claims for the invention of Man. It was in the writings of Shakespeare that the forest became the home of the spirits, the place the spirits return to regularly—their haunt. As I demonstrate in the first chapter of this study, with the dawn of the Enlightenment in Puritan America, these spirits in the forest materialized as racialized bodies, turning race into the demarcation line between the natural and the supernatural. The important Puritan concept of the Invisible World became increasingly visible in representations of the Other as figurations of the devil. Or was it a ghost?

At the same time, prompted by the writings of Thomas Hobbes and the ensuing discussions concerning the role of imagination in seeing ghosts, spectrality slowly shifted out of its religious context to questions concerning morality and ethics. In the late eighteenth century, an increasing number of scholars from Germany, England, and France expanded this scope as they followed their interest in ghosts in an Enlightenment effort to advance their understanding of metaphysical questions. Mostly they did so within the confines of the new sciences without aiming to enter into a conversation with adversaries of the occult. Allowing themselves to consider the possibilities of immaterial agents in conjunction with the promise of experiment, these scholars and writers amplified the Enlightenment's call to observe rather than to prescribe. Even the most hesitant treatises on ghosts, such as Immanuel Kant's anonymously published *Dreams of a Spirit-Seer,* advocated for an open-minded investigation; or, to use the term of spirit-theorist Joseph Glanvill, a "free philosophy" to replace the dogmatism of disbelief (*Essays* 63). These writers and scholars acted out of a shared recognition that envisioning progress based on reason alone is deficient. By way of spectrality, they found a footing in morality. Yet, how does the racialization of the irrational fit into this theorization of morality?

As a large number of fiction writers followed the philosophical discussion on nonreason and morality, interpreting their writing can advance our understanding of what it meant to be human in the early stages of establishing national identity patterns in the United States. Spectrality, or rather spectrology, as it was called at the time—the study of the seeing of ghosts—became a welcome instrument in the effort of reaching a more complete understanding of the less obvious demonstrations of being human. Irrational behavior and deception of the senses are only the most obvious mysteries of the human mind that spectrality was able to tackle. Prompted by the success of the fictional study of ghost-seeing in Germany that was inaugurated with the publication of Schiller's *The Ghost-Seer* and Tschink's *Victims of Magical Delusion* (first published in German as *Geschichte eines Geistersehers* [*History of a Spirit-Seer*])—both of which were fictional responses to Kant's *Dreams of a Spirit-Seer* (Träume eines Geistersehers)—Charles Brockden Brown set a standard for the American gothic by deploying spectrality to explore questions of morality. Along the lines of his predecessors in Germany, his ghost-seeing addressed the politics of the new republic and the incongruencies involved in living in a democracy under the auspices of genocide and slavery. However, as my analysis demonstrates, ghosts were helpful narrative devices in constructing a settler colonial imaginary that could be used for dehumanization processes that, in turn, would enable justification for genocide and land appropriation.

Writers of the early period followed Brown's lead and responded with ghost stories that serve the function of either rejecting or affirming dominant racial discourses, but only seldom did they depart from the humanist narrative of white settler supremacy. As a domain of the dead, the ghost story became for settler colonial writers the space where they could securely infix the living Indigenous population without compromising their own situatedness in what was conveniently termed the New World, suggesting regeneration and new life as a cyclical continuation of death. For this purpose, a recoding of the forest that was already established as a restricted space for the Invisible World was necessary. As a spectral space where death and life are entangled in a cyclical structure of regeneration, the forest could eventually function as a cleansing space for settler colonials to unburden their conscience.

At the center of these tales of the supernatural is a concept of reason that successfully poses as universal while constructing an exclusive "community of thinking beings," to use the famous phrase introduced by Kant in his moral theory. In his only book on ghosts, Kant used a more obviously exclusive phrase to cover a similar concept; "one great republic" that connects "all thinking beings" through their "moral state" offers a more explicit theorization of exclusive human communities on the account of reason. Reason in this theory is achievable by all and accessed by some. Similarly, antebellum ghost stories circumscribe a racially marked other side of reason that is inhabited by racialized characters. In this racial imaginary, embedded within highly popular gothic novel narrative structures harking back to Ann Radcliffe's "supernatural explained" (Clery) or Enlightenment "reformist novels" (Davidson), reason poses as a universal human capacity that is questioned only in relation to its insufficiency to be instrumentalized at all times.

The insistence on reason as a settler colonial domain is only affirmed in characters who have lost their minds, as can be seen in the popularity of twentieth-century literary and cinematic framings such as, for example, Stephen King's *The Shining*. In fact, there is a direct line between Brown's Wieland and King's Jack Torrance. In this highly popular novel that was adopted to an even more famous film directed by Stanley Kubrick, one will find the very landscape infused with dead Indigenous bodies somehow strangely connected to the faith of the settler characters without warranting the appearance to any Indigenous ghosts. The blackened spectral informant also appears in this recapitulation of traditional US American ghost stories, in the character of "the big black cook" Hallorann (King 140). Neither the novel nor the film can be interpreted as a call to action or in any way as speaking up for the rights of the dispossessed Indigenous population. On the contrary, the landscape suggestively haunted by the Indigenous dead serves the very same purpose it already had in Washington Irving's, John Neal's, and Lydia Maria Child's narratives; it frames the settler colonial violence as inevitable, acceptable, and accepted. And it creates a space separate from the settler civilization, to which Wendy, just like Child's Mary Conant, can safely return. Happy that the vulnerable, the woman and the child, survived, readers and viewers can forget about settler colonialism's violent policies of dispossession and land appropriation.

Particularly the Puritan concept of the Invisible World continued to serve as a blueprint for early American settler writers to construct colonial framings and fine-tune settler colonial fantasies. In the forest constructed in the writings of settler colonial authors of the early republic, the Puritan Invisible World was transformed into a space where Indigenous characters dematerialize without disappearing, as they would regularly rematerialize as components that design nature. In some cases, Puritan tropes were simply reproduced. Irving's forests, supposedly haunted by Indigenous spirits, feature materializations of the devil as "a black man" who resembled "an Indian" (Irving, *Tales* 657). Yet, in the end, even those spirits are replaced. The forest in Irving's writing repeatedly featured a denouement in a setting where spirits of the colonized dead are replaced by the spirit of the colonizer, thus successfully recodifying land as ancestral in relation to European settlers rather than the Indigenous population.

The antebellum ghost story was a forum for affirming white supremacy. The widespread interest in "spectrology" led to speculations about inter-psychic energies and spiritual networks that are at the base of modern conceptualizations of subjectivity. The aural ghosts in the writings of Charles Brockden Brown mark an attempt at paying tribute to the US American version of intersubjectivity as a premise for transcultural society. Yet, even Brown constructs a cultural hierarchy that suppresses the presence of non-Europeans through fantasies of incorporation. Irving's spectral tales expose the struggle to disentangle Man from his environment by demarcating a forceful separation from the (natural) Other. The literary history of ghosts in the United States is a history of relationality that promotes intimacy based on racial hierarchy. This tradition is countered in texts such as Hannah Crafts' slave narrative, in which ghosts appear as affective mediums that work in accord with their environment, offering narratives of stewardship instead.

To conclude, ghosts in US American history are more complex devices than literary scholarship has hitherto assumed, as this work has demonstrated in several ways. First, US American ghosts do not simply mark the return of the repressed or suppressed. Understanding the history of ghosts in terms of distributive energies, this work has offered an alternative to the guilt narrative that is prevalent in contemporary literary critique. Ever since Leslie Fiedler's 1960 monograph *Love and Death in the American Novel,* in which he reads American gothic literature as a response to the national feeling of guilt and repressed anxiety induced by the trauma of slavery and racial conflict, critics have been quick to interpret anything ghostly as a manifestation of settler colonial guilt over slavery. As Fiedler put it, "in the United States, certain special guilts awaited projection in the gothic form," and these "guilts" included the slave trade and the "slaughter of the Indians" (130). Consequently, Freudian psychological readings of ghosts in the US American gothic abound.[3] My interpretation of spectral narratives departs from these Freudian readings and consequently from the guilt theory. I contend that ghost stories were complicit in the colonial effort to eradicate the original American cultures.

Second, I have suggested that ghosts are not merely servants of the individual ghost-seer. Rather, ghostly figurations in literature commonly point at networks of distributive agency. So far, the psychological interpretation of ghosts in US American literature has relied on an understanding of ghosts as messengers engaged in revealing a transcendental truth that is communicated to the living through the spectral (suppressed) channel. This reading puts the ghost in the service of the ghost-seer in a way that constructs subjectivity on the premise of individualism and function. In this ego psychology, the human subject is a disentangled unity battling its own daemons. Yet, as the examples taken from Simms, Irving, Neal, Child, Hawthorne, and Crafts have shown in this work, ghosts often work in accord with nonhuman actors. As is demonstrated in the previous chapters, these writers borrowed more from Indigenous cosmologies and West African cultures' understandings of spirits than has been acknowledged in scholarship so far.

Sigmund Freud's continual return to inheritance questions in the context of haunting is certainly a helpful guide when trying to understand traumatic relations to previous generations, but it fails to explain spectral constellations that relate to alterity, morality, and embodiment. The focus on spectrality in Irving's tales of the supernatural reveals that haunted nature has often been the matrix through which racial subordination has been put in the service of subject formation. This narrative style is revised in Hawthorne's "Roger Malvin's Burial," Child's "She Waits in the Spirit Land" (1846), and Crafts' *The Bondwoman's Narrative* in their respective installments of transcorporeality, within which the dead human body acts in accord with the material it fuses with: the earth, the tree, and the wind. Freudian interpretations of a suppressed guilt are not applicable to a reading of these spectral matters, given that guilt is not suppressed in these narratives. If at all, guilt features as a conscious call to action, but it is neither colonial guilt nor does following this call involve retribution. Furthermore, the numerous more-than-human references create ethical relations that depart from the centrality of the subject, a fundamental aspect of Freudian interpretations.

In the third chapter of this study, the Hungarian-French psychoanalysts Nicolas Abraham and Maria Torok's theory of the transgenerational phantom proved useful for exploring national anxieties about non-European Americans in the early republic, because it pronouncedly departs from the Freudian transference theory of suppression. This theory of transgenerational inheritance demonstrates how the concept of the ghost can point out how traumas that have never been conscious or suppressed continue to determine the actions of the living. The ghost points not at one's own but somebody else's secret. This theory thus refers to the network structure of spectral relations and to the intrinsic alliance between ghosts and secrets. No association is required between the ghost and the haunted. In this way, the undisclosed traumas of previous generations become part of one's own psychology without any exposure or contact. In other words, the ghosts of the past determine the present, but no one seems to be accountable. Not only Brown's but also John Neal's investments in exposing the dangers of monocultural politics in his literature through the language of spectrality demonstrates a similar transference within social constellations.

Abraham and Torok's theory is helpful because it is a theory that relies on the power of intrapsychic energy. It is exactly this interlocking nature of spectral matters that has driven scholars and writers to repeatedly revert to the language of spectrality. Yet, this is certainly not a connection that was invented by Abraham and Torok, nor by Western psychology. The concept of ghosts in this context is closer to, for example, Apache cosmovisions or Lakota ethnoastronomical theories of connectedness than it is to Freudian theories of inheritance.[4] When applied to a reading of ghost stories in early American literature in general, ultimately even Abraham and Torok's theory is inadequate because of its exclusion of more-than-human interactions. Western psychology does not have the capacity to explain the persistence of ghosts in settler colonial literatures, where ghostly figurations often point at complementarity between the material and the immaterial. Therefore, new ways of reading ghosts are necessary.

American settler colonial writers have always written under the simultaneous influence and exclusion of Indigenous and West African cosmologies that extend the scope of influence to natural environments and human and nonhuman entanglements. I read the insistent recollection of European mystics such as Paracelsus, Böhme, and Swedenborg in relation to "Indian manners" in antebellum writings as a conscious avoidance of acknowledging non-European sources. Furthermore, all of the named mystics were influenced by what they term "heathen" sources, in what remains an instance of colonial appropriation of Indigenous philosophies.[5] As ghosts in European American settler literary narratives are imagined in the form of a specific energy with distributive agency, they can better be understood with the help of theories that do not dichotomize between human and nonhuman, natural and supernatural. European mysticism provides this necessary epistemic turn, yet so do most Native North American cosmologies and West African animism, omnipresent in the early republic. These unacknowledged sources left a significant mark on what came to be recognized as early *American* literature. Brown was familiar with the Lenape or the Delaware, Neal was familiar with the Lakota, Child was accustomed to the traditions of the Pequot, to name only the most obvious connections. All three cultures promoted a view of the reciprocal relations between the living and the dead as well as among the human and the nonhuman. Thus, one of the central aspects in mysticism—the interconnectedness that reaches beyond life and death as well as beyond human and nonhuman materialities—is also central to Indigenous cultures that the analyzed writers were familiar with. Given the fact that both Neal and Child demonstrated a life-long interest in what is today Haudenosaunee cultures (particularly Cayuga and Oneidas), and taking into consideration Brown's sporadic interest in Iroquois cultures and Irving's capitalizing on what he presented as "Native American" topics throughout his writing career, it is important to reflect on how persistently early American literature relates to Indigenous theories not only as a moment of appropriation but also as a constitutive element. As Christian Michael Gonzales convincingly argued in a different context: "Natives thus embedded or 'planted' Indigeneity into the cultural structures that the settler state supposed would erode Native cultures and eventually erase Indigenous people" (3).

Nancy Bonnivillain reports about an interesting tradition among the Hopi. After a person dies, it is traditional to place a white cotton mask over the face, which symbolizes clouds (5). The prayers for rain that will nourish the crops are thus concomitantly a reverence for the dead, who are believed to be part of this much-needed water supply. This ceremony presents a metaphysical interlocking that includes more-than-human elements in narratives of death and dying and proposes theories of the circularity of materialities that survive the living body of the human. Reading about this Hopi tradition, it is hard not to recall the strong correspondences with the gothic trope of the veil, so important to Poe and Hawthorne. Furthermore, the material remains of human bodies have a central place in both writers' oeuvres. Could the many white veils that spook through early American writing and that were elevated to a central element of American spiritualism be referencing Hopi traditions? Kucich convincingly argued that American spiritualism borrowed from both West African and Indigenous traditions. It is time to reconsider those important influences in early American writing as well.

Indigenous philosophies have thus played a much more important role in establishing modern ideas of subjectivity and morality through spectrality in early American writing than has been acknowledged so far. Circumscribing a different set of references, metaphysical questions like the ones provided by the Iroquois, the Lakota, or the Hopi cannot be applied directly to a reading of settler colonial narratives in the early republic; but they can inform the therein often included interpretation of the ontology of relationality. These transcultural intersections and traditional accordance were as influential to establishing the US American gothic as were the writings of Ann Radcliffe and William Godwin. A careful reading of spectrality in settler literary narratives of the early republic attests to a consistent search to understand and situate a broken, conflicting, and insufficient subject at the center of US American society. Often, a nonhuman environment provides the means for situating this broken Self. Ghosts function as mediums that hold the promise of fulfillment in spiritual connection to one's environment. As such, they could easily be instrumentalized by writers who sought to express natural relation to a place they knew was stolen.

Despite such congruencies, monocultural lineage and a recourse to European literary traditions is still the dominant mode of interpretation when it comes to the US American gothic and particularly ghost stories. Maisha L. Wester's research that demonstrates the firm standing of African American gothic narratives in antebellum cultures was only the first step in decolonizing US American literature. The epistemic erasures of Indigenous knowledge in settler colonial engagements with the supernatural led to a focus on British influences on the establishment of transculturality as a defining element of early American spectral narratives that is still in place. This focus, however, occludes not only the colonial structures within which spectral narratives were produced and the colonial purposes they have served but also the transcultural effect that they have engendered. Rather than replicating European gothic structures, the focus on spectrality in early American narratives demonstrates the entanglement of Indigenous, European, and enslaved people's cultures and the implications of this conjunction for transformations in European epistemologies.

Finally, can the ghost help to solve contemporary philosophical quandaries? The answer is yes. To follow the ghost means to acknowledge the entanglement of subjectivities, human and otherwise. Today we encounter a recourse to nonhuman agency that often reveals contours of free or magic philosophy. Many scholars are looking for subversive responses to a scientific community that is still indebted to the heritage of the Enlightenment. The unaccounted-for flow of energy is at the center of attention yet again. Schools such as New Materialism and critical posthumanism propose that more-than-human forces account for the processual nature of life. In many ways, interpreting ghosts as intrapsychic agents that question the separation between life and death but also between human and nonhuman relates to current theories of New Materialism and ecocriticism. This might be surprising, because ghosts, enveloped in their poststructuralist psychoanalytic cloak, appear to be the opposite of material structures. For this reason, ghosts feature rather seldom in more recent critical theoretical attempts at countering the humanist exclusivity of the Western subject. Yet, looking into transcultural figurations of ghosts as a certain type of energy that survives after the body's demise promises at the very least to provide a usable vocabulary for developing ideas that concern the process of decentering the human and establishing alternatives to classic humanist views. At their very best, ghosts might be able to help conceptualize much-needed alternative visions of planetary life without leaving the confines of science.

As conceptual tools, ghosts can also rehabilitate the connection between Indigenous knowledge systems and current ideas of new vitalist theories emerging in a transatlantic context. Just like eighteenth-century Eurocentric moral philosophy, the new vitalist theories have so far made insufficient recourse to Indigenous genealogies in spite of obvious congruencies between the two. In his introduction to *The Universe of Things: On Speculative Realism,* for example, Steven Shaviro writes: "The only way to outfox correlationism, and reach the great outdoors, without simply falling back into what Kant rejected as 'dogmatism' is to proceed obliquely through the history of philosophy, finding its points of divergence and its strange detours, when it moves beyond its own anthropocentric assumptions" (9). Presented as universal, this history of philosophy excludes not only Indigenous but all non-Western philosophies, most of which have elaborate concepts that can "outfox correlationism." Shaviro's statement demonstrates the ways in which current scholarship has limited the understanding not only of the supernatural but also of the natural. Zoe Todd's blog that overnight received 30,000 views and in 2016 was published under the title "An Indigenous Feminist's Take on the Ontological Turn: 'Ontology' Is Just Snother Word for Colonialism" exposes the extent to which dominant discourses in New Materialism function under the structural exclusion of Indigenous thinking.

Nonhuman ontology and ethics are at the center of most Indigenous cosmologies. The idea that life on earth is dictated by planetary boundaries and that humans are radically entangled with nonhuman environments is central to this line of thinking. The sense of the biological and nonbiological world as vital and alive is central to most if not all Indigenous conceptions of what could be called ghosts. New vitalist theories emerging in the context of posthumanism should thus find a helpful resource in Indigenous epistemologies and ontologies. Furthermore, as this study argued in the last chapter, Yoruba configurations of mediums and the study of the spread of Vodoun among enslaved communities, provides the much-sought-after vocabulary to address the agency of the past in the present.

Acknowledging Indigenous cosmologies and West African traditions as constitutive rather than corrective to early US American literature and culture effectively opposes stereotypical images of the "ecological Indian" and Indigenous people(s) as advocates of a transparent and pure spirituality rooted in nature and the long history of associating people abducted from Africa with the occult. In *The Ecological Indian,* Shepard Krech convincingly argued that the theory of Indigenous peoples living in harmony with their natural environment is a colonial hegemonic myth. Addressing inscriptions of Indigeneity and animism in colonial depictions of sentient nature is therefore also a small step towards decolonizing the naturalized production of "Man" as a scholarly imperative. Hopefully, in the future,

more studies will be devoted to exploring the rich cultural history of Indigenous spirits and ghosts as well as West African traditions of animism and,
in so doing, acknowledge their steady if occluded presence in US American
mainstream culture. Such studies necessarily expose the complex relationships between colonial temporalities, environmental degradation, subjectivity formation, and late capitalism. They therefore hold the promise of a
much-needed radical change in humanities.

As with any threshold, the new paradigm bares its own dangers. Now
that settler cultures are compelled by environmental forces to acknowledge their intrinsic inscription in their ecologies, the demand for epistemo-
logically distinct narratives that provide access to current realities grows.
Warning against the danger of silencing Indigenous voices, Vanessa Watts
writes in the context of theories of relationality in the twenty-first century:
"These types of historical Indigenous events [. . .] are increasingly becoming
not only accepted by Western frameworks of understanding, but sought
after in terms of non-oppressive and provocative or interesting interfaces
of accessing the real" (26). In a time when politics is turning into ecology
and the world is preparing for the sixth extinction (Kolbert), Indigenous
storytelling functions as a reminder that "the resources of the earth do not
belong to humankind; rather, humans belong to the earth" (Henare 202).
This also means that literature is once again in danger of returning to cultural appropriation. Just like the postrevolutionary United States, the current geological epoch is haunted most of all by the ghosts of an imperialist
ontology and the metaphysical essentialism of Enlightenment Man. My
study only traces ways in which Indigenous cosmologies and West African
traditions have been appropriated and put in the service of colonization. As
such, it marks only a small step in acknowledging these sources as genera-
tive conceptions for much of contemporary US American popular culture.
A lot more work needs to be done to break away from this tradition. Yet,
whatever the next step might be, it must begin with new parameters for the
category of the human. This reconceptualization must be done as much in
life as in death—and ghosts are formidable assistants mediating between
the two.

NOTES

Introduction

1. In *Dialectic of Enlightenment,* Adorno and Horkheimer include a section entitled "A Theory of Ghosts," in which they explain ghosts merely as an unsublimated fear of the dead; in *Ghostly Matters,* Gordon studies ghosts and haunting as a constituent element of modern social life; in the introduction to *Arts of Living on a Damaged Planet,* Tsing et al. use the concept of ghosts to explore "the traces of more-than-human histories through which ecologies are made and unmade" (G1).

2. This story initially appeared in *The Gift* in 1842 under the title "Murder Will Out." The same text under the title "Grayling; or, 'Murder Will Out'" was published in October 1845 in the Library of American Books series as part of the collection *The Wigwam and the Cabin.* In-text quotes are taken from the 1845 edition of the text.

3. *Spectral America: Phantoms and the National Imagination* is an important essay collection that seeks to attest to a spectral turn in literary and cultural studies in 2006 already (Weinstock, *Spectral America* 3). While the many turns that have been proposed more recently in the humanities are making the concept somewhat questionable, there is certainly an upsurge in spectral matters in literature and culture that calls for interpretation.

4. Most academic publications dedicated to the American Renaissance begin with Edgar Allan Poe's writing (Reynolds), which is why this study ends with the entrance of Poe onto the US American literary scene. Poe's first published short story, "Metzengerstein," appeared in Philadelphia's *Saturday Courier* in 1832. Yet, only with the publication of "The Narrative of Arthur Gordon Pym" in 1848 and "The Fall of the House of Usher" in 1840 would he reach great acclaim. The prime time for Poe's tales of the supernatural happens shortly after the period demarcated in this study.

5. American spiritualism is a popular religious and cultural movement that emerged in the late nineteenth-century United States and centered on various forms of communication with the spirits of the dead and shifted the public discourse on ghosts by serving as both a forum for personal expression and a subject for ridicule (see Braude; McGarry).

1. Instrumentalizing Ghosts

1. The annotated bibliography published in 2008 in K. David Goss' reference guide for the Salem witch trials counts thirty-one secondary print sources alone. See also Roach.

2. Norton writes in *In the Devil's Snare* about the focus on "strange noises" and "ghostly visitations" for the persecutions, which inevitably interlaces ghosts with witches. The mutual influence on the concepts of *ghost* and *witch* is explored by Gillian Bennett in "Ghost and Witch in the Sixteenth and Seventeenth Centuries." Bennett confirms that from the late sixteenth to the early eighteenth century, "the two were so closely allied that for over a hundred years they constituted virtually a single subject."

3. In 2010 Owen Davies edited a highly informative five-volume series entitled *Ghosts: A Social History* that collects a wide range of scholarly texts on ghosts published in Britain and the United States from the Reformation to the early twentieth century. This large editorial project also confirms the beginning of scholarly discussion on ghosts and related concepts in the midst of the seventeenth century.

4. More recent scholarship on Hobbes' *Leviathan,* such as Parkin's, reveals that in spite of the official condemnation of this publication and the discrediting of Hobbes as an atheist by influential clergy, the book was widely discussed, forwarding a whole range of religious and political debates in the second part of the seventeenth century.

5. Noel Malcolm writes in his introduction to a definitive edition of *Leviathan*— an introduction that was called "truly a masterpiece of scholarship" and takes up the complete first volume (Hammond)—that the "question of the motives or reasons for the writing of *Leviathan* is [...] the most vexed issue surrounding the work" and goes on in making the argument that the work was conceived by this political philosopher in order to teach how to govern and how to educate people (Malcolm 12). Teaching narrative techniques was part of this education.

6. On the relation between the Royal Society in its early years and magic in general as well as witchcraft in particular, see Hunter's informative study "The Royal Society and the Decline of Magic." Informative discussions on colonial fellows of the Royal Society of London can be found in Brasch.

7. The theory of ghost-seeing being a contagion in Hobbes' text resonates with Freud's theory of ghosts as a form of "mental conservatism" (Freud *Totem* 24). In *Totem und Taboo* (1913, first English edition published by George Routledge and Sons in 1919; I quote from the 1950 translation by James Strachey), Freud writes about taboos as an objectified fear of a demonic power and how this fear is passed to the next generation. He continues: "And thereafter it itself became the route of our moral precepts and of our laws" (Freud, *Totem* 24). Taking a

closer look at demons and ghosts, both Hobbes and Freud expose how moral laws are inherited and not questioned.

8. In "The Pathology of Reading: The Novel as an Agent of Contagion," Michel Fournier writes about "the pathology of reading" and the novel "as an early agent of contagion" (195). This discourse on reading and the danger of contagion relates to the concept of seeing ghosts as a contagious disease.

9. On Glanvill's career as a philosopher and questions concerning empirical criticism, see Popkin. Popkin argues that Glanvill was a precursor of David Hume.

10. The Royal Society was initiated by a group of English natural philosophers in London in 1660. Thomas Sprat was commissioned to write the story about the society only a few years later, which was published as *History of the Royal Society* in 1667.

11. "To the Royal Society" was published as a preface to *Scepsis Scientifica* in 1665. It was presented to the Royal Society in December 1664. I quote from the 1885 edition. The main part of the text was first published as *The Vanity of Dogmatizing* in 1661, the first work of Joseph Glanvill in print.

12. Another telling example of the instrumentalization of ghost stories as a means of writing against the spread of atheism is Baxter's *The Certainty of the Worlds of Spirits* (1691). For an overview of the seventeenth century link between atheism and disbelief in spirits and witches, see M. Prior.

13. Hunter explains in *The Decline of Magic* that "'Sadducism' is the word used to describe scepticism about the reality of spiritual beings, derived from the Sadducees of the New Testament—Acts 23:8" (14). A comprehensive study of social roles, beliefs, and values of the Sadducees can be found in Botha. The spelling and titles with the word "Sad(d)ucees" are here replicated from the original. In most secondary literature, the word "Sadducees" is spelled with a double *d,* whereas the first edition of Glanvill's book was published with the title *Saducismus Triumphatus.*

14. It is the first story in the chapter "Proof of Apparitions, Spirits, and Witches, from a choice Collection of Modern Relations," published under the title "Relation I: Which Is the Enlarged Narrative of the Daemon of Tedworth, or of the Disturbances at Mr. Mompesson's House, Caused by Witchcraft, and the Villainy of the Drummer."

15. On the individual versions since its first publication until today, see Hunter "New Light."

16. In *Religion and the Decline of Magic,* Keith Thomas also quoted a ghost story featuring an incident with a poltergeist and subsequent exorcism via sword. There, a sword was taken to the grave and "run into the middle part of the grave during which time of conjuration the doctor told the said wife of the sick person that she would hear strange noise in and about the house" (710). According to Thomas, running the sword through the buried corpse was the legally

required method of burial for suicides until 1823 (710). Here, too, the evil is imagined to have a corporeal existence that can be fought with a weapon.

17. Another famous ghost story often retold in spite of it being debunked from the beginning was recorded most prominently by Daniel Defoe under the title "A True Relation of the Apparition of One Mrs. Veal, the Next Day after Her Death: To One Mrs. Bargrave at Canterbury. The 8th of September, 1705." For a discussion about the "truthfulness" of this relation, see G. Cruikshank's *A Discovery Concerning Ghosts*. According to Cruikshank, the story was written by Defoe after the translator and publisher of *Drelincourt on Death* asked him to help the scarce sales, with his name and a story that would sell. Defoe wrote the story as a preface to *Drelincourt on Death*. Sasha Handley in "Ghosts, Gossip, and Gender in Eighteenth-Century Canterbury" demonstrates that ghost stories throughout the seventeenth and eighteenth century have been functionalized for purposes of justice in the context of gender.

18. Famous ghost stories from this period that were collected by scholars and can be found in print in various versions are, for example, the ghost of Anne Walker presented by More in a letter to Glanvill in *Saducismus Triumphatus* (1681); the Daemon of Spreyton presented in John Aubrey's *Miscellanies upon the Following Subjects Collected* (1696); the poltergeist of Isabel Heriot presented by George Sinclair in *Satan's Invisible World Discovered* (1685); or the possession of the Merideth children presented in Richard Bovet's *Pandaemonium* (1684).

19. The American Scientific Society, or Boston Philosophical Society, was established in Boston in 1683 by Increase Mather. It does not appear to have lasted very long; see Brasch; E. S. Morrison. For contributions by Cotton Mather, see especially Kittredge.

20. The first version of this manuscript was published in 1658 under the title *Remarkable Providences Illustrative of the Earlier Days of American Colonisation*. All quotes are taken from the 1684 reprint.

21. Lorraine Daston and Katharine Park write in their captivating study about a "coherent and long-lived cluster of wonders persisting from antiquity through at least Enlightenment" (10) confirming that Mather's collection was not unusual for the times.

22. This is still a widely acknowledged definition of rumors that was introduced by Shibutani in 1966. See Daston and Park about the ways in which "wonders" became the dominant form of discourse in seventeenth-century England and New England.

23. Numerous studies have already been conducted on the Salem witchcraft trials. Among various recent publications on the concept of "spectral evidence" particularly, and for an overview on current scholarship and ideas on reasons for the untiring fascination with the Salem witchcraft trials as a research topic, see Rivett, "Our Salem, Our Selves."

24. The marriage of rumors with spectral matters as a way to enter the court is not restricted to the seventeenth century. Jean-Noël Kapferer began his still-influential study of rumors, *Gerüchte: Das älteste Massenmedium der Welt* (translated by Ulrich Kunzmann as *Rumors: Uses, Interpretation and Necessity*) with the story of a court trial in which the large American corporation Procter and Gamble was accused of signing a contract with the devil in 1981. The source was a rumor that originates somewhere "West of Mississippi" (Kapferer 7).

25. According to Nancy Ruttenburg, the Salem witch trials nearly exclusively relied on spectral evidence (35). Wendel D. Craker on the other hand, claimed that no one was sent to trial, let alone hanged, on the basis of spectral evidence alone (333). The actual trial is not at stake here; important is the use of spectral evidence in court.

26. Matthew Wynn Sivils pointed out the connection between the gothic and the captivity narrative in his analysis of the Frontier Gothic, which in his opinion was the result of a "melding of Indian captivity tales, local history, wilderness environments, and select conventions of European works" (84). I would like to specify that the European element in this context often reverts to ghost-story conventions.

27. Recently, more sensibility is noticeable in critical theory and literary studies. Norton's *In the Devil's Snare* offers the first thorough analysis of the Salem witch trials based on their connections to the Second Indian War. Her conclusions differ strongly from those of her predecessors, as the often lethal accusations are presented as rooted in the animosity against the Indigenous population and not simply in the misogynistic Puritan ideology. Before Norton's seminal work, Karlsen had already made some significant remarks about this connection in her study of the North American witch trials in *The Devil in the Shape of Woman.*

28. "The Tryal of G. B. at a Court of Oyer and Terminer, Held in Salem, 1692."

29. See, for example, Ravalli; Gasser.

30. Among many others, Tamara Shefer and Kopano Ratele write about the construction of Black male bodies as physically and sexually dangerous as a way of entrenching and rationalizing white male power and privilege all the way into the twenty-first century. See also Hill Collins.

31. In the still influential study from 1987, *The Devil in the Shape of a Woman*, Karlsen makes the convincing argument that most witches (either serving the devil or possessed by the devil) in early American society were women because they either stood in the way of men's property inheritance or owned property themselves.

32. See also Chadwick Hansen, "The Metamorphosis of Tituba, or Why American Intellectuals Can't Tell an Indian Witch from a Negro."

2. Counter-Enlightenment

1. In *Das Andere der Vernunft,* Hartmut and Gernot Böhme present a philosophy of modernity that is based not on rationalism but on the other side of reason, which is mainly discussed in the context of the body (*Leib*), desire, feelings, imagination, and nature.

2. For eighteenth-century studies on counter-Enlightenment, see McMahon; Garrard. For an analysis of the politics of the counter-Enlightenment, see Wolin's study, *The Seduction of Unreason.* As the title of his book makes plain, Wolin argues that a shared suspicion of rationality crosses the boundary that is usually understood to be separating the political right from the academic left during the twentieth century. For studies questioning the one-sidedness of Horkheimer and Adorno's *Dialektik der Aufklärung,* see Bronner.

3. Following is merely a selection of representative articles published in the first years of the 1760s alone. They confirm a more focused attention on the public representation of ghosts in the second part of the eighteenth century. The selection includes articles published in the context of religion, public life, literature, public spectacle, and theater: "Dissertations upon the Apparitions of Angels, Daemons, and Ghosts, and Concerning the Vampires of Hungary, Bohemia, Moravia, and Silesia" in *Monthly Review* (1759); "The Apparition to a Great Man," also in *Monthly Review* (1760); "Relation of an Astonishing Apparition, from the Voyages and Cruises of Commodore WALKER," *Imperial Magazine; or, Complete Monthly Intelligencer* (1760); "PROLOGUE to THE DRUMMER; OR, HAUNTED HOUSE," *Universal Magazine of Knowledge and Pleasure* (Smith, 1762); "An Account of a Pretended Apparition in Kent," *Gentleman's Magazine* (Atticus, 1762); "Of Apparitions, Witches, & C." in *London Magazine; or, Gentleman's Monthly Intelligencer* (1762); "On the Subject of Apparitions," *London Magazine; or, Gentleman's Monthly Intelligencer* (1763); "The Affair of the Supposed GHOST in Cock-lane, Weft-Smithfield," *Universal Magazine of Knowledge and Pleasure* (1762).

4. Rush's writings on the senses are collected in *Benjamin Rush's Lectures on the Mind.* On Franklin's important trip to Paris in 1784 and his subsequent report on mesmerism, see McConkey and Perry.

5. All original citations to Kant's works are according to the standard practice of parenthetical references to the page of *Werkausgabe,* volume 2, Suhrkamp 1977. Unless otherwise noted, all translations are from the 1992 volume of *The Cambridge Edition of the Works of Immanuel Kant* and marked in the text as (*Dreams*). *Dreams of a Spirit-Seer, Elucidated by Dreams of Metaphysics* can be found in the first volume, *Theoretical Philosophy, 1755–1770.* This translation by David Walford in collaboration with Ralf Meerbote is, to date, the most accurate one. The first complete English translation, by Emanuel F. Goerwitz, was published in 1900 and edited by Frank Sewell, both US American

Swedenborgian ministers, under the title *Dreams of a Spirit-Seer, Illustrated by Dreams of Metaphysics.* The second translation, by John Manolesco, a Canadian author of books on astrology and the occult, was published in 1969 as *Dreams of a Spirit Seer by Immanuel Kant and Other Related Writings.* In 2002 the Swedenborg Foundation published a new (fourth) translation, by Gregory R. Johnson and Alexander Magee, under the title *Kant on Swedenborg: Dreams of a Spirit-Seer and Other Writings,* with the intention of providing an affordable edition that contains various letters and manuscripts.

6. Davis is not alone in crediting Derrida with the inauguration of ghost studies. In the introduction to *The Spectralities Reader: Ghosts and Haunting in Contemporary Cultural Theory,* María del Pilar Blanco and Esther Peeren write that Jacques Derrida's *Spectres de Marx* (1993) and the English translation of the book the following year are "commonly considered the catalyst for what Luckhurst has called 'the spectral turn'" (2).

7. On this unresolved dispute see McQuillan.

8. Three years before publishing his treatise on ghosts, on August 10, 1763, Kant writes to Charlotte von Knobloch: "I await with longing the book that Swedenborg will publish in London. I have made every provision for receiving it as soon as it leaves the press" (Kant, *Kant on Swedenborg* 158).

9. I am grateful for the input from and discussions with the German research group on "Emmanuel Swedenborg's Position within the European Enlightenment and Esoteric Discourse of the 18th Century," which explored the connection between Kant and Swedenborg as part of the Interdisciplinary Center for European Enlightenment Studies at Martin Luther University Halle-Wittenberg. The best overview can be found in the collection *Kant and Swedenborg,* edited by Stengel. See also Weissberg.

10. On Kant's troubling relation to Swedenborg, see Florschütz, *Swedenborgs verborgene Wirkung auf Kant: Swedenborg und die okkulten Phänomene aus der Sicht von Kant und Schopenhauer* and *Emmanuel Swedenborgs mystisches Menschenbild und die Doppelnatur des Menschen bei Immanuel Kant.*

11. I have discussed the connection between Kant's early publication on ghosts and his later work on morality in "Immanuel Kant's 'One Great Republic': From Spirit Theory to Moral Philosophy" (Blažan).

12. In the original text, "pneumatische" and "organische Regeln" (Kant, *Werkausgabe* 928).

13. All translations of *Grundlegung zur Metaphysik der Sitten* are from the 1996 *The Cambridge Edition of the Works of Immanuel Kant* volume on *Practical Philosophy* edited and translated by Mary J. Gregor. Further referenced in text as (Kant *Groundwork*).

14. Kant's famous "silent decade" is a period of eleven years (1770–81) during which he supposedly refused to publish (Werkmeister). He, indeed, did publish, notably, on human cognition, but this is not of any relevance

to my argument. On Kant's publications during the "silent decade," see Allison.

15. I owe thanks to John McCarthy for pointing this out in our correspondence per email (J. McCarthy, "Re: Christoph Martin Wieland in the United States"); see also Haney. A general introduction to Wieland's reception in the United States can be found in McCarthy "'An Indigenous and Not an Exotic Plant': Towards a History of Germanics at Penn."

16. All quotes are from Wieland, *Sämmtliche Werke.* The source for the translation is the much more famous 1796 version of the essay. I owe thanks to Viia Ottenbacher and Wieland Stiftung Bieberach for access to original documents. Translations from French and German are my own unless otherwise noted. I accept full responsibility for any errors.

17. The text was first translated in London only one year after the original publication in 1792 and reprinted several times but with some liberties that the author did not approve of. Jefferson considered the text to be extremely important and decided to translate it himself, albeit anonymously for fear of compromising his public office. For reasons of time, Jefferson was not able to finish the last four chapters. Volney asked Joel Barlow to finish the text, and Barlow accepted (Caron). The entire work appeared in two volumes in 1802 under the title *A New Translation of Volney's Ruins.* I quote from the so-called Jefferson-Barlow translation, further referenced in text as (*Ruins*). Levrault of Paris published two editions: 1802 and 1817. Bossange frères of Paris also published an edition in 1820, the year of Volney's death. In the United States, Dixon and Sickles of New York published the first American edition of the Jefferson-Barlow translation in 1828. The Jefferson-Barlow translation then went through several reprints during the nineteenth and twentieth centuries, including by Gaylord of Boston (1830s), Calvin Blanchard of New York (no date), Josiah Mendum of Boston (1880s), Peter Eckler of New York (1890s and 1910s-1920s) and the Truth Seeker Press of New York (1950).

18. Volney stayed in the United States from 1795 to 1798 conducting research, which he published in 1803, printed and translated in Philadelphia by Charles Brockden Brown in 1804 as *A View of the Soil and Climate of the United States of America, with Supplementary Remarks upon Florida; on the French Colonies on the Mississippi and Ohio, and in Canada; and on the Aboriginal Tribes of America.*

19. On the Self and the novel in the eighteenth century, see Julie Park, *The Self and It: Novel Objects and Mimetic Subjects in Eighteenth-Century England.*

20. Mary Shelley famously set out to write a ghost story when she sat down to write *Frankenstein.* The narrator in the novel repeatedly refers to the creature as a ghost, spirit, or apparition.

21. The earliest phantasmagoria shows took place in Paris in 1798, the most famous ones conducted by Etienne-Gaspard Robertson. His shows featured revolutionaries such as Rousseau, Voltaire, Robespierre, and Marat. On phantasmagoria

shows, see also Marina Warner's *Phantasmagoria*. For ghost shows in the US, consult Barber.

22. See also *The Flushing Phantasmagoria—or—Kings Conjurors Amuseing John Bull,* a print in which a magician explains politics to John Bull with a phantasmagoria device.

3. The Voice of Conscience

1. All references to the text are from *Three Gothic Novels,* published by the Library of America in 1998. The text in this edition is a reprint of the original print published in New York in 1798 by T. & J. Swords for Hocquet Caritat. Further references in the text under (C. Brown, *Three Gothic*). Shortly after publication, Brown's novels were translated into German (1802), French (1808), and Spanish (1818). He was thus the first US American author to appear in multiple translations and join a transatlantic community of literary voices. On the translations of Brown's work and his reception in Europe at the time, see Cody.

2. Edward Cahill writes that "Brown's German poet [Wieland] suggests the gothic sensibility of Goethe, Schiller, or Christoph Wieland" yet considers their work to be "of no significance," because any story "that represented genteel romance reading and stirred the delicate passions of educated Americans like the Wielands would have sufficed" (31). Sydney J. Krause asserts that "Wieland very likely had a bearing on Brown's composition of Wieland" (97); Friedrich Schiller's *The Ghost-Seer* and Cajetan Tschink's *The Victim of Magical Delusion* have been acknowledged as reference points for *Wieland* but without further analysis.

3. All references are taken from the article entitled "On Apparitions. *In a Letter from a Country Gentleman to his Friend in Town,*" published in the April 1799 issue of the *Monthly Magazine* and signed as "F. R." Further referenced in text as (F. R.).

4. The article is listed in the Charles Brockden Brown Electronic Archive and Scholarly Edition, run by scholars from the University of Central Florida, which was initiated with the aim of collecting and transcribing Brown's uncollected writing. The article is listed in their collection and marked with a "B," since Brown does not use the signature "F. R." anywhere else. However, "On Apparitions" was reprinted in *Lady's Monitor* in 1802, a periodical published in New York. Brown was going back and forth between New York and Philadelphia at the time. A few of his other pieces that were reprinted from *Monthly Magazine* in *Lady's Monitor* are "Trials of Arden" and "Lesson on Concealment" (both in multiple installments), "On the Prevailing Ignorance of Geography," "Portrait of an Emigrant," and "On a Taste for the Picturesque." This, at the very least, confirms that he had ties to the journal. It is, thus, very likely that "On Apparitions" is a piece written by Charles Brockden Brown.

5. For Brown's interest in ghost shows and spectral performance see Schmidt and Schweighauser.

6. Schiller's publication was a success throughout Europe and the United States. *Der Geisterseher, aus den Papieren des Grafen von O* was first published in the journal *Thalia* in 1787. The first English translation appears only a short time after its original publication: Friedrich Schiller, *The Ghost-Seer; or, Apparitionist: An Interesting Fragment, Found among the Papers of Count O***, translated by Daniel Boileau, London, Vernor and Hood, 1795. Tschink's novel was first published as *Geschichte eines Geistersehers: Aus den Papieren des Mannes mit der eisernen Larve* in three volumes from 1790–94. The first translation (by Peter Will) of Tschink's novel was published in book form also right after the original publication: Cajetan Tschink, *The Victim of Magical Delusion; or, The Mysteries of the Revolution of P—l.* London, printed for G. G. and J. Robinson, Peter-Noster-Row, 1795.

7. Brown took German classes and demonstrated a continual interest in German literature and culture throughout his career as a writer, publisher, and editor. The earliest English version of *The Ghost-Seer* was republished serially in New York in 1795–96 under the title *The Apparitionist* and read with great interest by Brown's New York circle, who compared it favorably with Tschink's *The Victim of Magical Delusion.*

8. The many correspondences between the Hungarian and the Armenian are yet another indication that might confirm Brown's authorship. Brown's contemporaries have recognized the correspondences between Brown's and Schiller's work. John Keats wrote in a letter to Richard Woodhouse in September 1819 about having read Brown's novel *Wieland* and describes it as "very powerful—something like Godwin—Between Schiller and Godwin—A domestic prototype of Shiller's [sic] Armenian."

9. For informed readings of Schiller's influence on the English gothic, see Conger; Hall.

10. See for example, Peter Kafer, who writes in *Charles Brockden Brown's Revolution and the Birth of American Gothic:* "At the age of twenty-seven Charles Brockden Brown invented the American Gothic novel [. . .]" (xi).

11. This early reception of Immanuel Kant's philosophy in English by one of his students is an often-overlooked reference in Kant scholarship: F. A. Nitsch's 1796 *A General and Introductory View of Professor Kant's Principles Concerning Man, the World, and the Deity, Submitted to the Consideration of the Learned.* Most critics refer to René Wellek's 1931 *Immanuel Kant in England, 1793–1838* as the first thorough exploration of Kant's reception in English.

12. The article appeared under the title "Memoirs of Immanuel Kant" in the *Literary Magazine and American Register.* The same text was first printed in the *London Monthly Magazine,* May 1, 1805, 354–61. The first part of the article was reprinted in the *European Magazine and London Review,*

no. 48, October 1805, 257–58. In all three versions, the article was published anonymously.

13. This article has not been discussed in Brown's scholarship so far. I owe thanks to the members of the Charles Brockden Brown Society for helping me verify the authorship of this text.

14. The most influential philosophers in this transatlantic context were Lord Shaftesbury, Francis Hutcheson, David Hume, and Adam Smith; see Taylor. On philosophical sources on sensationalism in the US American context, see Cahill.

15. Brown published all his seven novels between 1798 and 1801.

16. Brown refers himself to the James Yates murder case in Tomhanick in New York State in 1796, which was well known at the time ("Explanatory Notes" 290).

17. The response from January 15, 1800, can be found in the Thomas Jefferson Papers at the Library of Congress, Series 1: General Correspondence. 1651–1827, Microfilm Reel: 022. Contemporary scholarship on *Wieland* prefers a reading of *Wieland* as a commentary on the politics of the early Republic. In addition, critics such as Judson and Wolfe are two prominent scholars among many who offer a psychoanalytic reading of colonial guilt. Violence and anxieties about secret societies are also often assumed to be behind the story of *Wieland,* as in Galluzzo's or Bradshaw's readings.

18. Historical readings of *Wieland* can be found in Weldon, Christopherson, Rombes Jr., Looby, Samuels, and Clark. On Locke's sensational psychology in *Wieland,* see Voloshin.

19. In following this trace, Brown not only identifies himself as a child of his time but also proves his long-lasting love for Shakespeare, as he highlights the supernatural with the colors of the political. On the supernatural in Shakespeare's work, see Garber. The second chapter on *Richard III* and the shape of history is particularly interesting in the current context. Wayne Franklin has filled the gap on Shakespeare's influences on Brown's *Wieland* if only considering *Hamlet* and *Much Ado about Nothing.*

20. The word *depression* in the context of low spirits was first used in the 1660s, but in the current clinical sense it has been around only since the 1890s, a whole century after Brown's publication (Solomon). It is another Brown, William Hill Brown, who first structured a novel around what today would be considered depression. In his *Power of Sympathy,* he developed a very similar narrative that focuses on low spirits and incest. In fact, depression as a state of low mood and state of inactivity that affects one's behavior is at the center of early American literature and, in this context, still an understudied topic.

21. In his *Studies in Classic American Literature,* D. H. Lawrence called the new country a vast republic of fugitives from slavery, as even the Pilgrim Fathers "came so gruesomely over the black sea" (5).

22. For an exception, see Galluzzo. Eric Savoy rightly proposes that the American gothic troubles "the locus of cultural and political authority after the revolution

and the perfectibility of human beings in a democracy," yet he does not further specify ways in which this history was written into the narratives via spectrality (168).

23. Note that anxiety was not distinguished from depression until the 1980s.

24. An informative article concerning typical elements of exorcism can be found in Kallendorf.

25. This form of death was widely accepted as a natural phenomenon in the eighteenth century, although since the early nineteenth century, scientists have repeatedly expressed their skepticism. However, Arnold writes about twentieth-century cases of spontaneous combustion. Like ventriloquism, it seems to be a somatic occurrence that is often interpreted in relation to magic. Other famous literary representations can be found in Charles Dickens' *Bleak House*, Nikolaj Gogol's *Dead Souls*, and Herman Melville's *Redburn*. The earliest reference to spontaneous combustion that could be found in a newspaper published in the North American continent was from 1779, signed with the cryptic signature A. B. C. In 1815 spontaneous combustion seems to have been an extremely popular topic to discuss in daily newspapers.

26. An interesting parallel can be found in a footnote in *Dreams of a Spirit-Seer*, where Kant wrote about "surreptitious concepts" as conceptions that cannot be drawn from experience (43). Urging the reader to keep an open mind in spite of better judgment, Kant contended, just like Brown, that "many conceptions arise in secret and obscure conclusions incidental to experiences, and afterwards are transmitted to other minds without even the consciousness of that experience or conclusion which has first established the conception" (*Dreams* 43).

27. See Bennett's article for the first scholarly analysis of the architecture of the temple built by enslaved people, in which the author connects Thomas Jefferson's Monticello to the structures on the Mettingen estate in Brown's *Wieland* ("Silence").

28. Notice that John Adams, the president at the time when Brown wrote the novel, modeled much of his writing on Cicero's work and was known to compare the lack of public acknowledgment for his work to the stature of Cicero. On Cicero in *Wieland*, see Nichols.

29. In *Haunting Legacies*, Schwab uses Abraham and Torok's theory of transgenerational phantoms, with the help of current trauma theory, in order to analyze "how both victims and perpetrators pass on the ineradicable legacies of violent histories through generations" in the context of traumatic memories of World War II, particularly the Holocaust experience (1).

30. Various details relating to Abraham and Torok's theory of the transgenerational phantom are problematic. For a discussion of some of the pertinent problems, see Kamuf. I particularly disagree with Abraham and Torok's idea of exorcism, although this concept is not pertinent to the argument in this study. The theory

of the transgenerational phantom and of the crypt was expanded by critics such as Jacques Derrida, Laurence Rickels, and Avital Ronell.

31. The centrality of the connection between the death of the father and the death of the son in mystery and horror has been a subject of scholarly consideration. Larzer Ziff addresses the transgenerational connection in death as an "inherited depravity" passed from the father to the son ("A Reading" 54). Ringe writes that there was an "important element" in the children's past "which they can never escape, and an unexpected and unforeseen future waits to test them severely" (*Charles Brockden* 28); while Hinds calls the Wieland's house "haunted."

32. On the birth of psychology in the US, see the excellent introduction by Evans.

33. In *Playing in the Dark,* Morrison discusses the African presence that commonly marks an empty space that structures all of early American literature. The presence of the Indigenous population was widely discussed in early American literature and culture, producing a variety of cultural imaginaries that served the purpose of recoding their presence as an absence.

34. In his famous thesis of "regeneration through violence," Slotkin proposed in 1973 that violence towards Native Americans "as a structuring metaphor of the American experience" is constitutive to the inauguration of the US American nation (5).

35. One can find this interpretation in numerous readings, most recently in James Goho's "A Portrait of Charles Dexter Ward as a Haunted Young Man."

36. All references to *Memoirs of Carwin* are from the 2011 Norton Critical Edition edited by Waterman; further referenced in text as (Brown, *Wieland and Memoirs*).

37. While Brown's work has been either criticized for the lack of Indigenous characters or praised for the centrality of the character of Old Deb in *Edgar Huntly,* the spectral presence of the Indigenous population in his work has received much less attention. In a short review article with the title "The Spectral Indian Presence in Early American Literature," Sarah Rivett recently proposed that there is a "spectral presence of American Indians" in *Wieland* ("Spectral Indian" 625). On the significance of ventriloquism in *Wieland,* see also Fliegelman.

38. Whether or not Carwin is the source of the mysterious voices that Wieland hears continues to be a debate among critics.

39. Recently, critics have started contextualizing Brown's work in a wider US colonial discourse. See most notably Kazanjian; Burgett; Cahill; Hsu; Kamrath; Kutchen; Luciano; Mackenthun; Rowe, *At Emerson's Tomb;* Ruttenburg.

40. A thorough history of ventriloquism can be found in Connor.

41. On white settlers impersonating Native Americans, see in particular Deloria. The author traces historical references of cross-dressing as Native American, such as in the notorious Boston Tea Party all the way to current "Indian

hobbyists," people who meet to dress and behave as "Indians" (Deloria 128). See Seeman on the intersection of speaking with the dead and Indigenous rites, particularly on Shaker visions.

42. Quote from *Live and Let Live,* published by the Society of Indian Dead (quoted in Deloria 181).

43. In the introduction to this novel published in 1826, Cooper describes the "native warriors of America" in the following manner: "In war, he is daring, boastful, cunning, ruthless, self-denying, and self-devoted; in peace, just, generous, hospitable, revengeful, superstitious, modest, and commonly chaste" (7). This and similar descriptions of Indigenous characters in his novels drown any sense of individualism in stereotypical superhuman images. While Brown is certainly guilty of avoiding Indigenous characters in his text, he is exploring a more complex subjectivity based on interpersonal exchanges between the Native and the immigrant population. His writing cannot be subsumed under the same heading as Cooper's.

44. Taking a slightly different perspective, Snyder-Körber detects a similar affinity between Charles Brockden Brown's development of his character Theodore Wieland and Immanuel Kant's examination of enthusiasm in his *Critique of Judgement* (1790). Her study supports the proposal that a comparison of Kant and Brown offers "analytical profitable parallels" between the two concepts of "reasoning enthusiast[s]" (66).

45. The *Oxford English Dictionary* cites Brown as the source for the word *biloquist,* defined as "one who can speak with two different voices," whereas "ventriloquism" is defined as "the art or practice of speaking or producing sounds in such a manner that the voice appears to proceed from some person or object other than the speaker, and usually at some distance from him." Whereas DuBois writes about a double consciousness in an African American context, in a sense of looking at oneself through the eyes of the other, who looks with contempt and pity, Bakhtin is preoccupied with heteroglossia in human communication in general. I use "the torments of dubbing" in order to position Brown's biloquism somewhere between the two theories. "The torments of dubbing" ("Les souffrances du 'dubbing'") is a posthumously published article by Antonin Artaud, in which he set out to criticize French actors who engaged with American companies for small remuneration in "dubbing." Suitably, it was written in response to his own script for a film titled *The Dybbuk,* about a malicious possessing spirit believed to be the dislocated soul of a dead person in Kabbalistic and European Jewish tradition.

46. Freud famously interprets the uncanny (the German *unheimlich*) as the return of something formerly familiar, now estranged (Freud 1919/1963). In his much-quoted study *The Fantastic: A Structural Approach to a Literary Genre,* Tzvetan Todorov reads the ambivalence between the real and unreal as a characteristic of the fantastic.

47. The critical reception of Charles Brockden Brown's oeuvre is complicated, to say the least. Most famously, Nina Baym attacked the quality of the work. Simultaneously, critics have to justify why Brown was so highly regarded by notable literary figures such as Margaret Fuller, William Godwin, or Percy Bysshe Shelley and why he continues to be admired, read, and taught in literature classes to this day.

48. Some critics talk about a recent boom in Brown scholarship (Kazanjian; Weinstock, *Charles Brockden Brown*). The Charles Brockden Brown Society keeps a secondary sources website that is regularly updated by members, which clearly demonstrates that there has always been a strong interest in Brown's work: brockdenbrown.cah.ucf.edu/bibliography.php#secondary.

49. Davison calls Brown "the godfather of the American gothic" (Davison, "Charles Brockden Brown"; see also among many others Kafer, Chase, Warfel, Weinstock). Chapter 6 in Leslie Fiedler's much quoted *Love and Death in the American Novel* is entitled "Charles Brockden Brown and the Invention of the American Gothic" (126).

4. The Politics of Absence

1. It was during this gathering that Mary Shelley began writing her novel *Frankenstein; or, The Modern Prometheus,* which was published two years later, in 1818.

2. All references to the text are from the Library of America collection with the title *History, Tales, and Sketches* published in 1983.

3. An early version of this chapter has been published as "Silencing the Dead: Washington Irving's Use of the Supernatural in the Context of Slavery and Genocide" (Blažan 2013).

4. Particularly Irving's tale "The Legend of Sleepy Hollow" but also "The Devil and Tom Walker" and "Rip van Winkle" have repeatedly been adopted for cinema and TV. All three tales are regularly taught in literature classes in schools and universities today.

5. All references to the text are from the Library of America collection with the title *History, Tales, and Sketches* published in 1983.

6. All in text quotations refer to the reprints of the original editions by the Library of America. Further editions were published by Irving himself at several points in his life; see Michael L. Black and Nancy Black's "Introduction" in *A History of New York.*

7. American literature of the formative period was nationalized just as much through the distancing on the side of the English reception as it was through patriotic writings published in the new republic itself. See also McLamore.

8. Even today in the states of New York, New Jersey, Massachusetts, and Minnesota, it is necessary to disclose the reputation of a house as haunted when selling it. In *Stambovsky v. Ackley,* the New York State Supreme Court, Appellate

Division, ruled in 1991 that a seller must disclose that a house has a reputation for being haunted, because such a reputation may impair the value of the house (Lawlor).

9. In *Playing Indian*, Philip J. Deloria explains how US Americans molded narratives of national identity "around the rejection of an older European consciousness and an almost mystical imperative to become new" by "playing Indian" (2).

10. On the essential role of Blackness for the construction of whiteness, see Shelley Fisher Fishkin's now classic treatment of the topic in *Was Huck Black? Mark Twain and African-American Voices*.

11. On racism and interracial friendship, see also Jackman and Crane. In *Death, Mourning and American Affinity*, Christopher Peterson proposes the qualification of spectrality as implicated in but not reducible to "the social effects of racism, sexism and homophobia that engender a field of unlivable, abject beings" (10).

12. On gender and patriarchy in Irving's work, see Hurst.

13. Irving's misogynistically rendered white settler female characters such as Katharina van Tassel or Dame van Winkel only appear as antagonists that serve the purpose of affirming the free spirit of the protagonists.

14. On American gag rules and reactions in the public, see Holmes.

5. The Voice of Nature

1. On the ideology of the Vanishing Indian, see, among others, Deloria, *Playing Indian;* Bergland; Huhndorf; Bird; Berkhofer; Kerber; Dippie; O'Brien. How the frontier gothic aided the project of the Vanishing Indian has already been addressed by various scholars; Smith-Rosenberg's *This Violent Empire* is the prime, more recent example. In *The American Imperial Gothic*, Höglund charts a literary imperialism beginning with Brown's frontier gothic all the way into the twenty-first century and the popular Justin Cronin trilogy *The Passage* (2010–16).

2. Jefferson's note dated May 23, 1793, is quoted in Philip Marsh's *The Prose of Philip Freneau* (5).

3. The Indigenous population as the obvious Americans and the investment of European-American settlers to construct a myth that would excuse their colonizing efforts hold a special place in Smith-Rosenberg's account of the early years of the United States: "To fear and dehumanize alien Others, to ruthlessly hunt them down, is truly American" (x).

4. In "Satanizing the American Indian," Lovejoy offers a comprehensive overview of settler colonial images of satanic Indigenous characters produced throughout the seventeenth century.

5. The book was first published in Philadelphia by H. C. Carey & I. Lea in 1822 with the title *Logan, a Family History*. Unless otherwise noted, all further in-text references are taken from this edition. The novel was republished in

London by J. Cunningham, Crown-Court, Fleep-Street, in 1840 under the title *Logan, the Mingo Chief: A Family History.* More recently there has been considerable interest in Neal's writing. See, most of all, the edited collection by Watts and Carlson; Elmer, *On Lingering;* Richter.

6. The entry in *American National Biography* refers to James Logan (1725–80) as a "Mingo Indian, famous in his own time as an ally of English colonials, succeeding generations remember the tragedy that befell him and the lament he made in response. He was probably born at the village of Shamokin (Sunbury, Pa.), the son of the Oneida chief Shikellamy and a Cayuga woman. Known as Soyechtowa, Tocaniadrogon, or Logan the Mingo, historians have incorrectly called him Tah-Gah-jute" (Jennings).

7. In *The Indian Chief as Tragic Hero,* Sayre documents a long history of framing Native leaders as tragic heroes in the United States all the way into the end of the twentieth century. Seeber points out that the speech was reprinted numerous times in colonial newspapers as early as 1775 (130). Eastman demonstrates how representations "of the eloquent Indian in print and in schoolroom performance throughout the twentieth century helped Americans identify as national subjects on several levels," mainly by forming "collective responsibility" (537).

8. Knowing how much is at stake when rewriting a national myth, Neal published the novel anonymously; see Elmer, "John Neal and John Dunn Hunter."

9. For various invocations of the "Indian problem" throughout the nineteenth century, see Hayes.

10. The first version of "Roger Malvin's Burial" was completed in 1829 and published in *The Token* in 1831. It was republished in *Democratic Review* (1843) and *Mosses from an Old Manse* (1846).

11. The story reappeared in *The Snow-Image, and Other Twice-Told Tales,* published by Ticknor, Reed & Fields in 1852.

12. For an informative article that explores the intersection between Indigenous knowledges and the recent ontological turn in literary and cultural studies towards animism, see Anderson.

13. On mesmerism in Hawthorne see Coale.

14. For a good overview of secondary literature concerning this topic and a complication of the question of guilt, see Erlich.

15. See Povinelli, J.; Cruikshank; Kohn; Bacigalupo; Gordillo.

16. For an extensive overview of Hoffmann's and Tieck's influences on Hawthorne from the perspective of his contemporaries such as Poe, see Thompson.

17. On Hawthorne's thorough knowledge of alchemy, see Swann; Clack.

18. See Clack for the fundamental influence of alchemy on Hawthorne and North American literature of the nineteenth century in general.

19. Watts writes about John Neal's oeuvre and "the Indian Hater Tradition," demonstrating that Neal explicitly responded to a cultural trope constructed in the

1820s, that of the "Indian Hater." Constructed at least a century before, this cultural trope of "a righteous victim carrying out the necessary clearing of the frontier for the preordained white settlement," according to Watts, acquired a "status of allegory" during the 1820s (Watts, "He Could Not Believe" 209).

20. See, for instance, Bercovitch; Herbert.

21. Huhndorf theorizes "going native" as a social practice and a narrative formation within which usually a white cisgender male withdraws from his colonial setting to join the "Natives" (2–5).

22. This view is expressed particularly in *On the Study of Greek Poetry* (written in 1795 and published in 1797) and in *Dialogue on Poetry* (1799). On German early Romantic aesthetics in the context of literary theory, see Bowie; Lacoue-Labarthe and Nancy; Frank.

23. "Je nun, eine gute Verwirrung ist mehr wert, als eine schlechte Ordnung" (Tieck, *Verkehrte Welt*). My translation.

6. Feminist Colonialism

1. The feminist efforts in this novel are well recorded. In her introduction, Karcher calls *Hobomok* a "radical revision of patriarchal script" (Karcher quoted in Child x). Mary Kelley's introduction labels it an "alternative history" (xxx), a phrase Ross also adopts (323). Kaag revises Leonard Harris' assessment of Child's writings and political activism as insurrectionist philosophy and understands it rather as "subversion" (46). Marshall claims that Child "manipulates anti-feminist rhetoric through her male narrator and characters" (2).

2. In his article "In Praise of Extra-Vagant Women: *Hope Leslie* and the Captivity Romance," Christopher Castiglia writes about Sedgwick's novel *Hope Leslie* and ways in which it rejects "the agency of men" and overcomes "the limitations imposed on women" with the captivity romance that, in his opinion, "creates the first expression of female extra-vagance in America" (3).

3. John Winthrop's "Model of Christian Charity" (1630) is a sermon offered to his fellow travelers as they arrived from England to settle in Boston. Trying to balance out the insecurities, Winthrop proposed: "we shall be a city upon a hill [and] the eyes of all people are upon us," which eventually became a Puritan foundational paradigm (2:13). The "howling wilderness" is a phrase from the Bible, the Book of Moses, which was much repeated in Puritan writings to designate a hostile natural environment, as in Mary White Rowlandson's *Narrative of the Captivity and Restoration of Mrs. Mary Rowlandson* (103).

4. With "Domestic Frontier Romance; or, How the Sentimental Heroine Became White," Ezra Tawil was the first to refute the body of scholarship that promotes an interpretation of Child's and Sedgwick's frontier romances as simply progressive, pointing out that the heroines' choices to marry white men were complying with the racially exclusive narratives of the time.

5. On feminism in both Child's and Sedgwick's work, see, for example, Nany F. Sweet's "Dissent and the Daughter in *A New England Tale* and *Hobomok*," in which the author proposes that Child and Sedgwick introduced a new type of self-determined heroine as a sign of the success of Enlightenment feminist efforts in the young republic.

6. In her introduction to Child's writing, with a focus on "Native American" topics, Karcher argues that women writers in the 1820s often sympathized and identified with other excluded groups, which led to their imagining "alternatives to race war, genocide, and white male supremacy as modes of resolving the contradictions that riddled their society" (Karcher quoted in Child, *Hobomok* xvii). This interest often shifted the setting into the forest, which came to represent an alternative and oppositional space to the domestic settlement. Both *Hobomok* and *Hope Leslie* write the forest as a space for rebellious daughters to live out their ideas of freedom.

7. In *From Gift to Commodity: Capitalism and Sacrifice in Nineteenth-Century American Fiction,* Hildegard Hoeller interprets this scene with the help of Derrida's theory of sacrifice as a sacrificial rite, because Mary Conant has to shed her blood for the right husband.

8. That female subordination was considered to be part of a natural order in early Puritan settlements is discussed, for example, in Kathleen M. Brown's *Good Wives, Nasty Wenches, and Anxious Patriarchs: Gender, Race, and Power in Colonial Virginia.*

9. Wilderness as a space of female liberation has been explored before, but the centrality of the supernatural to many of these narratives has been neglected. *Hope Leslie* and Harriet Vaughn Cheney's *A Peep at the Pilgrims,* published the same year as *Hobomok,* in 1824, by Hannah Webster Foster's daughter, are two novels named by Castiglia as texts that, by reformulating captivity narratives, challenged the separate sphere of domestic and extradomestic spaces. Castiglia does not mention that both are set in spectral forests. In her much-quoted introduction to *Hobomok, and Other Writings on Indians,* Karcher argues that Child's along with Sedgwick's writings formed alliances between heroines and "Native Americans" in the service of female agency. Bergland and Tawil confirm this interpretation in their more thorough analysis of racial hegemony in the oeuvres of both writers.

10. There is not much information as to Child's activities in the Boston New Church on Beacon Hill. According to the membership register, she joined this Swedenborgian church in 1822 (Anders). See also the Swedenborg Foundation webpage on Lydia Maria Child: https://swedenborg.com/scholars-maria-child-visionary-antislavery-crusader-changed-a-church/.

11. Karcher also suggests that the poisoning of the fox in the short story "Chocorua's Curse," for example, signifies a "white settlers' hostile relationship to nature, which they treat as an enemy to be subjugated, rather than as a source of life to be venerated or propitiated" (Karcher quoted in Child, *Hobomok* 161).

12. The Indian Removal Act was passed by Congress in 1830 during Andrew Jackson's administration.

13. In *Made from This Earth: American Women and Nature,* published in 2002, Vera Norwood was already warning her readers that the "utopian focus" and its "lack of historical perspective" are a major problem in ecofeminism (xx).

14. On the formation of the "noble savage," see Jentz.

15. In a slightly different context, Audre Lorde writes about white women defining the category *women* based on their own experience and thus relegating Black women to an outsider position "too 'alien' to comprehend" (117).

16. More on Harriet Beecher Stowe's activities as a spiritualist can be found in Rugoff.

7. The Politics of Presence

1. As has been well documented, Crafts most likely had access to the private library of her master, John Hill Wheeler. A catalog with titles held by this library was compiled by the literary studies scholar Bryan C. Sinche and can be found in Appendix C of *The Bondwoman's Narrative* (Crafts). Sinche compiled this list while a doctoral student at the University of North Carolina. See "Introduction" and "Textual Annotations" in Crafts.

2. Many critics have pointed out the relation between the gothic genre and the slave narrative; see Winter; Malchow.

3. In "Decentralized Power and Resistance in *The Bondwoman's Narrative,*" Dong L. Isbister defends Crafts' "clear sense of resistance against ignorance, dehumanization, and polarization of racial and social relations" against similar claims, particularly Nina Baym's claim that Hannah Crafts was not a rebel (173).

4. On Gates' misplaced insistence on "authenticating" Crafts' "racial identity," see Ballinger, Lustig, and Townshend. On the dominating presence of Gates Jr.'s authority over this text see Bernier and Newman.

5. In *Sister Outsider,* Audre Lorde famously called for a refusal of "the master's tools" when attempting to "dismantle the master's house" (112).

6. See, for example, Daniel Hack on what he calls Crafts' "African Americanization of *Bleak House.*"

7. On black magic in general, see Chireau.

8. For an overview of how the Gothic "other" gets racialized, see Anolik and Howard; Wester, *African American Gothic.*

9. Scott is listed in the catalog compiled by Sinche.

10. The intertextuality between *The Bondwoman's Narrative* and Charles Dickens' *The Bleak House,* a book Crafts probably had access to in her enslaver's library, has been discussed by various critics. Warning that reading *The Bondwoman's Narrative* as an "authentic" document of slavery, as Gates Jr. had

initially done, might be misleading, Ballinger, Lustig, and Townshend high-light Crafts' reworking of Dickens' description of Tom-all-Alone in chapter 16 of *Bleak House* (209). The authors suggest that the skillful relocation of a London slum to a North Carolina plantation extends rather than constricts the narrative. For Dickens' influences and the influence of the gothic genre in general on this text, see also Kirkpatrick; Mantel; Castronovo, "Art of Ghost-Writing"; Gleason; Robbins; Sánchez-Eppler.

11. There is another parallel to be drawn between the reception of Crafts' and Jackson's work. Read as a ghost story, Jackson's *The Haunting of Hill House* appears as a psychological study of the harm inflicted upon the main protagonist by society. Reading the text as gothic horror shifts the emphasis to effects intended to shock the readers and away from what has caused them.

12. This classic distinction between terror and horror was drawn by one of the original gothic novel writers, Ann Radcliffe, in her article "On the Supernatural in Poetry" published in 1825.

13. Recently, scholars have broadened the scope of agency in the context of slavery and its afterlife. See Camp; Fett; T. Hunter.

14. In "The Death of the Author," the French literary scholar Roland Barthes argues against an integration of the author's intentions in literary interpretation. If this theory is not applicable in the context of a literary work such as *The Bondwoman's Narrative,* it cannot claim universality. If it is applicable, there is no reason to not read the text as literature.

15. On haunting in African American literature, see Parham.

16. Priscilla Wald opens her essay on *The Bondwoman's Narrative* with the provocative sentence: "This essay is about the absence of ghosts in *The Bondwoman's Narrative*" (213).

17. Henry David Thoreau publicly left the city for a "life in the woods" in 1845. It is thus even possible that the cabin in the woods is a reference to *Walden.*

18. Melvin Dixon writes in *Ride Out the Wilderness* about "the wilderness, the underground, and the mountaintop" as "broad geographical metaphors for the search, discovery, and achievement of self" (4–5).

19. The absence of African Americans in the scholarship on transcendentalism has been noted by various scholars. Eric Gardner's important recovery of Edmonia Goodelle Highgate's work as a contribution to US American transcendentalism offers yet another example of an African American woman developing a relational and communal type of transcendentalism.

20. In his study *Race and Nature from Transcendentalism to the Harlem Renaissance,* Paul Outka even claims that race is at the center of the transcendentalist understanding of nature: "I read transcendentalism's Romantic sublime embrace of the wilderness and its emphasis on freedom and individual self-creation as an attempt to reconstitute whiteness' identification with nature in the context of slavery" (8).

21. *The Cambridge Companion to the American Gothic,* edited by Jeffrey Weinstock and published in 2017, dedicates a chapter to "Race and the American Gothic" by Ellen Weinauer, which includes *The Bondwoman's Narrative* in her overview of representative texts (85–98).

22. The vast majority of enslaved people had little to no exposure to Christianity prior to the Jacksonian candidacy. The most comprehensive study of religion among those enslaved in North America remains Raboteau's *Slave Religion,* a comprehensive anthology of primary sources from early colonial religious rituals through the nineteenth century that includes African American vision stories, supernaturalism, and healing.

23. As opposed to Indigenous spirituality, for example, which was studied as a religion or a mythology. As has been explained in previous chapters, while Indigenous characters were subject to spectralization, African Americans were often represented as experts in the field of spectrality, as numerous examples in Irving's tales testify.

24. Cudjo is also the first character who speaks the dialect of Southern enslaved people in John Leacock's *The Fall of British Tyranny* (1776). It is also the name of the man known as the last survivor of the last recorded slave ship to the United States, the *Clotilda,* Cudjo Lewis. Zora Neale Hurston filmed Lewis, turning him into the only enslaved person whose moving image exists; see Diouf as well as Hurston.

25. For two excellent studies of Crafts' intertextual use of the Bible and Christian symbolism, see Sinche; Buell, "Bondwoman Unbound."

26. A predecessor for these discussions are early New England intellectual debates that often included discussion of the materialism in Thomas Hobbes' theories. These debates might have provided a fertile ground for the spread of mesmerism and animism in the United States. For an interpretation of Hobbes' work that argues that he developed a form of incorporeal materialism, see Duncan.

27. See the collection of ghost stories told by enslaved people in Rhyne.

28. Sharla Fett also describes communication with the spirits of the dead as an art of resistance to slavery in the antebellum South. Newbell Niles Puckett's published doctoral thesis from 1923 *Folk Beliefs of the Southern Negro,* which can be found in the holdings of the New York Public Library's Schomburg Center for Research in Black Culture, is also an important resource. During his fieldwork, Puckett identified cases of Afro-American practices that are guided by superstitions found in tales.

29. Walter C. Rucker has even demonstrated a direct connection between African conjuring practices and rebellion against slavery. This study shows that "powerful supernatural forces beyond the comprehension of their contemporaries" are elemental to anti-slavery resistance movements (84).

30. To name only a few studies: Goddu, *Gothic America;* Goddu, "African American"; Edwards, *Gothic Passages;* Haslam; Smith-Rosenberg; Soltysik-Monnet, *Poetics and Politics;* Wester, *African American Gothic.*

31. The list of library books compiled by the enslaver John Wheeler includes an entrance on "animal magnetism" (Crafts 354).

Conclusion

1. In the edited collection *Sylvia Wynter: On Being Human as Praxis,* Katherine McKittrick collects a representative body of work that builds on Wynter's oeuvre, undertaking the difficult task of "situating our intellectual questions outside our present system of knowledge" (x). The collection demonstrates that redefining the category of the human is at the center of efforts to decolonize the humanities.

2. In "Unsettling the Coloniality of Being/Power/Truth/Freedom," Sylvia Wynter proposes that future cultural struggles will be geared towards securing a conception of the human, "Man, which overrepresents itself as if it were the human itself," asserting "the central ethnoclass Man vs. Human struggle" (9–10).

3. See Berthin; Crow; Davis; Goddu, *Gothic America;* Savoy; Edwards, *Gothic Passages;* Lloyd-Smith; Punter.

4. Ethnoastronomy combines ethnography with astronomy and practices an interest in myths, legends, and beliefs. An overview of Lakota ethnoastronomy and Apache cosmovision can be found in Hollabaugh.

5. A corrective to the Eurocentrism in Swedenborg studies can be found in Garcia; Allen G. Debus locates Paracelsus' influences for his religious-vitalistic outlook toward nature in "Islamic and Indian authors" without specifying their names (86).

Works Cited

A. B. C. "Spontaneous Combustion." *Gentleman's Magazine,* vol. 49, Dec. 1779, p. 631.

Adams, John. *Papers of John Adams, May 1775–Jan. 1776.* Vol. 3, Belknap Press of Harvard UP, 1977.

Adéèkó, Adéléké. *Arts of Being Yorùbá: Divination, Allegory, Tragedy, Proverb, Panegyric.* Indiana UP, 2017.

Adorno, Theodor W., and Max Horkheimer. *Dialectic of Enlightenment: Philosophical Fragments.* 1947. Translated by Edmund Jephcott, Stanford UP, 2002.

"Advertisement." *New York Evening Post,* Nov. 4, 1803, p. 3.

"The Affair of the Supposed Ghost in Cock-Lane, Weft-Smithfield, Having Been Variously Talked of; by Some, as an Imposture; by Other, as a Reality." *Universal Magazine of Knowledge and Pleasure,* vol. 30, no. 205, 1762, pp. 48–49.

Alaimo, Stacy. *Bodily Natures: Science, Environment, and the Material Self.* Indiana UP, 2010.

———. *Undomesticated Ground: Recasting Nature as a Feminist Space.* Cornell UP, 2000.

Anders, Tisa M. "L. Maria Child: Visionary Antislavery Crusader Changed a Church by Leaving It." Swedenborg Foundation, https://swedenborg.com/scholars-maria-child-visionary-antislavery-crusader-changed-a-church/. Accessed May 15, 2020.

Anderson, Benedict. *Imagined Communities: Reflections on the Origin and Spread of Nationalism.* Verso, 1983.

Anderson, Elizabeth. "Reading the World's Liveliness: Animist Ecologies in Indigenous Knowledges, New Materialism and Women's Writing." *Feminist Modernist Studies,* vol. 3, no. 2, 2020, pp. 205–16, https://doi.org/10.1080/24692921.2020.1794458.

Andrews, William L. *To Tell a Free Story: The First Century of Afro-American Autobiography, 1760–1865.* U of Illinois P, 1986.

Anna. "St. Herbert.—A Tale." *New-York Weekly Magazine or Miscellaneous Repository,* vol. 1, no. 31, Feb. 1796, pp. 246–47.

Anolik, Ruth Bienstock, and Douglas L. Howard. *The Gothic Other: Racial and Social Constructions in the Literary Imagination.* McFarland and Co., 2004.

Allison, Henry E., *The "Silent Decade," Kant's Transcendental Deduction: An Analytical-Historical Commentary.* Oxford, 2015, online ed., https://doi.org/10.1093/acprof:oso/9780198724858.003.0004.

Arendt, Hannah. *The Origins of Totalitarianism.* Schocken Books, 2004.

Aristotle. *De anima.* Translated by Hugh Lawson-Tancred, Penguin, 1986.

Arnold, Larry E. *Ablaze! Spontaneous Human Combustion.* M. Evans, 1995.

Artaud, Antonin. *Ouvres complètes.* Vol. 3, Gallimard, 1978.

Atticus. "An Account of a Pretended Apparition in Kent." *Gentleman's Magazine,* vol. 32, 1762, pp. 114–15.

Aubrey, John. *Miscellanies upon the Following Subjects Collected.* London, 1696.

Bacigalupo, Ana Mariella. "Subversive Cosmopolitics in the Anthropocene: On Sentient Landscape and the Ethical Imperative in Northern Peru." *Climate Politics and the Power of Religion,* edited by Evan Berry, Indiana UP, 2021, pp. 176–205.

Bakhtin, M. M. *The Dialogic Imagination.* U of Texas P, 1981.

Ballinger, Gill, Tim Lustig, and Dale Townshend. "Missing Intertexts: Hannah Crafts's *The Bondwoman's Narrative* and African American Literary History." *Journal of American Studies,* vol. 39, no. 2, 2005, pp. 207–37.

Barber, X. Theodore. "Phantasmagorical Wonders: The Magic Lantern Ghost Show in Nineteenth-Century America." *Film History,* vol. 3, no. 2, 1989, pp. 73–86.

Barnard, Philip, and Shapiro, Stephen. Introduction. *Wieland; or, the Transformation, with Related Texts,* edited by Philip Barnard and Stephen Shapiro, Hackett, 2009, pp. ix–xlvi.

Barnard, Philip, et al. *The Oxford Handbook of Charles Brockden Brown.* Oxford UP, 2019.

Barthes, Roland. *Image, Music, Text.* Hill and Wang, 1977.

Basso, Keith. *Wisdom Sits in Places: Landscape and Language among the Western Apache.* U of New Mexico P, 1996.

Baxter, Richard. *The Certainty of the Worlds of Spirits,* London, 1691.

Baym, Nina. "A Minority Reading of 'Wieland.'" *Critical Essays on Charles Brockden Brown,* edited by Bernard Rosenthal, G. K. Hall, 1981, pp. 87–103.

Beddoes, Thomas. "To the Editor of the *Monthly Magazine.*" *Monthly Magazine or British Register,* no. 4, 1796, pp. 265–67.

Bennett, Bridget. "The Silence Surrounding the Hut: Architecture and Absence in Wieland." *Early American Literature,* vol. 53, issue 2, 2018, pp. 369–404.

Bennett, Gillian. "Ghost and Witch in the Sixteenth and Seventeenth Centuries." *Folklore,* vol. 97, no. 1, 1986, pp. 3–14.

Bennett, Jane. "Agency, Nature and Emergent Properties: An Interview with Jane Bennett." Interview by Gulshan Khan. *Contemporary Political Theory,* 2009, pp. 90–105.

Bergen, Fanny D. "Louisiana Ghost Story." *Journal of American Folklore,* vol. 12, no. 45, 1899, pp. 146–47.

Bercovitch, Sacvan. *The Office of the Scarlet Letter.* Johns Hopkins UP, 1991.

Bergland, Renée L. *The National Uncanny: Indian Ghosts and American Subjects.* UP of New England, 2000.

Berkhofer, Robert F. *The White Man's Indian: Images of the American Indian from Columbus to the Present.* Knopf, 1978.

Berlin, Isaiah. *The Proper Study of Mankind: An Anthology of Essays.* Chatto and Windus, 1997.

Bernier, Celeste-Marie, and Judie Newman. "*The Bondwoman's Narrative:* Text, Paratext, Intertext and Hypertext." *Journal of American Studies,* vol. 39, no. 2, 2005, pp. 147–65.

Berthin, Christine. *Gothic Hauntings: Melancholy Crypts and Textual Ghosts.* Palgrave Macmillan, 2010.

Bird, S. Elizabeth. *Dressing in Feathers: The Construction of the Indian in American Popular Culture.* Westview Press, 1996.

Blackstock, Michael. "Water: A First Nations' Spiritual and Ecological Perspective." *Perspectives: B.C. Journal of Ecosystems and Management,* vol. 1, no. 1, 2001, pp.1–14.

Blanco, Maria del Pilar, and Esther Peeren, editors. *The Spectralities Reader: Ghosts and Haunting in Contemporary Cultural Theory.* Bloomsbury, 2013.

Blažan, Sladja. "Immanuel Kant's 'One Great Republic': from Spirit Theory to Moral Philosophy." *Discovering the Human: Life Science and the Arts in the Eighteenth and Early Nineteenth Centuries,* edited by Ralf Haeckel and Sabine Blackmore, Vandenhoeck and Ruprecht UP, 2013, pp. 69–84.

———. "Lithic Corporeality: Elemental Philosophy in Nathaniel Hawthorne's Short Stories." *Nathaniel Hawthorne Review,* vol. 46, issue 2, 2021, pp. 155–73.

———. "Silencing the Dead: Washington Irving's Use of the Supernatural in the Context of Slavery and Genocide." *Arizona Quarterly,* vol. 69, no. 2, 2013, pp. 1–24.

Bonnivillain, Nancy. *Hopi: Indians of North America.* Chelsea House, 2005.

Böhme, Hartmut, and Gernot Böhme. *Das andere der Vernunft: Zur Entwicklung von Rationalitätsstrukturen am Beispiel Kants.* Suhrkamp, 1983.

Botha, Pieter J. J. "History and Point of View: Understanding the Sadducees." *Neotestamentica,* vol. 30, no. 2, 1996, pp. 235–80, http://www.jstor.org/stable /43048268.

Bovet, Richard. *Pandaemonium, or, the Devil's Cloyster Being a Further Blow to Modern Sadduceism, Proving the Existence of Witches and Spirits.* London, 1684.

Bowden, Mary Weatherspoon. *Washington Irving.* Twayne Publishers, 1981.

Bowie, Andrew. *From Romanticism to Critical Theory: The Philosophy of German Literary Theory.* Routledge, 1997.

Bradshaw, Charles C. "The New England Illuminati: Conspiracy and Causality in Charles Brockden Brown's *Wieland.*" *New England Quarterly,* vol. 76, no. 3, 2003, pp. 356–77.

Brasch, F. E. "The Royal Society of London and Its Influence upon Scientific Thought in the American Colonies." *Scientific Monthly,* vol. 23, 1931, pp. 337–55.

Braude, Ann. *Radical Spirits: Spiritualism and Women's Rights in Nineteenth-Century America.* Indiana UP, 1989.

Breslaw, Elaine G. *Tituba, Reluctant Witch of Salem: Devilish Indians and Puritan Fantasies.* New York UP, 1996.

Brewster, Scott, and Luke Thurston. *The Routledge Handbook to the Ghost Story.* Routledge, 2017.

Brogan, Kathleen. *Cultural Haunting: Ghosts and Ethnicity in Recent American Literature.* UP of Virginia, 1998.

Bronner, Stephan E. *Reclaiming the Enlightenment: Towards a Politics of Radical Engagement.* Columbia UP, 2004.

Brown, Charles Brockden. *Collected Writings of Charles Brockden Brown.* Edited by Philip Barnard, Elizabeth Hewitt, and Mark L. Kamrath, Bucknell UP, 2013.

Brown, Kathleen M. *Good Wives, Nasty Wenches, and Anxious Patriarchs: Gender, Race, and Power in Colonial Virginia.* U of North Carolina P, 2012.

Brown, Joseph Epes, and Emily Cousins. *Teaching Spirits: Understanding Native American Religious Traditions.* Oxford UP, 2001.

Brown, William Hill, and Hannah Webster Foster. *The Power of Sympathy* and *The Coquette.* Penguin Classics, 1996.

Buell, Lawrence. "Bondwoman Unbound: Hannah Crafts's Art and Nineteenth-Century U.S. Literary Practice." *In Search of Hannah Crafts: Critical Essays on "The Bondwoman's Narrative,"* edited by Henry Louis Gates Jr. and Hollis Robbins, Basic Books, 2004, pp. 16–29.

Burgett, Bruce. *Sentimental Bodies: Sex, Gender, and Citizenship in the Early Republic.* Princeton UP, 1998.

Burke, Edmund. *Reflections on the Revolution in France, and on the Proceedings in Certain Societies in London Relative to That Event.* 1790. New York, 1791.

Butler, Judith. "The Force of Fantasy: Feminism, Mapplethorpe, and Discoursive Excess." *Differences: A Journal of Feminist Cultural Studies,* vol. 2, no. 2, 1990, pp. 105–25.

———. *Precarious Life: The Powers of Mourning and Violence.* Verso, 2004.

———. *Gender Trouble.* Routledge, 1999.

Cahill, Edward. "An Adventurous and Lawless Fancy: Charles Brockden Brown's Aesthetic State." *Early American Literature,* vol. 36, no. 1, 2001, pp. 31–70.

Calef, Robert. *More Wonders of the Invisible World; or, the Wonders of the Invisible World Display'd in Five Parts.* 1700. Salem, 1823.

Calmet, Rev. Fr. Dom Augustin. "Dissertations upon the Apparitions of Angels, Daemons, and Ghosts, and concerning the Vampires of Hungary, Bohemia, Moravia, and Silesia." *Monthly Review,* vol. 20, 1759, p. 564.

Camp, Stephanie M. H. *Closer to Freedom: Enslaved Women and Everyday Resistance in the Plantation South.* U of North Carolina P, 2004.

[Candidus]. "Walstein's School of History: From the German of Krants of Gotha." *Monthly Magazine and American Review,* vol. 1, no. 5, 1799, pp. 335–38.

Caron, Nathalie. "Friendship, Secrecy, Transatlantic Networks and the Enlightenment: The Jefferson-Barlow Version of Volney's *Ruines* (Paris, 1802)." *Mémoires du livre / Studies in Book Culture,* vol. 11, no. 1, 2019, https://doi.org/10.7202/1066940ar.

Castiglia, Christopher. "In Praise of Extra-Vagant Women: *Hope Leslie* and the Captivity Romance." *Legacy,* vol. 6, no. 2, 1989, pp. 3–16.

———. *Interior States: Institutional Consciousness and the Inner Life of Democracy in the Antebellum United States.* Duke UP, 2008.

Castle, Terry. "Phantasmagoria: Spectral Technology and the Metaphorics of Modern Reverie." *Critical Inquiry,* vol. 15, no. 1, 1988, pp. 26–61.

———. *The Female Thermometer: Eighteenth-Century Culture and the Invention of the Uncanny (Ideologies of Desire).* Oxford UP, 1999.

Castronovo, Russ. "The Art of Ghost-Writing: Memory, Materiality, and Slave Aesthetics." *In Search of Hannah Crafts: Critical Essays on "The Bondwoman's Narrative,"* edited by Henry Louis Gates Jr. and Hollis Robbins, Basic Books, 2004, pp. 195–212.

Cavarero, Adriana. *Horrorism: Naming Contemporary Violence.* Columbia UP, 2011.

Cave, Alfred A. "Abuse of Power: Andrew Jackson and the Indian Removal Act of 1830." *The Historian,* vol. 65, issue 6, December 2003, pp. 1330–53.

Chase, Richard. *The American Novel and Its Tradition.* Doubleday, 1957.

Child, Lydia Maria. *The First Settlers of New-England; or, Conquest of the Pequods, Narragansets, and Pokanokets.* Boston, 1828.

———. *Hobomok and Other Writings on Indians.* 1824. Rutgers UP, 1986.

Chireau, Yvonne Patricia. *Black Magic: Religion and the African American Conjuring Tradition.* U of California P, 2003.

Chitakure, John. *African Traditional Religion Encounters Christianity: The Resilience of a Demonized Religion.* Pickwick, 2017.

Clack, Randall A. *The Marriage of Heaven and Earth: Alchemical Regeneration in the Works of Taylor, Hawthorne, and Fuller.* Greenwood, 2000.

Clark, Michael. "Charles Brockden Brown's *Wieland* and Robert Proud's *History of Pennsylvania.*" *Studies in the Novel,* vol. 20, 1988, pp. 239–48.

Clery, E. J. *The Rise of Supernatural Fiction, 1762–1800.* Cambridge UP, 1995.

Coale, Samuel Chase. *Mesmerism and Hawthorne: Mediums of American Romance.* U of Alabama P, 1998.

Cody, Michael A. "Brown's Early Biographers and Reception, 1815–1940s." *The Oxford Handbook of Charles Brockden Brown,* edited by Hilary Emmett, Philip Barnard, and Stephen Shapiro, Oxford UP, 2019, pp. 522–36.

Coleridge, Samuel Taylor. *Aids to Reflection in the Formation of a Manly Character, on the Several Grounds of Prudence, Morality, and Religion.* Edited by James Marsh, Burlington, 1829.

Conger, Sydney McMillen. "A German Ancestor for Mary Shelley's Monster: Kahler, Schiller, and the Buried Treasure of Northhanger Abbey." *Philological Quarterly,* vol. 59, no. 2, 1980, pp. 216–32.

Connor, Steven. *Dumbstruck: A Cultural History of Ventriloquism.* Oxford UP, 2000.

Cooper, James Fenimore. *The Last of the Mohicans.* Oxford UP, 1998.

Crafts, Hannah. *The Bondwoman's Narrative,* edited by Henry Louis Gates Jr. Warner Books, 2002.

Craker, Wendel D. "Spectral Evidence: Non-Spectral Acts of Witchcraft, and Confession at Salem in 1692." *Historical Journal,* vol. 40, no. 2, 1997, pp. 331–58.

Christopherson, Bill. "Picking Up the Knife: A Psychohistorical Reading of Wieland." *American Studies,* vol. 27, no. 1, 1986, pp. 115–26, http://www.jstor.org /stable/40642098.

Crow, Charles L. *History of the Gothic: American Gothic.* U of Wales P, 2009.

Cruikshank, George. *A Discovery Concerning Ghosts, with a Rap at the "Spirit-Rappers."* London, 1863.

Cruikshank, Julie. "Glaciers and Climate Change: Perspectives from Oral Tradition." *Arctic,* vol. 54, no. 4, 2001, pp. 377–93.

Danforth, Samuel. "A Brief Recognition of New England's Errand into the Wilderness." Sermon 1670, edited and transcribed by Paul Royster, Faculty Digital Publications, UNL Libraries, paper 35, 2006.

Darwin, Erasmus. *Zoönomia; or, The Laws of Organic Life.* London, 1794.

da Silva, Denise Ferreira. *Toward a Global Idea of Race.* U of Minnesota P, 2007.

Daston, Lorraine, and Katharine Park. *Wonders and the Order of Nature 1150–1750.* Princeton UP, 2001.

Davidson, Cathy N. *Revolution and the Word: The Rise of the Novel in America.* Oxford UP, 2004.

Davies, Owen. *Ghosts: A Social History.* Pickering and Chatto, 2010. 5 vols.

Davis, Colin. *Haunted Subjects: Deconstruction, Psychoanalysis and the Return of the Dead.* Palgrave Macmillan, 2007.

Davison, Carol Margaret. "American Gothic Passages." *Romantic Gothic: An Edinburgh Companion,* edited by Angela Wright and Dale Townshend, Edinburgh UP, 2015, pp. 267–86.

———. "Charles Brockden Brown: Godfather of the American Gothic." *A Companion to American Gothic,* edited by C. L. Crow, 2013, https://onlinelibrary.wiley .com/doi/abs/10.1002/9781118608395.ch9.

Debus, Allen G. "History with a Purpose: The Fate of Paracelsus." *Pharmacy in History,* vol. 26, no. 2, 1984, pp. 83–96.

Deloria, Philip J. *Playing Indian.* Yale UP, 1998.

Derrida, Jacques. *Specters of Marx: The State of Debt, the Work of Mourning, and the New International.* Translated by Peggy Kamuf, Routledge, 1994.

Derrida, Jacques, and Bernard Stiegler. *Echographies of Television: Filmed Interviews.* Polity Press, 2002.

Diala-Ogamba, Blessing. "Gothic Elements in Toni Morrison's 'Beloved' and Elechi Amadi's 'The Concubine.'" *CLA Journal,* vol. 54, no. 4, 2011, pp. 410–24.

Diouf, Syviane Anne. *Dreams of Africa in Alabama: The Slave Ship* Cotilda *and the Story of the Last Africans Brought to America.* Oxford UP, 2007.

Dippie, Brian W. *The Vanishing American: White Attitudes and U.S. Indian Policy.* Wesleyan UP, 1982.

Dixon, Melvin. *Ride Out the Wilderness: Geography and Identity in Afro-American Literature.* U of Illinois P, 1987.

Dolar, Mladen. *A Voice and Nothing More.* MIT P, 2006.

Douglas, Ann. *The Feminization of American Culture.* Knopf, 1977.

Douglass, Frederick. *Narrative of the Life of Frederick Douglass, an American Slave.* 1845. Modern Library, 2000.

Doyle, Laura. *Freedom's Empire: Race and the Rise of the Novel in Atlantic Modernity, 1640–1940.* Duke UP, 2008.

Du Bois, W. E. B. *The Negro Church: Report of a Social Study Made under the Direction of Atlanta University.* 1903. Altamira, 2003.

DuCille, Ann. *The Coupling Convention: Sex, Text, and Tradition in Black Women's Fiction.* Oxford UP, 1993.

Duncan, Stewart. "Hobbes's Materialism in the Early 1640s." *British Journal for the History of Philosophy,* vol. 13, no. 3, 2005, pp. 437–48, https://www.tandfonline.com/doi/abs/10.1080/09608780500157171.

Easlea, Brian. *Witch Hunting, Magic, and the New Philosophy: An Introduction to Debates of the Scientific Revolution, 1450–1750.* Harvester, 1980.

Eastman, Carolyn. "The Indian Censures the White Man: 'Indian Eloquence' and American Reading Audiences in the Early Republic." *William and Mary Quarterly,* vol. 65, no. 3, 2008, pp. 535–64, https://doi.org/10.2307/25096813.

Edwards, Justin D. *Gothic Passages: Racial Ambiguity and the American Gothic.* U of Iowa P, 2003.

Elmer, Jonathan. "John Neal and John Hunter." *John Neal and Nineteenth-Century American Literature and Culture,* edited by Edward Watts and David J. Carlson, Bucknell UP, 2012, pp. 145–58.

———. "Melancholy, Race, and Sovereign Exemption in Early American Fiction." *Novel,* vol. 40, nos. 1–2, 2007, pp. 151–70, DOI: 10.1215/ddnov.040010151.

———. *On Lingering and Being Last: Race and Sovereignty in the New World.* Fordham UP, 2008.

Emerson, Ralph Waldo. *The Collected Works of Ralph Waldo Emerson.* Vol. 2, Harvard UP, 1971–2011.

———. *The Essential Writings of Ralph Waldo Emerson.* Modern Library, 2000.

Erlich, Gloria Chasson. "Guilt and Expiation in 'Roger Malvin's Burial.'" *Nineteenth-Century Fiction,* vol. 26, no. 4, 1972, pp. 377–89, https://doi.org/10.2307/2933271.

Evans, Rand B. "The Origins of American Academic Psychology." *Explorations in the History of Psychology in the United States,* edited by Josef Brozek, Bucknell UP, 1983, pp. 17–60.

"Explanation and Vindication of the Kantian Tenets." *New-York Magazine or Literary Repository,* vol. 8, 1797, pp. 365–66.

"Explanatory Notes." *Wieland; or, the Transformation and Memoirs of Carwin, the Biloquist,* edited by Emory Elliott, Oxford UP, 2009, pp. 290–94.

"Familiar, *N.*" *OED Online,* Oxford UP, 2020, www.oed.com/view/Entry/186096.

Faulkner, William. *Requiem for a Nun.* 1950. Vintage International, 2011.

Federal Writers' Project. "Slave Narratives: A Folk History of Slavery in the United States from Interviews with Former Slaves." Library of Congress, https://lccn.loc .gov/41021619.

Fett, Sharla M. *Working Cures: Healing, Health, and Power on Southern Slave Plantations.* U of North Carolina P, 2002.

Fiedler, Leslie. 1960. *Love and Death in the American Novel.* Dalkey Archive Press, 1982.

Fisher Fishkin, Shelley. *Was Huck Black? Mark Twain and African-American Voices.* Oxford UP, 1993.

Fliegelman, Jay. *Prodigals and Pilgrims: The American Revolution against Patriarchal Authority, 1750–1800.* Cambridge UP, 1982.

Florschütz, Gottlieb. *Emmanuel Swedenborgs mystisches Menschenbild und die Doppelnatur des Menschen bei Immanuel Kant.* Swedenborg Foundation, 1993.

———. *Swedenborgs verborgene Wirkung auf Kant: Swedenborg und die okkulten Phänomene aus der Sicht von Kant und Schopenhauer.* Königshausen und Neumann, 1992.

The Flushing Phantasmagoria—or—Kings Conjurors Amuseing John Bull. Cornhill, 1809. Digital Collection. The Lewis Walpole Library. Yale University. Aug. 15, 2019.

Fortes, Meyer. *Oedipus and Job in West African Religion.* Octagon, 1981.

Foucault, Michel. *Society Must Be Defended: Lectures at the Collège de France, 1975–76.* Picador, 2003.

Fournier, Michael. "The Pathology of Reading: The Novel as an Agent of Contagion." *Imagining Contagion in Early Modern Europe,* edited by Claire Carlin, Palgrave Macmillan, 2005, pp. 195–211.

F. R. "On Apparitions." *Monthly Magazine and American Review,* vol. 1, no. 1, Apr. 1799, pp. 3–8.

Frank, Manfred. *Unendliche Annäherung: Die Anfänge der philosophischen Frühromantik.* Suhrkamp, 1997.

Franklin, Wayne. "Tragedy and Comedy in Brown's 'Wieland.'" *NOVEL: A Forum on Fiction,* vol. 8, no. 2, Winter 1975, pp. 147–63.

Freneau, Philip. "The Dying Indian; or, The Last Words of Shalum." *American Museum; or, Repository of Ancient and Modern Fugitive Pieces, &c. Prose and Poetical,* vol. 3, no. 2, Feb. 1788, pp. 190–91.

———. "The Indian Student; or, The Force of Nature." *American Museum; or, Repository of Ancient and Modern Fugitive Pieces, &c. Prose and Poetical,* vol. 2, no. 4, Oct. 1787, pp. 413–14.

———. "Lines Occasioned by a Visit to an Old Indian Burying Ground." *American Museum; or, Repository of Ancient and Modern Fugitive Pieces, &c. Prose and Poetical,* vol. 2, no. 5, Nov. 1787, pp. 515–16.

———. "On the Emigration to America, and Peopling the Western Country." *American Museum; or, Repository of Ancient and Modern Fugitive Pieces, &c. Prose and Poetical,* vol. 1, no. 2, Feb. 1787, pp. 159–60.

Freud, Sigmund. *Totem and Taboo: Some Points of Agreement between the Mental Lives of Savages and Neurotics.* Translated by James Strachey, Norton, 1989.

———. *The Uncanny.* 1919. Hogarth, 1963. Vol. 17 of *The Standard Edition of the Complete Psychological Works of Sigmund Freud.*, translated by James Strachey, edited by James Strachey and Anna Freud.

Galluzzo, Anthony. "Charles Brockden Brown's *Wieland* and the Aesthetics of Terror: Revolution, Reaction, and the Radical Enlightenment in Early American Letters." *Eighteenth-Century Studies,* vol. 42, no. 2, 2009, pp. 255–71.

Garber, Marjorie. *Shakespeare's Ghost Writers: Literature as Uncanny Causality.* Methuen, 1987.

Garcia, Humberto. "Blake, Swedenborg, and Muhammad: The Prophetic Tradition, Revisited." *Religion and Literature,* vol. 44, no. 2, 2012, pp. 35–65.

Gardner, Eric. "'Each Atomic Part': Edmonia Goodelle Highgate's African American Transcendentalism." *Toward a Female Genealogy of Transcendentalism,* edited by Jana L. Argersinger and Phyllis Cole, U of Georgia P, 2014, pp. 277–99.

Garrard, Graeme. *Rousseau's Counter-Enlightenment: A Republican Critique of the Enlightenment.* State U of New York P, 2003.

Garuba, Harry. "Explorations in Animist Materialism: Notes on Reading/Writing African Literature, Culture, and Society." *Public Culture,* vol. 15, 2003, https://doi.org/10.1215/08992363-15-2-261.

Gasser, Erika. *Vexed with Devils: Manhood and Witchcraft in Old and New England.* New York UP, 2017.

Gates, Henry Louis, Jr. *The Signifying Monkey: A Theory of African-American Literary Criticism.* Oxford UP, 1989.

Ghost Story. Directed by David Lowery, performances by Casey Affleck and Rooney Mara, Universal Pictures, 2017.

Gilmore, Paul. "John Neal, American Romance, and International Romanticism." *American Literature,* vol. 84, no. 3, 2012, pp. 477–504, https://doi.org/10.1215/00029831-1664692.

Glanvill, Joseph. *A Blow at Modern Sadducism, in Some Philosophical Considerations about Witchcraft.* London, 1668.

———. *Essays on Several Important Subjects in Philosophy and Religion by Joseph Glanvill.* London, 1676.

———. *Saducismus Triumphatus; or, Full and Plain Evidence Concerning Witches and Apparitions.* London, 1681.

———. *Scepsis Scientifica; or, Confest Ignorance, the Way to Science.* Edited by John Owen, London, 1885.

Gleason, William. "'I Dwell Now in a Neat Little Cottage': Architecture, Race and Desire in *The Bondwoman's Narrative.*" *In Search of Hannah Crafts: Critical Essays on "The Bondwoman's Narrative,"* edited by Henry Louis Gates Jr. and Hollis Robbins, Basic Books, 2004, pp. 145–74.

Goddu, Teresa A. "The African American Slave Narrative and the Gothic." *A Companion to American Gothic,* edited by Charles L. Crow, Wiley, 2013, https://onlinelibrary.wiley.com/doi/abs/10.1002/9781118608395.ch6.

———. *Gothic America: Narrative, History, and Nation.* Columbia UP, 1997.

Goho, James. "A Portrait of Charles Dexter Ward as a Haunted Young Man." *Lovecraft Annual,* no. 15, 2021, pp. 167–82. https://www.jstor.org/stable/27118867.

Gonzales, Christian Michael. *Native American Roots: Relationality and Indigenous Regeneration under Empire, 1770–1859.* Routledge, 2020.

Gordillo, Gaston. "The Power of the Terrain: The Affective Materiality of Planet Earth in the Age of Revolution." *Dialogues in Human Geography,* vol. 11, issue 2, 2021, pp. 190–94.

Gordon, Andrew M., and Vera Hernán. *Screen Saviors: Hollywood Fictions of Whiteness.* Rowman and Littlefield, 2003.

Gordon, Avery F. *Ghostly Matters: Haunting and the Sociological Imagination.* U of Minnesota P, 1997.

Goss, David K. *The Salem Witch Trials: A Reference Guide.* Greenwood, 2008.

Greenblatt, Stephen. *Hamlet in Purgatory.* Princeton UP, 2001.

Hack, Daniel. "Close Reading at a Distance: The African Americanization of Bleak House." *Critical Inquiry,* vol. 34, no. 4, 2008, pp. 729–53, https://doi.org/10.1086/592542.

Hall, Daniel. "The Gothic Tide: Schauerroman and Gothic Novel in the Late Eighteenth Century." *The Novel in Anglo-German Context: Cultural Cross-Currents and Affinities,* Rodopi, 2000, pp. 51–60.

Hamilton, James E. "Review: Elihu Palmer's *Principles of Nature.*" *Transactions of the Charles S. Peirce Society,* vol. 27, no. 3, 1991, pp. 389–92, http://www.jstor.org/stable/40320338.

Hammond, Paul. "Noel Malcolm, Thomas Hobbes, Leviathan." *Seventeenth Century,* vol. 28, no. 1, 2013, pp. 91–92, https://doi.org/10.1080/0268117X.2012.760938.

Handley, Sasha. "Ghosts, Gossip, and Gender in Eighteenth-Century Canterbury." *Ghosts, Stories, Histories: Ghost Stories and Alternative Histories,* edited by Sladja Blažan, Cambridge Scholars Press, 2007, pp. 10–20.

Haney, John Louis. "German Literature in England before 1790." *Americana Germanica,* vol. 4, no. 2, 1902, pp. 130–54.

Hansen, Chadwick. "The Metamorphosis of Tituba; or, Why American Intellectuals Can't Tell an Indian Witch from a Negro." *New England Quarterly,* vol. 47, 1974, pp. 3–12.

Harrison, Robert Pogue. *Forests: The Shadow of Civilization.* U of Chicago P, 1992.

Hartman, James D. *Providence Tales and the Birth of American Literature.* John Hopkins UP, 2003.

Haslam, Jason. "'The Strange Ideas of Right and Justice': Prison, Slavery and Other Horrors in *The Bondwoman's Narrative.*" *Gothic Studies,* vol. 7, no. 1, 2005, pp. 29–40.

"haunt, n." *OED Online,* Oxford UP, 2019, https://www.oed.com/search/dictionary/?scope=Entries&q=Haunt.

Hawthorne, Nathaniel. "The Birth-Mark." *Mosses from an Old Manse,* Ohio State UP, 1977, pp. 36–56. Vol. 10 of *The Centenary Edition of the Works of Nathaniel Hawthorne.*

———. *The Elixir of Life Manuscripts.* Ohio State UP, 1977. Vol. 13 of *The Centenary Edition of the Works of Nathaniel Hawthorne.*

———. "The Great Carbuncle." *Twice-Told Tales.* Ohio State UP, 1974, pp. 149–65. Vol. 9 of *The Centenary Edition of the Works of Nathaniel Hawthorne.*

———. "The Great Stone Face." *The Snow-Image and Uncollected Tales.* Ohio State UP, 1974, pp. 26–48. Vol. 11 of *The Centenary Edition of the Works of Nathaniel Hawthorne.*

———. "Roger Malvin's Burial." *Nathaniel Hawthorne's Tales: Authoritative Texts, Backgrounds, Criticism.* Norton, 1987, pp. 17–31.

———. *The Scarlet Letter.* Ohio State UP, 1964. Vol. 1 of *The Centenary Edition of the Works of Nathaniel Hawthorne.*

Hayes, Robert G. *A Race at Bay: New York Times Editorials on 'The Indian Problem,' 1860–1900.* Southern Illinois Press, 1997.

Hazlitt, William. *The Spirit of the Age; or, Contemporary Portraits.* London, 1825.

Henare, M. "Tapu, Mana, Mauri, Hau. Wairua: A Maori Philosophy of Vitalism and The Cosmos." *Indigenous Traditions and Ecology: The interbeing of Cosmology and Community.* Edited by J. A. Grim. Harvard University Press, 2001, pp. 197–221.

Herbert, Walter T. *Dearest Beloved: The Hawthornes and the Making of the Middle-Class Family.* U of California P, 1993.

Herndon, William Henry. *Herndon's Life of Lincoln, the History and Personal Recollections of Abraham Lincoln as Originally Written.* 1930. World Pub. Co., 1949.

High, Jeffrey L. "Schiller, Coleridge, and the Reception of the 'German (Gothic) Tale.'" *Colloquia Germanica,* vol. 42, no. 1, 2009, pp. 49–66.

Hill Collins, Patricia. *Black Sexual Politics: African Americans, Gender, and the New Racism.* Routledge, 2004.

Hinds, Elizabeth Jane Wall. "American Frontier Gothic." *The Cambridge Companion to American Gothic,* edited by Jeffrey Andrew Weinstock, Cambridge UP, 2017, pp. 128–40, https://www.cambridge.org/.

Hobbes, Thomas. *Leviathan.* 1651. Edited by David Johnston, Norton, 2019.

Hochfield, George. *Selected Writings of the American Transcendentalists.* Yale UP, 2004.

Hoeller, Hildegard. *From Gift to Commodity: Capitalism and Sacrifice in Nineteenth-Century American Fiction.* U of New Hampshire P, 2012.

Hoffer, Peter. *The Devil's Disciplines: Makers of the Salem Witchcraft Trials.* Johns Hopkins UP, 1996.

Hofmannsthal, Hugo von. "Gedankenspuk." In *Die Gedichte 1891–1898 / Die Gedichte 1924.* Edited by Michael Holziger, CreateSpace, 2017, pp. 14–16.

Höglund, Johan. *The Imperial Gothic: Popular Culture, Empire, Violence.* Routledge, 2016.

Hollabaugh, Mark. *The Spirit and the Sky: Lakota Visions of the Cosmos.* U of Nebraska P, 2017.

Holland, Sharon Patricia. *Raising the Dead: Radings of Death and (Black) Subjectivity.* Duke UP, 2000.

Holmes, Stephen. "Gag Rules or the Politics of Omission." *Constitutionalism and Democracy,* edited by Jon Elster and Rune Slagstad, Cambridge UP, 1988, pp. 19–58.

Howe, Julia Ward. "The Results of the Kantian Philosophy." *Journal of Speculative Philosophy,* vol. 15, no. 1, 1881, pp. 274–92.

Hsu, Hsuan L. "Democratic Expansionism in 'Memoirs of Carwin.'" *Early American Literature,* vol. 35, 2000, pp. 137–56.

Huhndorf, Shari M. *Going Native: Indians in the American Cultural Imagination.* Cornell UP, 2001.

Hunter, Michael. *The Decline of Magic: Britain in the Enlightenment.* Yale UP, 2020.

———. "New Light on the 'Drummer of Tedworth': Conflicting Narratives of Witchcraft in Restoration England." *Historical Research,* vol. 78, no. 201, 2005, pp. 311–53.

———. *Robert Boyle: Between God and Science.* Yale UP, 2009.

———. "The Royal Society and the Decline of Magic." *Notes and Records of the Royal Society of London,* vol. 65, no. 2, 2011, pp. 103–19, https://doi.org/10.1098/rsnr.2010.0086.

Hunter, Tera W. *To 'Joy My Freedom: Southern Black Women's Lives and Labors after the Civil War.* Harvard UP, 1997.

Hurst, Michael C. "Reinventing Patriarchy: Washington Irving and the Autoerotics of the American Imaginary." *Early American Literature,* vol. 47, no. 3, 2012, pp. 649–78, https://www.jstor.org/stable/41705694.

Hurston, Zora Neale. *Barracoon: The Story of the Last "Black Cargo."* Amistad, 2018.

Insko, Jeffrey. "Diedrich Knickerbocker, Regular Bred Historian." *Early American Literature,* vol. 43, 2008, pp. 605–43.

Irving, Washington. *Bracebridge Hall.* In *History, Tales, and Sketches,* edited by Andrew B. Myers, Library of America, 1991, pp. 1–378.

———. *History of New-York, from the Beginning of the World to the End of the Dutch Dynasty, by Diedrich Knickerbocker.* In *History, Tales, and Sketches,* edited by James Tuttleton, Library of America, 1983, pp. 363–730.

———. *The Sketch Book of Geoffrey Crayon, Gent.* In *History, Tales, and Sketches,* edited by James Tuttleton, Library of America, 1983, pp. 731–.

———. *Tales of a Traveller.* In *History, Tales, and Sketches,* edited by Andrew B. Myers, Library of America, 1991, pp. 379–718.

Irwin, Robert. *For Lust of Knowing: The Orientalists and Their Enemies.* Allen Lane, 2006.

Isbister, Dong L. "Decentralized Power and Resistance in *The Bondwoman's Narrative.*" *Critical Insights: The Slave Narrative,* edited by Kimberly Drake, Grey House, pp. 162–74.

Jackman, Mary R., and Marie Crane. "'Some of My Best Friends Are Black': Interracial Friendship and White's Racial Attitudes." *Public Opinion Quarterly,* vol. 50, Winter 1986, pp. 459–86.

Jackson, Shirley. *The Haunting of Hill House.* Penguin, 1984.

James, Henry. *The Ghostly Tales of Henry James.* Rutgers UP, 1948.

Jefferson, Thomas. Letter. Thomas Jefferson to Charles Brockden Brown, Jan. 15, 1800, Thomas Jefferson Papers at the Library of Congress, Series 1: General Correspondence. 1651–1827, Microfilm Reel: 022.

———. *Notes on the State of Virginia.* 1785. Penguin, 1999.

Jennings, Francis. "Logan, James (1725–1780), Mingo Indian." *American National Biography,* Feb. 2000, https://doi.org/10.1093/anb/9780198606697.article.0100530.

Jentz, Paul. *Seven Myths of Native American History.* Hackett, 2018.

Jones, Donna V. *The Racial Discourses of Life Philosophy: Negritude, Vitalism, and Modernity.* Columbia UP, 2010.

Judson, Barbara. "A Sound of Voices: The Ventriloquial Uncanny in *Wieland* and *Prometheus Unbound.*" *Eighteenth-Century Studies,* vol. 44, no. 1, Fall 2010, pp. 21–37.

"A Jumbus, or Negro Wake." *Christian Inquirer,* vol. 1, no. 7, Feb. 1825, p. 28.

Jung, Carl G. *Collected Works of C. G. Jung: Spirit in Man, Art, and Literature,* vol. 15, edited by Erhard Adler and R. F. C. Hull, Princeton UP, 1971.

Kaag, John. "Transgressing the Silence: Lydia Maria Child and the Philosophy of Subversion." *Transactions of the Charles S. Peirce Society,* vol. 49, no. 1, 2013, pp. 46–53, https://doi.org/10.2979/trancharpeirsoc.49.1.46.

Kafer, Peter. *Charles Brockden Brown's Revolution and the Birth of American Gothic.* U of Pennsylvania P, 2004.

Kallendorf, Hilaire. "The Rhetoric of Exorcism." *Rhetorica: A Journal of the History of Rhetoric,* vol. 23, no. 3, 2005, pp. 209–37, https://doi.org/10.1525/rh.2005.23.3.209.

Kamrath, Mark. *The Historicism of Charles Brockden Brown: Radical History and the Early Republic.* Kent State UP, 2010.

Kamuf, Peggy. "Abraham's Wake." *Diacritics,* vol. 9, 1979, pp. 32–43.

Kant, Immanuel. *Critique of the Power of Judgement.* Edited and translated by Paul Guyer, translated by Eric Matthews, Cambridge UP, 2000.

———. *Dreams of a Spirit-Seer, Elucidated by Dreams of Metaphysics (1766): Theoretical Philosophy, 1755–1770.* Edited and translated by David E. Walford and Ralf Meerbote, Cambridge UP, 1992, pp. 301–59.

———. *Dreams of a Spirit-Seer, Illustrated by Dreams of Metaphysics.* Edited by Frank Sewall, translated by Emanuel F. Goerwitz, Macmillan, 1900.

———. *Dreams of a Spirit Seer, Illustrated by Dreams of Metaphysics.* Translated by Emanuel Goerwitz, New Church Press, 1915.

———. *Dreams of a Spirit Seer and Other Related Writings*. Translated by John Manolesco, Vantage Press, 1969.

———. *Groundwork of the Metaphysics of Morals: Practical Philosophy*. Edited and translated by Mary J. Gregor. Cambridge UP, 1996.

———. *Kant on Swedenborg: Dreams of a Spirit-Seer and Other Writings*. Translated by Gregory R. Johnson and Glenn Alexander Magee, Swedenborg Foundation, 2002.

———. "Observations on the Feeling of the Beautiful and Sublime (1764)." *Kant: Observations on the Feeling of the Beautiful and Sublime and Other Writings*. Edited by Patrick Frierson and Paul Guyer. Cambridge UP, 2011. 9–62.

———. "Physical Geography (1802)." *Kant: Natural Science*. Ed. Eric Watkins. Cambridge: Cambridge University Press, 2012. 434–679.

———. "Träume eines Geistersehers, erleutert durch Träume der Metaphysik." In *Werkausgabe,* edited by Wilhelm Weischedel, vol. 2, Suhrkamp, 1977, pp. 921–89.

"Kantian Philosophy." *Philadelphia Monthly Magazine,* vol. 2, no. 9, Sept. 1798, pp. 151–53.

"Kant's Project to Perpetual Peace: Zum ewigen Frieden; I. E. To Perpetual Peace, a Philosophical Project." *Monthly Review,* Aug. 2, 1796, pp. 486–90.

Kapferer, Jean-Noel. *Gerüchte: Das älteste Massenmedium der Welt*. Kiepenhauer, 1987.

Karcher, Carolyn L. *The First Woman in the Republic: A Cultural Biography of Lydia Maria Child*. Duke UP, 1994.

Karlsen, Carol F. *The Devil in the Shape of a Woman: Witchcraft in Colonial New England*. Norton, 1987.

Kazanjian, David. *The Colonizing Trick: National Culture and Imperial Citizenship in Early America*. U of Minnesota P, 2003.

Keats, John. "Letter to Richard Woodhouse, 21 and 22, September 1819." *The Major Works,* edited by Elizabeth Cook, Oxford UP, 2008, pp. 494–97.

Kelley, Mary. "Introduction." *Hope Leslie; or, Early Times in the Massachusetts,* by Catharine Maria Sedgwick, Rutgers UP, 1987, pp. ix–xi.

Kerber, Linda K. "The Abolitionist Perception of the Indian." *Journal of American History,* vol. 62, no. 2, 1975, pp. 271–95, https://doi.org/10.2307/1903255.

King, Stephen. *The Shining*. Doubleday, 1977.

Kirkpatrick, David D. "On Long-Lost Pages: A Female Slave's Voice," *New York Times,* 11 November 2001, A1.

Kittredge, G. L. "Cotton Mather's Scientific Communications to the Royal Society." *American Antiquarian Society Proceedings,* Worcester, 1916, 18–57.

Koester, Nancy. *Harriet Beecher Stowe: A Spiritual Life*. Eerdmans, 2014.

Kohn, Eduardo. *How Forests Think: Toward an Anthropology beyond the Human*. U of California P, 2013.

Kolbert, Elizabeth. *The Sixth Extinction: An Unnatural History*. Henry Holt, 2014.

Krause, Sydney J. "Charles Brockden Brown and the Philadelphia Germans." *Early American Literature,* vol. 39, issue 1, 2004, pp. 84–119.

Krech, Shepard. *The Ecological Indian: Myth and History.* Norton, 1999.

Krumholz, Linda. "The Ghosts of Slavery: Historical Recovery in Toni Morrison's *Beloved.*" *African American Review,* vol. 26, no. 3, 1992, pp. 395–408. https://www .jstor.org/stable/3041912.

Kucich, John J. *Ghostly Communion: Cross-Cultural Spiritualism in Nineteenth-Century American Literature.* Dartmouth College Press, 2004.

Kurth-Voigt, Lieselotte E. "Existence after Death in Eighteenth-Century Literature: Prolegomena to a Study of Poetic Visions of the Beyond and Imaginative Speculations about Continued Life in a Future State." *South Atlantic Review,* vol. 52, May 1987, pp. 3–14.

———. "The Reception of *Wieland* in America." *The German Contribution to the Building of the Americas: Studies in Honor of Karl J. R. Arndt.* Edited by John Richard et al., Clark UP, 1977, pp. 97–133.

Kutchen, Larry. "The 'Vulgar Thread of the Canvas': Revolution and the Picturesque in Ann Eliza Bleecker, Crèvecoeur, and Charles Brockden Brown." *Early American Literature,* vol. 36, 2001, pp. 395–425.

Lacan, Jacques. *Écrits: A Selection.* Edited by Bruce Fink, Norton, 2002.

Lacoue-Labarthe, Philippe, and Jean-Luc Nancy. *The Literary Absolute: The Theory of Literature in German Romanticism.* State U of New York P, 1988.

Latour, Bruno. *We Have Never Been Modern.* Translation by Catherine Porter, Harvard UP, 1993.

Lawlor, James D. "Seller Beware: Burden of Disclosing Defects Shifting to Sellers." *ABA Journal,* vol. 78, no. 8, 1992, p. 90.

Lawrence, D. H. *Studies in Classic American Literature.* Penguin, 1971.

Le Loyer, Pierre. *A Treatise of Specters or Straunge Sights, Visions and Apparitions Appearing Sensibly unto Men.* Translation by Zachary Jones, London, 1605.

Leacock, John. *The Fall of British Tyranny; or, American Liberty Triumphant.* 1776. http://name.umdl.umich.edu/N11731.0001.001.

Lemoine, Henry. "Phantasmagoria." *Gentleman's Magazine,* no. 72, part 1, June 1802.

Lessing, Gotthold Ephraim. *The Hamburg Dramaturgy,* edited by Natalya Baldyga, translated by Wendy Arons and Sara Figal, Routledge, 2019.

"Lessing's Dramaturgy." *Monthly Magazine or British Register,* vol. 12, no. 78, 1801, pp. 224–24.

Levine, Caroline. *Forms: Whole, Rhythm, Hierarchy, Network.* Princeton UP, 2015.

Levine, Robert S. "Trappe(d): Race and Genealogical Haunting in *The Bondwoman's Narrative.*" *In Search of Hannah Crafts: Critical Essays on "The Bondwoman's Narrative,"* edited by Henry Louis Gates and Hollis Robbins, BasicCivitas, 2004, pp. 276–94.

Lincoln, Abraham. *Abraham Lincoln: Speeches and Writings.* Vol. 1, Library of America, 1989.

Lloyd-Smith, Allan. *American Gothic Fiction: An Introduction.* Continuum, 2004.

Looby, Christopher. *Voicing America: Language, Literary Form, and the Origins of the United States.* U of Chicago P, 1996.

Lorde, Audre. *Sister Outsider: Essays and Speeches.* Crossing Press, 2007.

Lovejoy, David S. "Satanizing the American Indian." *New England Quarterly,* vol. 67, no. 4, 1994, pp. 603–21, https://doi.org/10.2307/366436.

Luciano, Dana. "'Perverse Nature:' *Edgar Huntly* and the Novel's Reproductive Disorders." *American Literature,* vol. 70, 1998, pp. 1–27.

Mackenthun, Gesa. "Captives and Sleepwalkers: The Ideological Revolutions of Post-Revolutionary Colonial Discourse." *European Review of Native American Studies,* vol. 11, 1997, pp. 19–26.

"Magic, *N.*" *OED Online,* Oxford UP, December 2020, https://www.oed.com /dictionary/spectrology_n.

Malchow, Howard L. *Gothic Images of Race in Nineteenth Century Britain.* Stanford UP, 1996. *Hobbes: Leviathan,* vol. 1, edited by Noel Malcolm, Oxford UP, 2014.

Mantel, Hilary. "The Shape of Absence." *London Review of Books,* vol. 24, no. 15, August 8, 2002, https://www.lrb.co.uk/the-paper/v24/n15/hilary-mantel/the -shape-of-absence.

Marker, Michael. "There Is no *Place of Nature;* There Is Only the *Nature of Place:* Animate Landscapes as Methodology for Inquiry in the Coast Salish Territory." *International Journal of Qualitative Studies in Education,* vol. 31, no. 6, 2018, pp. 453–64, https://doi.org/10.1080/09518398.2018.1430391.

Marsh, Philip Morin. *The Prose of Philip Freneau.* Scarecrow Press, 1955.

Marshall, Ian. "Heteroglossia in Lydia Maria Child's Hobomok." *Legacy,* vol. 10, no. 1, 1993, pp. 1–16, http://www.jstor.org/stable/25679095.

Martin, Robert K., and Eric Savoy. "Introduction." *American Gothic: New Interventions in a National Narrative,* edited by Robert K. Martin and Eric Savoy, U of Iowa P, 1998, pp. 3–20.

Mather, Cotton. *Good Fetch'd Out of Evil.* Printed by Bartholomew Green, 1706. Early American Imprint Collection. http://name.umdl.umich.edu/N15311.0001.001.

———. *Memorable Providences, Relating to Witchcrafts and Possessions.* Boston, 1689.

———. *A Voice from Heaven: An Account of a Late Uncommon Appearance in the Heavens. With REMARKS upon it.* Boston, 1719.

———. *The Wonders of the Invisible World: Observations as Well Historical as Theological, upon the Nature, the Number, and the Operations of the Devils,* Boston, 1693, https://digitalcommons.unl.edu/cgi/viewcontent.cgi?referer=https:// www.google.com/&httpsredir=1&article=1019&context=etas.

Mather, Increase. *Cases of Conscience Concerning Evil Spirits Personating Men, Witchcrafts, Infallible Proofs of Guilt in Such as Are Accused with That Crime, All Considered According to the Scriptures, History, Experience, and the Judgment of Many Learned Men.* Boston, 1693.

———. *An Essay for the Recording of Illustrious Providences: Narratives of the Witch-craft Cases, 1648–1706,* edited by George Lincoln Burr, C. Scribner's Sons, 1914, pp. 3–38.

———. *An Essay for the Recording of Illustrious Providences wherein an Account Is Given of Many Remarkable and Very Memorable Events, Which Have Hapned This Last Age, Especially in New-England.* Boston, 1684, https://www.proquest.com /books/essay-recording-illustrious-providences-wherein/docview/2240911880 /se-2?accountid=15156.

Martin, Harold C. "The Colloquial Tradition in the Novel: John Neal." *New England Quarterly,* vol. 32, no. 4, 1959, pp. 455–75.

Matthews, John. *A Voyage to the River Sierra-Leone: On the Coast of Africa.* London, 1788.

Mbembe, Achille. *Necropolitics.* Duke UP, 2019.

———. *On the Postcolony.* U of California P, 2001.

Mbiti, John S. *Introduction to African Religion.* Heinemann, 1991.

McCarthy, John. "'An Indigenous and Not an Exotic Plant': Towards a History of Germanistisch at Penn." *Teaching German in Twentieth-Century America,* edited by David B. Benseler et al., U of Wisconsin P, 2001, pp. 146–72.

McConkey, Kevin M., and Campbell Perry. "Benjamin Franklin and Mesmerism." *International Journal of Clinical and Experimental Hypnosis,* vol. 33, no. 2, 1985, pp. 122–30, https://doi.org/10.1080/00207148508406642.

McGarry, Molly. *Ghosts of Futures Past: Spiritualism and the Cultural Politics of Nineteenth-Century America.* U of California P, 2008.

McKittrick, Katherine. *Sylvia Wynter: On Being Human as Praxis.* Duke UP, 2015.

McLamore, Richard V. "The Dutchman in the Attic: Claiming an Inheritance in the Sketch Book of Geoffrey Crayon." *American Literature,* vol. 72, March 2000, pp. 31–57.

McMahon, Darrin. *Enemies of the Enlightenment: The French Counter-Enlightenment and the Making of Modernity.* Oxford UP, 2001.

McQuillan, J. Colin. "Reading and Misreading Kant's *Dreams of a Spirit Seer.*" 2015, pp. 178–203, https://kantstudiesonline.net/uploads/files/McQuillanColin02315 .pdf.

"Memoirs of Immanuel Kant." *Literary Magazine and American Register,* vol. 19, no. 128, 1805, pp. 354–61.

Mills, Charles. "Kant's *Untermenschen.*" *Race and Racism in Modern Philosophy,* edited by Andrew Valls, Cornell UP, 2005, pp. 169–93.

More, Henry. *An Antidote against Atheisme; or, an Appeal to the Natural Faculties of the Minde of Man, Whether There Be Not a God.* London, 1653.

Morrison, E. S. *The Puritans Pronaos: Studies in the Intellectual Life of New England in the Seventeenth Century.* New York UP, 1936.

Morrison, Toni. *Beloved.* Knopf, 2006.

———. *Playing in the Dark: Whiteness and the Literary Imagination.* Vintage, 1993.

Morton, Sarah Wentworth (Philenia, a Lady of Boston). "Ouâbi; or, The Virtues of Nature: An Indian Tale." *Massachusetts Magazine; or, Monthly Museum of Knowledge and Rational Entertainment*, vol. 2, no. 12, Dec. 1790, pp. 759–60.

M—R—E, J—L. "The Apparition." *Gentleman's Magazine; or, Monthly Intelligencer*, vol. 5, Mar. 1735, p. 160.

Murphy, Ryan, and Brad Falchuk. *American Horror Story*. FX, 2011–2021.

Murray, David. *Matter, Magic, and Spirit: Representing Indian and African American Belief.* U of Pennsylvania P, 2007.

Murray, Laura J. "The Aesthetic of Dispossession: Washington Irving and Ideologies of (De)Colonization in the Early Republic." *American Literary History*, vol. 8, no. 2, 1996, pp. 205–31.

Neal, John. *American Writers, a Series of Papers Contributed to Blackwoods Magazine (1824–1825)*, edited by Fred Lewis Patter, Duke UP, 1937.

———. "Critical Essays and Stories by John Neal. Edited, with an Introduction, by Hans-Joachim Lang. With a Note on the Authorship of 'David Whicher' and a Bibliography of John Neal by Irving T. Richards." *Jahrbuch für Amerikastudien*, vol. 7, Universitätsverlag Winter, 1962, pp. 204–319, http://www.jstor.org/stable/41155013.

———. *Logan, a Family History*. 2 vols., Philadelphia, 1822.

Nichols, Marcia. "Cicero's *Pro Cluentio* and the 'Mazy' Rhetorical Strategies of *Wieland*." *Law and Literature*, vol. 20, no. 3, 2008, pp. 459–76, https://doi.org/10.1525/lal.2008.20.3.459.

Nickerson, Cynthia D. "Artistic Interpretations of Henry Wadsworth Longfellow's 'The Song of Hiawatha,' 1855–1900." *American Art Journal*, vol. 16, no. 3, 1984, pp. 49–77.

Nitsch, F. A. *A General and Introductory View of Professor Kant's Principles Concerning Man, the World, and the Deity, Submitted to the Consideration of the Learned.* New York, 1796.

Norton, Mary Beth. *In the Devil's Snare: The Salem Witchcraft Crisis of 1692*. E-book edition, Knopf, 2002.

Norwood, Vera. *Made from This Earth: American Women and Nature*. U of North Carolina P, 2014.

O'Brien, Jean M. *Firsting and Lasting: Writing Indians Out of Existence in New England*. U of Minnesota P, 2010.

"Ode on Seeing a Negro Funeral." *New-York Magazine or Literary Repository*, vol. 7, 1796, pp. 165–66.

"Of Apparitions, Witches, & C." *London Magazine; or, Gentleman's Monthly Intelligencer*, vol. 31, 1762, pp. 583–84.

"Of Ghosts and Apparitions." *London Magazine; or, Gentleman's Monthly Intelligencer*, vol. 3, Nov. 1734, pp. 592–93.

"On the Subject of Apparitions." *London Magazine; or, Gentleman's Monthly Intelligencer*, vol. 32, 1763, pp. 14–15.

Outka, Paul. *Race and Nature from Transcendentalism to the Harlem Renaissance.* Palgrave Macmillan, 2008.

Palmer, Elihu. "Superstitious Terrors." *Prospect; or, View of the Moral World,* vol. 1, no. 1, 1803, pp. 5–7.

———. "To the Public." *Prospect; or, View of the Moral World,* vol. 1, no. 1, 1803, pp. 1–2.

———. "Your Old Men Shall Dream Dreams, Your Young Ones Shall See Visions." *Prospect; or, View of the Moral World,* vol. 1, no. 4, 1803, pp. 27–28.

Paracelsus, Philippus Theophrastus. *Astronomia Magna; oder, die ganze Philosophia sagax der großen und kleinen Welt* samt Beiwerk. In: Paracelsus:. Edited by Karl Sudhoff. München, 1929. Reprint: Olms 1996. Volume 12, pp. 1–507.

Parham, Marisa. *Haunting and Displacement in African American Literature and Culture.* Routledge, 2009.

Park, Julie. *The Self and It: Novel Objects and Mimetic Subjects in Eighteenth-Century England.* Stanford UP, 2010.

Parker, Elizabeth. *The Forest and the Ecogothic: The Deep Dark Woods in the Popular Imagination.* Palgrave Macmillan, 2020.

Parkin, Jon. "The Reception of Hobbes's Leviathan." *The Cambridge Companion to Hobbes's Leviathan,* edited by Patricia Springborg, Cambridge UP, 2007, pp. 441–59.

Patrick, Barbara. "Lady Terrorists: Nineteenth-Century American Women Writers and the Ghost Story." *American Women Short Story Writers: A Collection of Critical Essays,* edited by Julie Brown, Garland Publishing, 1995, pp. 73–84.

Patterson, Orlando. *Slavery and Social Death: A Comparative Study.* Harvard UP, 2018.

Pease, Donald. *Visionary Compacts: American Renaissance Writings in Cultural Context.* U of Wisconsin P, 1987.

Peterson, Christopher. *Kindred Specters: Death, Mourning, and American Affinity.* U of Minnesota P, 2007.

Philanthropist. *An Account of the Beginning, Transactions, and Discovery of Ransford Rogers Who Seduced Many by Pretended Hobgoblins and Apparitions, and Thereby Extorted Money from Their Pockets.* 1792. Newark, 1876.

Poe, Edgar Allan. "William Gilmore Simms." *The Works of the Late Edgar Allan Poe,* vol. 3, 1850, pp. 272–75.

Popkin, Richard H. "The Development of the Philosophical Reputation of Joseph Glanvill." *Journal of the History of Ideas,* vol. 15, no. 2, 1954, pp. 305–11, https://doi.org/10.2307/2707775.

Povinelli, Elizabeth. *Labor's Lot.* Chicago UP, 1993.

Pratt, Mary Louise. "Arts of the Contact Zone." *Profession,* 1991, pp. 33–40. *JSTOR,* http://www.jstor.org/stable/25595469.

Priestman, Martin. *Romantic Atheism: Poetry and Freethought, 1780–1830.* Cambridge UP, 1999.

Prior, Charles W. A. *Settlers in Indian Country: Sovereignty and Indigenous Power in Early America.* Cambridge UP, 2020, https://doi.org/10.1017/9781 108883979.

Prior, Moody E. "Joseph Glanvill, Witchcraft, and Seventheenth-Century Science." *Modern Philology,* vol. 30, Nov. 1932, pp. 167–93.

Pryse, Marjorie. "Stowe and Regionalism." *The Cambridge Companion to Harriet Beecher Stowe.* Ed. Cindy Weinstein. Cambridge UP, 2004. 131–153.

"Psyche, *n.*" *OED Online,* Oxford UP, September 2020, www.oed.com/view/Entry /153848.

Puckett, Newbell Niles. *Folk Beliefs of the Southern Negro.* U of North Carolina P, 1926.

Punter, David. *The Literature of Terror: A History of Gothic Fiction from 1765 to the Present Day.* Longman, 1996.

Raboteau, Albert J. *Slave Religion: The "Invisible Institution" in the Antebellum South.* Oxford UP, 2004.

Radcliffe, Ann. "On the Supernatural in Poetry." *New Monthly Magazine,* vol. 16, no. 1, 1826, pp. 145–52.

"Rannie's Exhibition." *Prospect; or, View of the Moral World,* vol. 1, no. 24, 1804, pp. 191–92.

Ravalli, Richard. "Cotton Mather, Levitation, and a Case for Wonders in History." *Christian Scholar's Review,* vol. 35, no. 2, 2006, pp. 193–204.

"Reason Proscribed by Superstition." *Prospect; or, View of the Moral World,* vol. 1, no. 1, 1803, pp. 3–4.

Reed, Kenneth T. "Washington Irving and the Negro." *Negro American Literature Forum,* vol. 4, no. 2, 1970, pp. 43–44.

"Register of Debates." 24th Congress, 1st session, vol. 12, May 18, 1836, https:// memory.loc.gov/ammem/amlaw/lwrdlink.html.

"Revenant, *N.* and *Adj.* (2)." *Oxford English Dictionary,* Oxford UP, March 2024, https://doi.org/10.1093/OED/4277736598.

Reynolds, Larry J. *The Routledge Introduction to American Renaissance Literature.* Routledge, 2021.

Rhyne, Nancy. *Slave Ghost Stories: Tales of Hags, Hants, Ghosts and Diamondback Rattlers.* Sandlapper, 2002.

Richards, Jason. *Imitation Nation: Red, White, and Blackface in Early and Antebellum U.S. Literature.* E-book. U of Virginia P, 2017.

Richter, Jörg Thomas. *Nationalität als literarisches Verfahren: Der amerikanische Roman (1790–1830).* Ferdinand Schöningh, 2004.

Rifkin, Mark. *Beyond Settler Time: Temporal Sovereignty and Indigenous Self-Determination.* Duke UP, 2017.

Ringe, Donald. *American Gothic: Imagination and Reason in Nineteenth-Century Fiction.* UP of Kentucky, 1982.

———. *Charles Brockden Brown.* Twayne, 1966.

Rivett, Sarah. "Empirical Desire: Conversion, Ethnography, and the New Science of the Praying Indian." *Early American Studies,* vol. 4, no. 1, 2006, pp. 16–45.

———. "Indigenous Metaphors and the Philosophy of History in Cooper's Leatherstocking Tales," *Unscripted America: Indigenous Languages and the Origins of a Literary Nation,* Oxford UP, 2017, pp. 238–72. https://doi.org/10.1093/oso/9780190492564.003.0009.

———. "Our Salem, Our Selves." *William and Mary Quarterly,* vol. 65, no. 3, 2008, pp. 495–502, https://doi.org/10.2307/25096811.

———. "The Spectral Indian Presence in Early American Literature." *American Literary History,* vol. 25, no. 3, 2013, pp. 625–37.

Roach, Marylinne K. *The Salem Witchcraft Trials: A Day-by-Day Chronicle of a Community under Siege.* Taylor Trade Publishing, 2004.

Roberts, Siân Silyn. *Gothic Subjects: The Transformation of Individualism in American Fiction, 1790–1861.* U of Pennsylvania P, 2014.

Robbins, Hollis. "Blackening Bleak House: Hannah Crafts's *The Bondwoman's Narrative.*" *In Search of Hannah Crafts: Critical Essays on "The Bondwoman's Narrative,"* edited by Henry Louis Gates and Hollis Robbins, BasicCivitas, 2004, pp. 71–86.

Rombes, Nichols, Jr. "'All Was Lonely, Darksome, and Waste': *Wieland* and the Construction of the New Republic." *Studies in American Fiction,* vol. 22, no. 1, 1994, p. 37–46. https://doi.org/10.1353/saf.1994.0021.

Ross, Cheri Louise. "Rewriting the Frontier Romance: Catharine Maria Sedgwick's *Hope Leslie.*" *CLA Journal* 39 (1996): 320–340.

Rousseau, Jean-Jacques. *Émile; or, On Education.* Translated by Allan Bloom, Basic Books, 1979.

Rowe, John Carlos. *At Emerson's Tomb: The Politics of Classic American Literature.* Columbia UP, 1996.

———. *Literary Culture and U.S. Imperialism: From Revolution to World War II.* Oxford UP, 2000.

Rowlandson, Mary White. *Narrative of the Captivity and Restoration of Mrs. Mary Rowlandson. Narratives of the Indian Wars, 1675–1699,* edited by Charles H. Lincoln, Scribner's, 1913.

Rucker, Walter. "Conjure, Magic, and Power: The Influence of Afro-Atlantic Religious Practices on Slave Resistance and Rebellion." *Journal of Black Studies,* vol. 32, no. 1, 2001, pp. 84–103.

Rugoff, Milton. *The Beechers: An American Family in the Nineteenth Century.* Harper Collins, 1981.

Rush, Benjamin. *Benjamin Rush's Lectures on the Mind.* Edited by Eric T. Carlson, Jeffrey L. Wollock and Patirica S. Noel, vol. 144, U of Pennsylvania P, vol. 144, 1981.

Ruttenburg, Nancy. *Democratic Personality: Popular Voice and the Trial of American Authorship.* Stanford UP, 1998.

Sade, Marquis de. *The Crimes of Love.* Bantam Books, 1993.

Samuels, Shirley. "'Wieland': Alien and Infidel." *Early American Literature,* vol. 25, no. 1, 1990, pp. 46–66, http://www.jstor.org/stable/25056795.

Sánchez-Eppler, Karen. "Gothic Liberties and Fugitive Novels: *The Bondwoman's Narrative* and the Fiction of Race." *In Search of Hannah Crafts: Critical Essays on "The Bondwoman's Narrative,"* edited by Henry Louis Gates Jr. and Hollis Robbins, Basic Books, 2004, pp. 254–75.

Saunders, George. *Lincoln in the Bardo.* Random House, 2017.

Savoy, Eric. "The Rise of American Gothic." *The Cambridge Companion to Gothic Fiction,* edited by Jerrold E. Hogle, Cambridge UP, 2002, pp. 167–88.

Sayre, Gordon M. "'Azakia,' Ouâbi, and Sarah Wentworth Apthorp Morton: A Romance of the Early American Republic." *Princeton University Library Chronicle,* vol. 64, no. 2, 2003, pp. 313–32, https://doi.org/10.25290/prinunivlibrchro.64.2.0313.

———. *The Indian Chief as Tragic Hero: Native Resistance and the Literatures of America, from Moctezuma to Tecumseh.* U of North Carolina P, 2005.

Sayre, Jillian. "The Necropolitics of New World Nativism." *Early American Literature,* vol. 53, no. 3, 2018, pp. 713–44, https://www.jstor.org/stable/90025277.

Schelling, F. W. J. *Über das Wesen der menschlichen Freiheit.* 1809. Suhrkamp, 1988.

Schiffman, Robyn. "Novalis and Hawthorne: A New Look at Hawthorne's German Influences." *Nathaniel Hawthorne Review,* vol. 38, no. 1, 2012, pp. 41–57.

Schiller, Friedrich. *The Ghost-Seer; or, Apparitionist: An Interesting Fragment, Found among the Papers of Count O**.* Translated by Daniel Boileau, London, 1795.

———. *The Robbers, A Tragedy.* Translated by Alexander Fraser Tytler, London, 1792.

———. *Schillers Werke.* In *Nationalausgabe,* vol. 24, edited by Lieselotte Blumenthal and Benno von Wiese, Bühlau, 1989.

Schlegel. *Dialogue on Poetry and Literary Aphorisms.* 1799. Translation by Ernst Behler and Roman Struc, Pennsylvania State UP, 1968.

———. *On the Study of Greek Poetry.* 1797. Translation by Stuart Barnett, State U of New York P, 2001.

Schmidt, Leigh Eric. "From Demon Possession to Magic Show: Ventriloquism, Religion, and the Enlightenment." *Church History,* vol. 67, no. 2, 1998, pp. 274–304. *JSTOR,* https://doi.org/10.2307/3169762.

———. *Hearing Things: Religion, Illusion, and the American Enlightenment.* Harvard UP, 2000.

Schwab, Gabriele. *Haunting Legacies: Violent Histories and Transgenerational Trauma.* Columbia UP, 2010.

Schweighauser, Philipp. *Beautiful Deceptions: European Aesthetics, the Early American Novel, and Illusionist Art.* U of Virginia P, 2016.

Scot, Reginald. *The Discoverie of Witchcraft, wherein the Lewde Dealing of Witches and Witchmongers Is Notablie Detected, the Knauerie of Coniurors, the Impietie of Inchantors, the Follie of Soothsaiers.* London, 1584, http://hdl.loc.gov/loc.rbc/mcyoung.45413b.1.

Scott, Sir Walter. *Letters on Demonology and Witchcraft.* 1830. London, 2001.

Sedgwick, Catharine Maria. *Hope Leslie; or, Early Times in the Massachusetts.* 1827. Edited by Mary Kelley, Rutgers UP, 1987.

———. *Tales and Sketches.* Philadelphia, 1835.

Seeber, Edward D. "Critical Views on Logan's Speech." *Journal of American Folklore,* vol. 60, no. 236, 1947, pp. 130–46, https://doi.org/10.2307/536695.

Seeman, Erik R. "Native Spirits, Shaker Visions: Speaking with the Dead in the Early Republic." *Journal of the Early Republic,* vol. 35, no. 3, 2015, pp. 347–73.

Sehgal, Parul. "The Ghost Story Persists in American Literature. Why?" *New York Times,* Oct. 22, 2018, www.nytimes.com/2018/10/22/books/review/ghost-stories.html.

Shaviro, Steven. *The Universe of Things: On Speculative Realism.* U of Minnesota P, 2014.

Shefer, Tamara, and Kopano Ratele. "Racist Sexualisation and Sexualised Racism in Narratives on Apartheid." *Psychoanalysis, Culture and Society,* vol. 16, 2011, https://doi.org/10.1057/pcs.2010.38.

Shibutani, Tamotsu. *Improvised News: A Sociological Study of Rumor.* Bobbs-Merrill, 1966.

The Shining, directed by Stanely Kubrick, starring Jack Nicholson, Shelley Duvall, and Danny Lloyd. Warner Bros, 1980.

Simms, William Gilmore. "Grayling; or, 'Murder Will Out.'" *The Wigwam and the Cabin.* New York, 1845, pp. 1–36.

———. "'Murder Will Out': A Genuine Ghost Story of the Old School." *The Gift.* Philadelphia, 1841, pp. 262–304.

Simpson, Leanne Betasamosake. *As We Have Always Done.* U of Minnesota P, 2017.

Sinche, Bryan. "Godly Rebellion in *The Bondwoman's Narrative.*" *In Search of Hannah Crafts: Critical Essays on "The Bondwoman's Narrative,"* edited by Henry Louis Gates Jr. and Hollis Robbins, Basic Books, 2004, pp. 175–94.

Sinclair, George. *Satan's Invisible World Discovered; or, a Choice Collection of Modern Relations Proving Evidently against the Saducees and Atheists of This Present Age, That There Are Devils, Spirits, Witches, and Apparition.* Edinburgh, 1685.

Sivils, Matthew Wynn. "Indian Captivity Narratives and the Origins of American Frontier Gothic." *A Companion to American Gothic,* 2013, pp. 84–95.

Skouen, Tina. "Science versus Rhetoric? Sprat's *History of the Royal Society* Reconsidered." *Rhetorica: A Journal of the History of Rhetoric,* vol. 29, no. 1, 2011, pp. 23–52, https://doi.org/10.1525/rh.2011.29.1.23.

Slotkin, Richard. *Regeneration through Violence: The Mythology of the American Frontier, 1600–1860.* Wesleyan UP, 1973.

Smeall, J. F. S. "Variants: 'The Indian Burying Ground' of Philip Freneau." *Papers of the Bibliographical Society of America,* vol. 75, no. 3, 1981, pp. 257–70.

Smith, Andrew. *The Ghost Story, 1840–1920: A Cultural History.* Manchester UP, 2010.

Smith, Mr. "PROLOGUE to THE DRUMMER; OR, HAUNTED HOUSE; Occasioned by the Cock-Lane Apparition." *Universal Magazine of Knowledge and Pleasure,* vol. 30, no. 206, Feb. 1762, p. 97.

Smith-Rosenberg, Carroll. *This Violent Empire: The Birth of an American National Identity.* U of North Carolina P, 2010.

Snyder-Körber, MaryAnn. "Perilous Performances: Picturing Occult Inheritance and Staging the Melodrama of the Mind in *Wieland.*" *Melodrama! The Mode of Excess from Early America to Hollywood,* edited by Frank Kelleter and Ruth Mayer, Winter, 2007, pp. 55–72.

Sobel, Mechal. *The World They Made Together: Black and White Values in Eighteenth-Century Virginia.* Princeton UP, 1987.

Sollors, Werner. "Dr. Benjamin Franklin's Celestial Telegraph, or Indian Blessings to Gas-Lit American Drawing Rooms." *American Quarterly,* vol. 35, no. 5, Winter 1983, pp. 459–80.

Solomon, Andrew. *The Noonday Demon.* Chatto and Windus, 2001.

Soltysik Monnet, Agnieszka. "Gothic Literature in America." *When Highbrow Meets Lowbrow: Popular Culture and the Rise of Nobrow,* edited by Peter Swirski and Tero Eljas Vanhanen, Palgrave Macmillan US, 2017, pp. 109–30, https://doi.org /10.1057/978-1-349-95168-0_6.

———. *The Poetics and Politics of the American Gothic: Gender and Slavery in the Nineteenth Century American Gothic.* Ashgate, 2010.

Soyinka, Wole. *Myth, Literature, and the African World.* Cambridge UP, 1976.

Spaulding, A. Timothy. *Re-Forming the Past: History, the Fantastic, and the Postmodern Slave Narrative.* Ohio State UP, 2005.

"Spectral, *Adj.*" *OED Online,* Oxford UP, December 2020, www.oed.com/view/ Entry/186096.

"Spectrology, *N.*" *OED Online,* Oxford UP, December 2020, www.oed.com/view/ Entry/186096.

Spence, Mark David. *Dispossessing the Wilderness: Indian Removal and the Making of the National Parks.* Oxford UP, 1999.

Spira, Andrew. *The Invention of the Self: Personal Identity in the Age of Art.* Bloomsbury, 2022.

Sprat, Thomas. *The History of the Royal-Society of London for the Improving of Natural Knowledge.* London, 1667.

Stengel, Freidmann, editor. *Kant und Swedenborg: Zugänge zu einem umstrittenen Verhältnis.* Niemeyer, 2008.

Stowe, Harriet Beecher. 1852. *Uncle Tom's Cabin,* edited by Elizabeth Ammons, Norton, 1994.

Stowe, Harriet Beecher. "The Ministration of Departed Spirits in This World." *Christian Inquirer,* vol. 3, no. 25, 1849, p. 98.

———. *Oldtown Folks.* In *Uncle Tom's Cabin, or, Life among the Lowly; the Minister's Wooing; Oldtown Folks,* Library of America, 1982, pp. 877–1468.

———. *Sam Lawson's Oldtown Fireside Stories.* Houghton, Mifflin and Company, 1891.

"Supernatural, *Adj.*" *An American Dictionary of the English Language.* Vol. 2, New Haven, 1841, p. 722.

"Superstitious Terrors." *Prospect; or, View of the Moral World,* vol. 1, no. 1, 1803, p. 5.

Swann, Charles. "Alchemy and Hawthorne's 'Elixir of Life Manuscripts.'" *Journal of American Studies,* vol. 22, no. 3, 1988, pp. 371–87.

Swedenborg, Emmanuel. *Arcana Coelestia: The Heavenly Arcana Contained in the Holy Scriptures, or Word of the Lord, Unfolded, Beginning with the Book of Genesis.* Translated by John F. Potts, Swedenborg Foundation, 1963.

———. *The Athanasian Creed.* Swedenborg Society, 1954.

———. *The Spiritual Diary of Emmanuel Swedenborg.* Translated by Bush, Smithson and Buss. 1747–1765. *Internet Sacred Text Archive.* https://sacred-texts.com/swd/sd/index.htm.

Sweet, Nancy F. "Dissent and the Daughter in a New England Tale and Hobomok." *Legacy,* vol. 22, no. 2, 2005, pp. 107–25.

Tawil, Ezra. "Domestic Frontier Romance; or, How the Sentimental Heroine Became White." *NOVEL: A Forum on Fiction,* vol. 32, no. 1, 1998, pp. 99–124, https://doi.org/10.2307/1346058.

Taylor, Barbara. "Enlightenment and the Uses of Woman." *History Workshop Journal,* no. 74, 2012, pp. 79–87.

Thomas, Keith. *Religion and the Decline of Magic.* Penguin, 1991.

Thompson, G. R. "Literary Politics and the 'Legitimate Sphere': Poe, Hawthorne, and the 'Tale Proper.'" *Nineteenth-Century Literature,* vol. 49, no. 2, 1994, pp. 167–95, https://doi.org/10.2307/2933980.

Thoreau, Henry D. *Walden, Civil Disobedience, and Other Writings.* Edited by William Rossi, Norton, 2008.

Thurston, Luke. *Literary Ghosts from the Victorians to Modernism: The Haunting Interval.* Routledge, 2012.

Tieck, Ludwig. *Die verkehrte Welt: Ein historisches Schauspiel in fünf Aufzügen.* 1800. Winkler, 1963.

Todd, Zoe. "An Indigenous Feminist's Take on the Ontological Turn: 'Ontology' Is Just Another Word for Colonialism." *Journal of Historical Sociology,* vol. 29, no. 1, 2016, pp. 4–22.

Todorov, Tzvetan. *The Fantastic: A Structural Approach to a Literary Genre.* Translated by Richard Howard, Cornell UP, 1975.

Tomc, Sandra. "'Clothes upon Sticks': James Fenimore Cooper and the Flat Frontier." *Texas Studies in Literature and Language,* vol. 51, no. 2, 2009, pp. 142–78, https://doi.org/10.1353/tsl.0.0026.

Tooker, Elisabeth. "Iroquois Culture, History, and Prehistory." In *Proceedings of the 1965 Conference on Iroquois Research.* Vol. 16, U of the State of New York / State Education Department / New York State Museum and Science Service, 1967.

Torok, Maria, and Nicolas Abraham. *The Shell and the Kernel: Renewals of Psycho-analysis.* Translated by Nicholas T. Rand, U of Chicago P, 1994.

Townshend, Dale. "Speaking of Darkness: Gothic and the History of the African American Slave-Woman in Hannah Crafts' *The Bondwoman's Narrative* (1855–1961)." *Victorian Gothic,* edited by Rosemary Mitchell Karen Sayer, U of Leeds P, 2003, pp. 141–54.

Tschink, Cajetan. *The Victim of Magical Delusion; or, The Mysteries of the Revolution of P—l.* London, 1795. 3 vols.

Tsing, Anna Lowenhaupt, et al. *Arts of Living on a Damaged Planet.* U of Minnesota P, 2017.

Twain, Mark. *The Best Short Stories of Mark Twain.* Modern Library, 2004.

"Universal Spectator, Oct. 7. No. 209. Of Ghosts, Daemons, and Spectres." *Gentleman's Magazine; or, Monthly Intelligencer,* vol. 2, Oct. 1732, pp. 1001–2.

Venables, Robert W. "The Clearings and The Woods: The Haudenosaunee (Iroquois) Landscape—Gendered *and* Balanced." *Archaeology and Preservation of Gendered Landscapes,* edited by Serene Baugher and Suzanne Spencer-Wood, Springer, https://doi.org/10.1007/978-1-4419-1501-6_2.

Vetere, Lisa M. "Horrors of the Horticultural: Charles Brockden Brown's *Wieland* and the Landscapes of the Anthropocene." *Dark Scenes from Damaged Earth,* edited by Justin D. Edwards, Rune Graulund, and Johan Höglund, U of Minnesota P, 2022, pp. 111–29.

Vial, Theodore. *Modern Religion, Modern Race.* Oxford UP, 2016.

Volney, C. F. *A New Translation of Volney's Ruins; or, Meditations on the Revolution of Empires.* Translated by Thomas Jefferson and Joel Barlow, Paris, 1802. 2 vols.

———. *A View of the Soil and Climate of the United States of America, with Supplementary Remarks upon Florida; on the French Colonies on the Mississippi and Ohio, and in Canada; and on the Aboriginal Tribes of America.* Translated with occasional remarks by C. B. Brown, Philadelphia, 1804.

Voloshin, Beverly R. "*Wieland:* 'Accounting for Appearances.'" *New England Quarterly,* vol. 59, no. 3, Sept. 1986, pp. 341–57.

Voltaire. *Philosophical Dictionary.* Translated by H. I. Woolf, Dover Publications, 2010.

Vox, Valentine. *I Can See Your Lips Moving: The History and Art of Ventriloquism.* Plato, 1996.

Wadström, Carl Bernhard. *Plan for a Free Community at Sierra Leona.* London, 1792.

Wagstaffe, John. 1669. *The Question of Witchcraft Debate; or, a Discourse against Their Opinion That Affirm Witches, Considered and Enlarged.* London, 1671.

Wald, Priscilla. "Hannah Crafts." *In Search of Hannah Crafts: Critical Essays on "The Bondwoman's Narrative,"* edited by Henry Louis Gates Jr. and Hollis Robbins, Basic Books, 2004, pp. 213–30.

Wall, Drucilla. *Identity and Authenticity: Explorations in Native American and Irish Literature and Culture.* 2006. PhD dissertation, U of Nebraska.

Warfel, Harry R. *Charles Brockden Brown: American Gothic Novelist*. U of Florida P, 1949.

Warner, Marina. *Phantasmagoria: Spirit, Visions, Metaphors and Media*. Oxford UP, 2006.

"Washington Irving Review." *Daily National Journal*, April 22, 1825.

Watts, Edward. "He Could Not Believe that Butchering Red Men Was Serving Our Maker." *John Neal and Nineteenth-Century American Literature and Culture*, edited by Edward Watts and David J. Carlson, Bucknell UP, 2011, pp. 209–226.

Watts, Edward, and David J. Carlson, editors. *John Neal and Nineteenth-Century American Literature and Culture*. Bucknell UP, 2011.

Watts, Vanessa. "Indigenous Place-Thought and Agency amongst Humans and Nonhumans (First Woman and Sky Woman Go on a European World Tour!)." *Decolonization: Indigeneity, Education and Society*, vol. 2, no. 1, 2013, pp. 20–34.

Wegner, Georg Wilhelm. *Philosophische Abhandlung von Gespenstern*. 1747. Edited by Catherine Theodorsen, Wehrhahn Verlag, 2006.

Weinauer, Ellen. "Race and the American Gothic." In *The Cambridge Companion to American Gothic*, edited by Jeffrey A. Weinstock, Cambridge UP, 2017, pp. 85–98.

Weinstock, Jeffrey Andrew. *Charles Brockden Brown*. U of Wales P, 2011.

———. *Scare Tactics: Supernatural Fiction by American Women*. Fordham UP, 2008.

———. *Spectral America: Phantoms and the National Imagination*. U of Wisconsin P / Popular Press, 2004.

Weissberg, Liliane. *Geistersprache: Philosophischer und literarischer Diskurs im späten achtzehnten Jahrhundert*. Königshausen and Neumann, 1990.

Weldon, Roberta F. "Charles Brockden Brown's *Wieland*: A Family Tragedy." *Studies in American Fiction*, vol. 12, no. 1, 1984, pp. 1–11, https://doi.org/10.1353/saf.1984.0018.

Wellek, René. *Immanuel Kant in England*. Princeton UP, 1931.

Werkmeister, W. H. *Kant's Silent Decade: A Decade of Philosophical Development*. UP of Florida, 1979.

Wester, Maisha L. *African American Gothic: Screams from Shadowed Places*. Palgrave Macmillan, 2012.

———. "The Gothic in and as Race Theory." *The Gothic and Theory: An Edinburgh Companion*, edited by Jerrold E. Hogle and Robert Miles, Edinburgh UP, 2019, pp. 53–70. http://www.jstor.org/stable/10.3366/j.ctvggx38r.6.

Whitman, Walt. *With Walt Whitman in Camden: July 16, 1988—October 31, 1888*. Rowman and Littlefield, 1961.

Wieland, Christoph Martin. "Betrachtung über den Standpunkt, worin wir uns in Absicht auf Erzählungen und Nachrichten von Geistererscheinungen befinden." *Teutscher Merkur*, no. 2, 1781, pp. 226–39.

———. *The History of Agathon*. Translated by John Richardson of York, London, 1773.

———. *Private History of Peregrinus Proteus, the Philosopher*. London, 1796.

———. "Über den Hang der Menschen an Magie und Geistererscheinungen zu glauben." In *Sämmtliche Werke,* vol. 24, Leipzig, 1796, pp. 71–92.

"Wieland" and "Memoirs of Carwin the Biloquist": Authoritative Texts, Sources and Contexts, Criticism. Edited by Bryan Waterman, Norton, 2011.

Wieland; or, The Transformation: Three Gothic Novels. Library of America, 1998.

Williams, Adebayo. "Review: Of Human Bondage and Literary Triumphs: Hannah Crafts and the Morphology of the Slave Narrative." *Research in African Literatures,* vol. 34, no. 1, 2003, pp. 137–50.

Willich, A. F. M. "Elements of the Critical Philosophy." *Monthly Review,* vol. 28, Jan. 1799, pp. 62–69.

Wilson, Colin. *Poltergeist: A Classic Study in Destructive Hauntings.* 1983. Llewellyn Publications, 2009.

Winter, Kari J. *Subjects of Slavery, Agents of Change: Women and Power in Gothic Novels and Slave Narratives 1790–1865.* U of Georgia P, 1992.

Winthrop, John. "Model of Christian Charity." 1630. *Winthrop Papers,* 5 vols., edited by Stewart Mitchell, Massachusetts Historical Society, 1931.

Wolfe, Eric A. "Ventriloquizing Nation: Voice, Identity, and Radical Democracy in Charles Brockden Brown's *Wieland.*" *American Literature,* vol. 78, no. 3, 2006, pp. 431–57.

Wolin, Richard. *The Seduction of Unreason: The Intellectual Romance with Fascism from Nietzsche to Postmodernism.* Princeton UP, 2004.

Wright, Angela, and Dale Townshend, editors. *Romantic Gothic: An Edinburgh Companion.* Edinburgh UP, 2016.

Wynter, Sylvia. "Unsettling the Coloniality of Being/Power/Truth/Freedom." *Postcolonialism and the Law: Critical Concepts in Law,* edited by Mark Harris and Denise Ferreira da Silva, Routledge, 2018, pp. 7–67.

Yellin, Jean Fagan. "Texts and Contexts of Harriet Jacobs' *Incidents in the Life of a Slave Girl: Written by Herself.*" *The Slave's Narrative,* edited by Henry Louis Gates Jr. and Charles T. Davis, Oxford UP, 1985, pp. 262–78.

Ziff, Larzer. "A Reading of Wieland." *PMLA,* vol. 77, no. 1, 1962, pp. 51–57.

Index

Abenaki people, 154
abolitionism, 53, 117, 132
Abraham, Nicolas, 83–86, 91, 218, 236–37nn29–30
absence: material, 51, 86; present, 8, 86, 93, 123, 131, 172, 194, 237n33; spectrality and, 11, 86
Adams, John, 79–80, 236n28
Adams, John Quincy, 60
Adorno, Theodor W., 3, 225n1, 230n2
African Americans: animalization of, 98, 109, 171; double consciousness and, 238n45; folk practices of, 199; funeral rites among, 206–7; as ghost-storytellers, 97–104, 113, 199–200; gothic literature and, 183, 184, 195; as the Other, 115; settler colonialism and, 100; silencing of, 86, 97–104; stereotypes of, 117; superstition and, 110, 117, 199, 246n28; transcendentalism and, 245n19; white American friendships with, 106, 109, 119; worship of nature by, 198. *See also* Blackness; slavery and enslaved people
African world view, 198
Alaimo, Stacy, 159, 195
alchemy, 145, 150, 153, 241nn17–18
American Renaissance, 5, 7, 225n4
American spiritualism, 7, 178, 209, 220, 225n5
ancestral spirits, 11, 15, 31, 32
Anderson, Benedict, 100
Andrews, William L., 180
animal magnetism. *See* mesmerism
animism: in *The Bondwoman's Narrative,* 182, 197–98, 201–2; enslaved people and, 10, 202; Indigenous peoples and, 145, 151, 241n12; mesmerism and, 146, 209; neomaterialist concept of, 210; slave narratives and, 181; spread in United States, 246n26; subjectivity and, 10; in West African traditions, 182, 209, 219, 223
Anna, *St. Herbert—A Tale,* 6, 121, 155
anxiety, 5, 49, 82, 158, 217–18, 235n17, 236n23
Apaches, 148, 218, 247n4

Apes, William, 115
apparitional tales: Hobbes on, 18, 23; instrumentalization of, 23; as natural history, 30–31, 98; origin of literature and, 20; providence tales and, 28–33, 36; Puritans and, 28–43, 98, 100, 113, 120; racialization of, 17, 37–43, 100–101; redefined as natural phenomena, 6; women as victims in, 29, 33, 35, 38–42
arboreal hauntings, 138–42, 193–95
Arendt, Hannah, 122, 149
Aristotle, 19, 105
Arnold, Larry E., 236n25
Artaud, Antonin, 238n45
atheism, 16, 20–23, 26, 28, 63, 226n4, 227n12

Bakhtin, M. M., 238n45
Ballinger, Gill, 190, 245n10
Barlow, Joel, 63, 232n17
Barthes, Roland, 137, 192, 245n14
Basso, Keith, 148
Baxter, Richard, *The Certainty of the Worlds of Spirits,* 227n12
Baym, Nina, 239n47, 244n3
Beecher, George, 176
Bennett, Bridget, 236n27
Bennett, Gillian, 15, 226n2
Bennett, Jane, 9
Bergland, Renée L., 123, 124, 143, 162–63, 243n9
Bergson, Henri, 9
Berlin, Isaiah, 44
biloquism, 93–94, 238n45
black magic, 183, 244n7
Blackness: in apparitional tales, 17, 37–43; in construction of whiteness, 109, 240n10; Kant on characterizations of, 57; sexual predation and, 41, 229n30. *See also* African Americans; slavery and enslaved people
Blanco, María del Pilar, 231n6
Böhme, Hartmut and Gernot, 44, 219, 230n1

Hoffmann, E. T. A., 96, 149–50, 241n16
Holt, Kerin, 134
Hopi people, 220
Horkheimer, Max, 3, 225n1, 230n2
horrorism, 185–92, 245n11
Hubbard, William, 115
Huhndorf, Shari M., 242n21
humanism, 18, 85, 215, 221–22
human overrepresentation of itself as Man, 213, 247nn1–2
Hume, David, 227n9
Hunter, Michael, 27, 28, 227n13
Hurston, Zora Neale, 246n24

imagination and imaginaries: attacks on, 23; defined, 110; ghosts and, 6, 16, 19–21, 31, 44–45, 60, 213; power of, 19–21, 26, 64; racial, 215; settler colonial, 36, 126, 214; social and cultural, 5, 110, 123, 237n33; spiritualism and, 177; theories of sight in relation to, 68. *See also* national imaginary
Indian Removal Act of 1830, 154, 168, 244n12
Indigenous peoples: animalization of, 131, 132, 172; animism among, 145, 151, 241n12; in captivity narratives, 35–37, 158, 229n26; cosmology of, 11, 145, 149–53, 217, 219, 222, 223; demonization of, 92, 123, 126, 240n4; dispossession of, 111, 113, 165, 169, 216; "ecological Indian" myth, 222; genocide against, 12, 118, 128, 149, 169; impersonations by white Americans, 92, 108–9, 125, 237–38n41, 240n9; "Indian problem," 143, 241n9; instrumentalization of, 5, 90; in Irving's ghost stories, 96–98; Kant's view of, 55; leaders framed as tragic heroes, 127–28, 241n7; miscegenation and, 154–58; in national imaginary, 143, 149; nature and, 110, 146, 222; noble savage trope, 120, 154, 159, 174, 244n14; as the Other, 81, 115, 125, 240n3; present absence of, 86, 93, 123, 131, 172, 237n33; religious rituals viewed as magic, 159; settler colonialism and, 5, 34–43, 125–26, 132, 240n4; silencing of, 223; spectralization of, 90, 92, 97, 113, 121–26, 131–32, 163, 237n37; spirits of, 11, 31, 96, 100, 110–16, 143; supernatural and, 27, 28; superstition and, 125, 138, 150, 153; Vanishing Indian trope, 123–26, 128, 130,

132, 160, 168, 170–71, 240n1; violence towards, 237n34; voice of, 89–94; white American friendships with, 106, 108, 109, 119; in *Wieland*, 80–81, 86. *See also specific groups of people*
individualism, 81–82, 168, 217, 238n43
Insko, Jeffrey, 99
interracial friendships, 106, 108–10, 119, 240n11
intersubjectivity, 1, 84, 89, 103, 216
intuition, 4, 50, 52, 57, 58
Invisible World: forests and, 16, 121, 157, 215, 216; gender and, 16; nature as visible part of, 4–5, 134; race and, 6, 16, 42, 213; recodification of, 195, 216; settler colonialism and, 4, 216
Iroquois, 89–92, 127, 130, 136–37, 159, 219–20
irrationality, 7–8, 30, 54, 65, 70, 79, 174, 214
Irving, Washington: "Adventures of the Black Fisherman," 111; *Bracebridge Hall*, 97, 100–109; "The Devil and Tom Walker," 110–13, 239n4; "Dolph Heyliger," 108–9, 126; exculpation narratives, 5, 112, 114; frontier gothic and, 121; gender in works by, 113, 116, 240nn12–13; "The Haunted House," 101–3, 105, 111; "The Historian," 101; *A History of New York*, 97–99, 102, 104–5, 113; "The Legend of Sleepy Hollow," 4, 96, 99, 126, 239n4; literary anachronisms of, 104–5; patriarchy in works by, 108, 240n12; prototypes for spectral narratives, 3, 4; Puritan influences on works by, 43, 98, 100, 113, 120; revised readings of texts by, 6; "Rip van Winkle," 96, 99, 239n4; scholarly engagement with, 116–17; *The Sketch Book of Geoffrey Crayon, Gent.*, 97, 99, 100, 105, 115; *Tales of a Traveller*, 97, 105, 110–13; "Traits of Indian Character," 115
Irwin, Robert, 63
Isbister, Dong L., 244n3

Jackson, Andrew, 117, 154, 244n12
Jackson, Shirley, *The Haunting of Hill House*, 188, 245n11
Jacobs, Harriet, *Incidents in the Life of a Slave Girl*, 180, 191
James, Henry, *The Turn of the Screw*, 104

Writing the Early Americas

Printed in the USA
CPSIA information can be obtained
at www.ICGtesting.com
LVHW042040251124
797601LV00004B/71

* 9 7 8 0 8 1 3 9 5 2 3 9 0 *